Useful Quantities in Vision Science

CORTEX

- Total *cortical area*: 1.3×10^5 mm^2; *cortical thickness*: 1.7 mm.

- *Cortical neurons*: total number, 10^{10}; average density, 10^5/mm^3.

- *Synapses*: average density, 5×10^8/mm^3; per neuron, 4×10^3.

- *Axons*: 3 km/mm^3.

- Number of *corpus callosum fibers*: 5×10^8.

- Number of *macaque visual areas*: 30.

- *Size of area V1* (each hemisphere): 3 cm × 8 cm. Half of area V1 represents the central 10 deg (2%) of the visual field.

- Width of *ocular dominance columns*: human, 0.5–1.0 mm; macaque, 0.3 mm.

SENSITIVITY

- *Minimum number of absorptions*: detectable electrical excitation of a rod, 1; scotopic detection, 1–5; photopic detection, 10–15.

- Following exposure to a sunny day, *dark adaptation* to a moonless night requires: photopic, 10 minutes; scotopic, 40 minutes; change in visual sensitivity, 6 log$_{10}$ units.

- *Highest detectable spatial frequency*: at high ambient light levels, 50–60 cpd; at low ambient light levels, 20–30 cpd.

- *Contrast threshold* ($\Delta L/L$) for a static edge at photopic luminances: 1%.

- *Highest detectable temporal frequency*: high ambient light, large field, 80 Hz; low ambient light, large field, 40 Hz.

- Typical *localization threshold*: 6 arc sec (0.5 μ on the retina).

- *Minimum temporal separation* needed to discriminate two small, brief light pulses from a single equal-energy pulse: 15–20 ms.

- *Stereoscopic depth discrimination thresholds*: step threshold, 3 arc sec; point threshold, 30 arc sec.

COLOR

- *Visible spectrum*: 370–730 nm.

- *Peak wavelength sensitivity*: scotopic, 507 nm; photopic, 555 nm.

- *Spectral equilibrium hues*: blue, 475 nm; green, 500 nm; yellow, 575 nm (no spectral equilibrium red).

- Number of basic *English color names*: 11.

- *Incidence of color deficiencies*: anomalous trichromacy, 10^{-2} (male), 10^{-4} (female); protanopia and deuteranopia, 10^{-2} (male), 10^{-4} (female); tritanopia, 10^{-4}; rod monochromacy, 10^{-4}; cone monochromacy, 10^{-5}.

FOUNDATIONS OF VISION

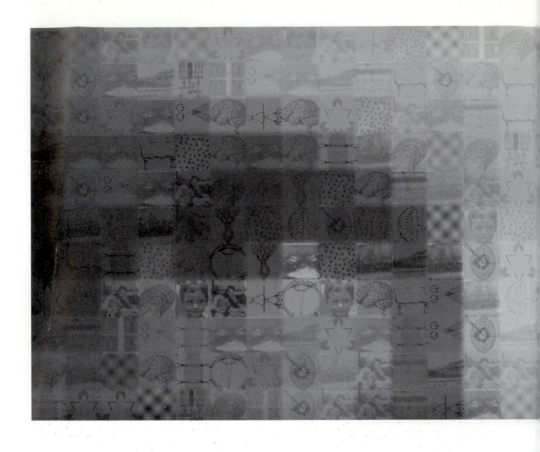

 Sinauer Associates, Inc.
Publishers
Sunderland, Massachusetts

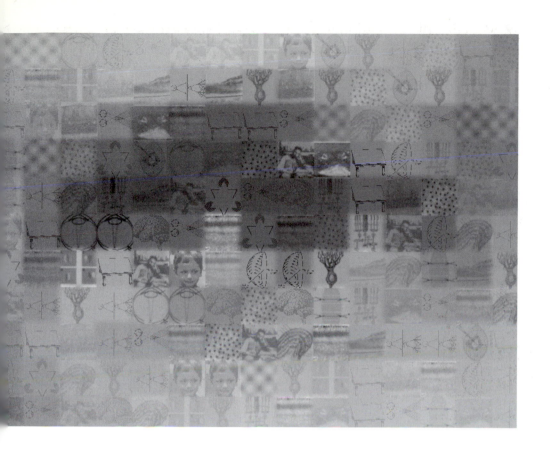

Foundations
of
Vision

Brian A. Wandell

STANFORD UNIVERSITY

The cover and frontispiece
The images were created by David Heeger, Hagit Hel-Or, and the author by combining images of human eyes with small versions of illustrations from this book. The images were all digitally created or scanned and combined using image processing tools written in Matlab. The contrast and color of the smaller images were adjusted by an automatic process to match that of the large image. Depending on the viewing distance, the large image or the smaller images will be more salient.

Foundations of Vision
© Copyright 1995 by Sinauer Associates, Inc.
For information or to order, address: Sinauer Associates, Inc., Sunderland, Massachusetts 01375–0407 U.S.A. FAX: 413–549–1118. Internet: publish@sinauer.com

Library of Congress Cataloging-in-Publication Data
Wandell, Brian A.
    Foundations of vision science / Brian A. Wandell.
      p. cm.
    Includes bibliographical references and index.
    ISBN 0-87893-853-2
    1. Vision.   2. Vision—Research—Methodology.   3. Visual cortex.
  4. Visual pathways.   I. Title.
    QP475.W32   1995
    612.8'4—dc20   94-42769
                                       CIP

Printed in U.S.A.

8 7 6 5 4 3 2 1

To my family

Table of Contents

Appendixes

Acknowledgments

While preparing this book, I received generous and wise advice from many people. I am especially grateful to Tony Movshon for reading and commenting on several chapters and answering many dozens of questions. Dave Marimont also read large portions of the manuscript thoroughly, and continually reminded me what this book should be about. E. J. Chichilnisky, Joyce Farrell, and David Heeger all spent many hours talking with me about aspects of this book, and they shared their views on many issues ranging from substance to style. They were all patient and cheerful through an endless series of interruptions, but I am sure that we are all relieved this project is complete.

Many other individuals were also a great help—reading and commenting on a chapter, suggesting a figure or providing one, or assisting with some part of the production process. Their efforts were essential to whatever merit this book may have. Many thanks to Ted Adelson, Al Ahumada, Denis Baylor, Gary Blasdel, Rick Born, Geoff Boynton, Dave Brainard, Patrick Cavanagh, Seung Choi, Christine Curcior, Dennis Dacey, Steve Engel, David Fleet, John Foley, Bill Geisler, Norma Graham, David Grossof, Hagit Hel-Or, Toni Haun, Anita Hendrickseyn, Don Kelly, Dan Kersten, Ken Knoblauch, Shirit Kronzon, Gordon Legge, Peter Lennie, Jennifer Lund, Don MacLeod, John Mollon, Vic Nalwa, Bill Newsome, Liddy Olds, Sandy Pentland, Geoff Phillips, Allen Poirson, John Robson, Bob Rodieck, Stan Schein, Bob Scott, Mike Shadlen, Bob Shapley, Roger Shepard, Luis Silveira, Eero Simoncelli, Patrick Teo, Peter Thompson, Shoji Tominaga, Nick Wade, Heinz Wässle, Beau Watson, Dave Williams, Jack Yellott, and Mei Zhang.

Special thanks are due to Dave Brainard, Gordon Legge, Dan Kersten, Jonathan Marshall, and Stephen Pizer, who all bravely agreed to teach from early versions of this book; I benefited a great deal from the comments they and their students provided. Likewise, I wish to thank all of the students at Stanford who offered me comments and encouragement during the years I taught from preliminary versions of this book. Their keen interest in vision science and their enthusiasm for learning in general were an inspiration, and their encouragement was often much needed.

I am deeply indebted to Jan Ruby for the many different things she has done for me during the last fifteen years. Jan's diligence and good spirits have been a great resource to me and to all the members of my laboratory who have had the good fortune to work with her.

Working with Peter Farley, my editor at Sinauer Associates, has been a pleasure. Many thanks to Peter for his support and for being direct and helpful at all times. Kathaleen Emerson, project editor, and Christopher Small, production manager, also worked hard and well to help realize this book, and I appreciate their efforts. Roberta Lewis and J. David Baldwin provided expert copy editing, and the book was much improved by their advice and attention to detail.

Several people arranged financial support so that I might suspend my teaching and committee responsibilities at Stanford and concentrate on writing. In this regard, I am grateful to Dave Marimont, Maureen Stone, and John S. Brown for arranging a one-quarter leave at Xerox Palo Alto Research Center in 1992, and to Gardner Lindzey and Robert Scott for making a special effort to arrange a sabbatical year for me in 1988–89 at the Center for Advanced Study in the Behavioral Sciences. During that year this project and my son were born.

Thanks also to the many people on CVNET who responded to my electronic query for useful numbers in vision science, many of which appear within the front cover of this book. A much larger posting of their work can be found on the World Wide Web at `http://vision.arc.nasa.gov`.

Finally, Hagit Hel-Or and David Heeger took time out from their work to help me create the cover image, and I thank them. Working on the cover gave us a chance to step back and see one big picture. Whenever I became too absorbed in writing this book, my son Adam reminded me that playing soccer, basketball, or taking a bike ride to the park are important too, and this helped me to step back and see another big picture. Thanks, Adam.

1

How to Study Vision

While working to bring this book together, I was inspired and overwhelmed by the breadth and vibrancy of vision science. Vision scientists solve problems across the fields of biology, psychology, and engineering. Our field takes on problems ranging from studying the nature of consciousness to creating a hurry-up-and-ship-it product needed to keep a company afloat. In selecting from the huge amount of material available, I decided to write this book for the student who wishes to know *how* to study vision: the pages are filled with measurements and facts, but my goal in writing this book is to explain to the student how we learned these facts, not the facts themselves. To organize the material, I have divided the book into three parts that reflect three of the basic problems of vision: encoding, representation, and interpretation.

Encoding

Part One describes how the retinal image is encoded by the visual pathways. The material in this section is particularly important for three reasons. First, how the visual system encodes light has implications for everything else the visual pathways do. Distortions that are introduced into the signal by poor optics, sparse and uneven spatial sampling of the image, or meager wavelength encoding become part of the signal that must be represented and interpreted by the central visual pathways. We cannot understand the role of the central nervous system in vision without understanding the quality of information encoded within the eye.

Second, the properties of visual encoding have implications for the design of instruments that display visual information. The quality of the representation of pattern and color in display media must be structured to satisfy, but not exceed, the limits of the human visual system. For example, the products of the color imaging industry, including visual displays, color film, and color printing, rely on the fact that human color vision uses three types of cone photopigments to encode light. As a result of this sparse representation of wavelength, color reproductions need not represent the wavelength composition of the original in order to provide a satisfactory appearance match. This is but one example of many in which the initial encoding of the image in the human eye defines practical limits whose properties determine the character of imaging devices.

Third, the methods and standards of proof that are used to understand image encoding set an important example concerning the standards of explanation we aim to achieve at all levels of vision science. The questions of methods and standards of proof are very important in a field like vision science, which draws on expertise from many different disciplines. Part One contains several examples that combine physical calculations, biological experiments, and behavioral studies. By examining how these fields come together when we measure the quality of the retinal image formed by the optics of the eye, and again when we establish that human color vision is trichromatic, we see how these diverse fields can forge strong links that define important aspects of visual function. We can learn from these examples as we move on to other problems in vision science.

Representation

Part Two of this volume reviews how the encoded image is represented by the neural response within the peripheral and early cortical visual pathways. Our understanding of the neural representation is based on work in several different disciplines. This section begins with a review of the anatomical and electrophysiological measurements of the image representation within the retina and primary visual cortex. These measurements characterize the neural hardware of the visual representation and demonstrate that there are several distinct categories of neurons called visual streams. The neurons in these visual streams respond to light stimulation in different ways, and their signals are communicated to different destinations.

The second half of Part Two reviews behavioral and computational studies of image representation. The behavioral studies of image representation involve the simplest performances, such as detection, discrimination, and simple recognition. These experiments have led to various proposals about how pattern and color information is represented within the retina and early cortical areas. The computational studies review fundamental issues about the role of these representations in efficient image coding and other image operations.

Interpretation

Perception is an interpretation of the retinal image, not a description. Part Three contains examples of how we interpret the retinal image and assign perceptual properties such as color, motion, and shape to objects.

Information in the retinal image may be interpreted in many different ways. Because we begin with ambiguous information, we cannot make deductions from the retinal image, only inferences. When we create algorithms to interpret image data—say, to infer the color, motion, and shape of objects—we confront the same challenges as the visual pathways. The success of the visual system in interpreting image data represents a remarkable achievement.

By studying computations designed to infer object properties, we have learned that the visual system succeeds in interpreting images because of statistical regularities present in the visual environment and hence in the retinal image. These regularities permit the visual system to use the fragmentary information present in the retinal image to draw accurate inferences about the physical cause of the image. For example, when we make inferences from the retinal image, the knowledge that we live in a three-dimensional world is essential to the correct interpretation of the image. Often, we are made aware of the existence of these powerful interpretations and their assumptions when they are in error, that is, when we discover a visual illusion.

The Range of Material in This Book

The material I have chosen to include in this book comes from three sources: theory, data, and fruitful applications that are grounded in theoretical and empirical vision science. Portions of this book are written with the expectation that the reader has had some experience with linear algebra and calculus. In most sections of the book, however, I have tried to provide the reader with the basic ideas without using mathematical symbols or formal arguments.

Theory

Certain theoretical and empirical methods appear repeatedly within vision science. The most important theoretical method, which appears across all areas of vision science, is linear-systems theory. Whether characterizing optics, neurophysiology, color vision, spatial vision, image compression, or pattern analysis, linear systems play an important role. There is little possibility of understanding the current foundations of vision science without understanding linear systems. I introduce the principles of linear systems in the first chapter, and I refer to them throughout the book.

Linear methods are not a theory of vision; linear systems methods consist of a set of experiments and calculations that one should use to analyze a system. If the system's performance satisfies certain experimental properties, such as the principle of superposition, then we can use linear methods to characterize the system completely. Even if the system turns out to be nonlinear, it is useful to begin studying the system using summation experiments to obtain some insights as to the nature of the nonlinearities.

In part, the emphasis on linear systems methods is my choice; in part, this emphasis is inevitable because of a second choice I made in selecting the material. I have tried to include important problems that vision science has solved, or that I think are close to being solved. At present linear methods are much better understood than nonlinear methods. Consequently, we understand those problems which yield to linear analysis much better than we understand nonlinear problems.

A linear characterization of a system is rarely a complete scientific account of the system. There are usually many theoretical questions that require further explanation before the scientist is done. This will be evident in the first section on image encoding. Optical image formation, photoreceptor sampling, and color matching are all fundamentally linear, and thus we can characterize the performance of these system components. However, even when this work is done, we still must explain the measurements in terms of the purpose of these elements and how their properties serve the goals of visual perception.

While linear analyses are central, there are some significant examples of successful nonlinear analyses. The first example is the analysis of the relationship between color matching and the cone photocurrent treatment in Chapter 4. This system consists of an initial linear encoding followed by a fixed nonlinearity. These types of nonlinear systems can also be treated very thoroughly. The review of pattern sensitivity in Chapter 7 also includes models that begin with linear encodings followed by a nonlinear stage. In Appendix C, I treat the profoundly nonlinear act of classification. Applications of Bayesian classification to interpret image data are likely to be important in future research.

Data

The field of vision draws on experimental results from many separate disciplines, each with its own standards and methods. The tools of anatomy, electrophysiology, behavior, and computation are so different that no one can can be an expert in all of these disciplines. To be a good vision scientist, however, one must appreciate the standards and methods of each discipline. The psychologist must understand whether an anatomical measurement is sufficiently thorough to serve as a good standard for comparison in a behavioral experiment; the computational theorist must understand the generality of a result from electrophysiology.

I have included empirical studies from all of the disciplines of vision. I have tried to describe these results, and their theoretical implications, in enough detail so that the advanced student can learn something about the standards of each of the fields. By placing these results together in a single volume I hope to explain what is special about the interdisciplinary field of vision.

Applications

As I selected problems to review, I did not distinguish strongly between those that are called "basic" from those that are called "applied." I share Edwin Land's frustration with this distinction. After a theoretical lecture on color appearance, Land, who was both a brilliant inventor and entrepreneur, was asked to explain what applied problem his work would solve, and he replied quickly that the work had a wonderful application. He then paused while the audience leaned forward in anticipation of an answer that might help them decide whether to invest in Polaroid stock. "If the theory is right," Land whispered confidentially, "we'll finally understand what we are doing."

Vision science finds applications in at least three important areas that I will draw on throughout the book. The first is medicine. If we are to help the blind, we must understand how the visual portion of the brain functions, including the anatomy and functional properties of nerve cells. Equally important, we must understand how information represented within the brain results in behavior. The results of behavioral experiments can answer questions about the organization of information within the visual pathways that are inaccessible to the anatomist or the electrophysiologist. Together, these results can speed the development of medical diagnostic tools and prosthetic devices. Tom Cornsweet's (1970) beautiful book, *Visual Perception*, was a guide to most of my generation as we first learned about the systematic analysis of vision ranging from the visual pathways to behavior. In this book I hope to explain to the new student why so many of us found Cornsweet's presentation exhilarating and to build on Cornsweet's review.

A second area of application is the design of computer algorithms capable of analyzing information in an image. Typical applications range from part inspections in a factory to the identification of a tumor in a medical image. David Marr's (1982) book, *Vision*, stimulated the interest of many young scientists in this area. He presented a bold overview that related biological concepts and computer algorithms of visual processing. The contrast between the broad scope of Marr's imagination and the elegant, meticulous discussions by Cornsweet captures something of the creative tension that can arise when different disciplines contribute to a broad scientific endeavor.

The third area of application is the design of visual display devices to communicate information to the human visual system. When two electronic components communicate, the components must be designed to accommodate a set of communication protocols. In the case of communication between an electronic display medium (such as a television display) and the human visual system, the designer can only redesign one of the two components. To communicate information efficiently between the electronic system and the human visual system we must build displays that are matched to human capabilities. A remarkable harmony between vision science and applications technology has been achieved in some areas, such as color science. I hope that this book will contribute to the further coordination of our basic understanding of vision and the design of useful and efficient visual displays.

A Guide to the Principles of Vision

Much of vision science is based on the principle that the components of the visual system that limit or govern performance vary from task to task. In some experiments, performance is limited by the lens, while in other experiments performance is limited by a computation performed in visual cortex. Because different visual tasks may be limited by completely distinct components of the visual pathways, a static diagram of the visual pathways cannot adequately capture their flexibility and adaptability.

There are, however, several general principles that I found useful as I wrote and organized this volume. Some of these principles are embedded in the organization of the book, repeated in the introductions to the three sections, and repeated within the chapters themselves. Here I will introduce you to the principles, briefly, in one place.

The Inescapable Components of Image Encoding

The properties of image encoding, such as blurring by the lens, receptor sampling, and trichromacy, shape the information available to the rest of the nervous system. The first third of this book is devoted to describing these aspects of vision. The properties of image formation set the stage for what the rest of the nervous system must confront.

The limits of image encoding set limits on the image information available to the visual pathways. As we shall see, the encoded image is a very partial representation of the light that arrives at the eye: there is only a narrow region of high visual acuity in the fovea; the dynamic range of the sensors is very small; and the representation of wavelength is very coarse. You would never buy a camera with such poor optics and coarse spatial sampling. Yet, the visual algorithms can interpret the properties of objects from this poor encoding.

Whether you wish to study the eye or study algorithms embedded in the central nervous system, you will not go wrong by studying image encoding and thinking further about its implications for vision.

Adaptation and Flexibility

The visual pathways compensate for the poor quality of the image encoding by their flexibility. Nearly all of the peripheral elements of the visual pathways adapt in response to the viewing conditions: the lens accommodates; the eye moves to bring the high visual acuity portion of the retina into a favorable viewing position; and the retinal neurons adjust their sensitivity when the mean illumination changes. The flexible responses of the visual system overcome the mediocre image encoding.

The visual system's adjustments, or adaptations, to the environment are fundamental to its design. We see adaptation throughout the visual representation, not just in the peripheral components. Because adaptation is so widespread, it is impossible to characterize the visual system as a static device. The ability to adapt in response to a changing environment is a fundamental design principle of the visual pathways, beginning at the earliest stages and continuing into the central brain representations.

Image Representation: Visual Streams

As we review the visual representation of the image, we will find that the neural pathways are organized into several distinct pathways. These pathways, sometimes called visual streams, can be identified based on anatomical studies. Some cells have different shapes from others; some cells send their outputs in different directions from others.

Many of the most important discoveries about vision concern the the identification of visual streams. Many of the important contemporary challenges in vision concern explanations of the functional significance of these streams. Segregation of visual information into these visual streams begins with the photoreceptors (rods and cones). Clarifications concerning the visual streams within the optic nerve have revolutionized our understanding of the visual representation. Understanding the organization of visual information with respect to these visual streams is one of most hotly debated topics in modern visual neuroscience. Identifying new visual streams and understanding their function is an important challenge to vision scientists.

Image Interpretation: Statistical Inferences

To me, vision science is about how we see things: the interpretations of the image, or as Helmholtz called them, the unconscious inferences. I study vision in order to understand the methods of interpreting images and relating them to objects and their properties.

Since the retinal image is often ambiguous, the visual system's success in interpreting images must be because it makes good assumptions about the likely properties of objects in the world. Not all configurations of objects are equally likely; we exist in a three-dimensional world. Not all surface-reflectance functions are equally likely; there are regularities in the wavelength properties of surfaces and illuminants. Not all types of motion are equally likely; hard objects cannot pass through one another. The unequal probabilities of different interpretations make it possible to make informed guesses about the color, motion, position, and shape of objects. The probabilities of different events are sufficiently skewed so that the visual system succeeds at interpreting the image data. Understanding these regularities and understanding how to use them to interpret the retinal image are central to vision science.

My devotion to image encoding and representation, the first two parts of this volume, flows from my conviction that we will not understand visual interpretations of the image without understanding encoding and representation. Encoding and representation define the environment in which image interpretation takes place and must be structured to permit image interpretation to succeed. Thus, as you look through each section of this volume, you will find ideas about image interpretation. The material in this book will seem unified to you if you continue to ask how image encoding and image representation serve the ultimate goal of image interpretation.

*T*HE FIRST SECTION of this book describes the initial encoding of
light by the eye. Chapter 2 reviews the image-formation process,
that is, the process by which light incident at the eye is focused
onto the retina. Chapters 3 and 4 review some of the basic properties of the
conversion of light into a neural signal by the light-sensitive elements of the eye, the
photoreceptors. These early stages of image encoding establish essential limits on
vision; the consequences of the image-formation process can be found in many parts
of the visual neural representation.

In addition to the properties of image formation, the early chapters introduce
and make use of the principles of linear systems. Linear methods are fundamental
to vision science, as they are to much of science. Since the methods apply well to
image formation, it seems natural to introduce them as a solution to the problem of
measuring the properties of eye. I describe the principles of linear systems in the text
but I have placed most of the mathematical notation and derivations in Appendix A.

Image Formation

The quality and general properties of the image formed at the retina establish
the basic image parameters that the rest of the nervous system must use to make
inferences about objects. Because the image-formation process is linear, we can
characterize its properties fairly thoroughly. The image-formation process attenuates

PART ONE

Encoding

the contrast of patterns that vary rapidly across space. This leaves the nervous system with only a small contrast range available in the fine spatial detail of an image, while there is a substantial contrast range present in slowly varying spatial patterns. Finally, the precise meaning of high and low frequency varies with the wavelength of the incident light because the quality of the retinal image varies strongly with wavelength. Under ordinary viewing conditions the short-wavelength light (blue portion of the spectrum) is blurred strongly so that very little pattern information is available in this part of the spectrum compared to longer wavelengths of light (green, yellow, and red parts of the spectrum).

The Photoreceptor Mosaics

Chapter 3 reviews the the spatial arrangement of the light-sensitive elements of the photoreceptors. There are two fundamentally different types of receptors: rods and cones. The spatial organization of the rod and cone photoreceptor mosaics differ; each mosaic reflects the main goal of the visual stream it initiates.

The rod visual stream initiates vision under low-illumination conditions when relatively few quanta are available. The rods are present in high density to capture more quanta, not to achieve high spatial resolution. Indeed, the spatial resolution of the rod pathway is fairly coarse, since many rod photoreceptors converge their outputs onto single cells in the retina.

The visual streams initiated by the cone mosaic ordinarily operate at high light levels where there are plenty of quanta. The organization of the cone mosaic can be understood in terms of the goal of representing fine spatial detail, rather than capturing more quanta. This goal is reflected separately in the spatial arrangement of the separate mosaics of the three different types of cones, the L-, M-, and S-cones. The density of the short-wavelength-sensitive S-cones is lowest, matching the poor resolution of the optics in the short-wavelength region. Only the L- and M-cones are present in the very central fovea, where they have a very high sampling density and form a regular sampling grid. The sampling density of the L- and M-cones is also a good match to the quality of the image passed by the optics of the eye in the portion of the wavelength spectrum where they have their peak sensitivity. Signals from individual cones in the fovea do not converge onto retinal neurons, but instead these signals are communicated along private neural channels to the cortex.

Wavelength Encoding

Chapter 4 reviews how the visual pathways encode the wavelength of light, an encoding that has much to do with color appearance. The behavioral predictions that the eye contains three types of cones, as well as behavioral predictions of the way these cones encode wavelength, have been confirmed in a stunning set of experiments that represent an intellectual collaboration involving very different disciplines. The nexus of results from physics, psychology, and biology concerning wavelength encoding form one of most beautiful and satisfying stories in science. The successful interactions among these disciplines is a remarkable intellectual achievement. The facts concerning how the visual pathways encode wavelength has been important for all color-imaging technologies. The scientific methods that link the color-matching experiment to the cone photocurrents are important for all who wish to relate behavior and brain.

2

Image Formation

Visual perception results from a series of optical and neural transformations. Light arriving at the eye is first transformed by the cornea and lens, which focus light and create a retinal image. The retinal image is then transformed into neural responses by the light-sensitive elements of the eye, the photoreceptors. The photoreceptor responses are transformed into several neural representations within the optic nerve, and these are transformed into a multiplicity of cortical representations.

Many of these transformations occur in parallel streams within the visual pathways, so it is unlikely that every transformation has an influence on every visual experience. But the first visual transformation—the formation of the retinal image by the cornea and lens—is inescapable. Because it limits all of our visual experience, it deserves careful examination.

Studying Reflections from the Eye

Figure 2.1 is an overview of the imaging components of the eye. When light from a source arrives at the cornea, it is focused by the cornea and lens onto the **photoreceptors**, a collection of light-sensitive neurons that are part of a thin layer of neural tissue called the **retina**. The photoreceptors transform light into neural signals, which are communicated through the several layers of retinal neurons to those neurons whose output fibers make up the **optic nerve**. The optic nerve fibers exit

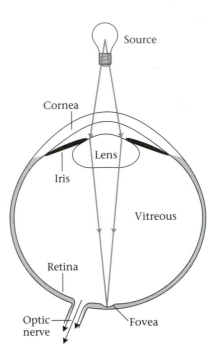

2.1 IMAGING COMPONENTS OF THE HUMAN EYE
seen in cross section. When light arrives at the eye, it enters
through the pupil, which is bordered by the iris. Light is
brought into focus on the retina by the cornea and lens,
but must pass through the transparent vitreous and several
retinal cell layers (see Figure 2.4) before reaching the
light-sensitive photoreceptors.

the eye through a hole in the retina called the **optic disk**,[1] and carry the
neural signals to the brain for further processing. This optical imaging
of light incident at the cornea into an image at the retinal photoreceptors is the first visual transformation, and all of our visual experience is
influenced by this transformation. So, we begin the study of vision by
analyzing the properties of image formation.

To study the optics of a human eye you will need an experimental
eye, so you might invite a friend to dinner. In addition, you will need a
light source, such as a candle, as a stimulus to present to your friend's
eye. If you look directly into your friend's eye, you will see a myste-
rious darkness that has beguiled poets and befuddled visual scientists.
The reason for the darkness can be understood by considering the problem illustrated in Figure 2.2A.

If the light source is behind you, so that your head is between the
light source and the eye you are studying, then your head will cast a
shadow that interferes with the light from the point source arriving at
your friend's eye. As a result, when you look in to measure the retinal
image you see nothing beyond what is in your heart. If you move to the
side of the light path, the image at the back of your friend's eye will be
reflected toward the light source, following a reversible path. Since you
are now on the side, out of the path of the light source, no light will be
sent towards your eye.

[1] Also known as the "blind spot"; see Figures 3.1 and 5.3.

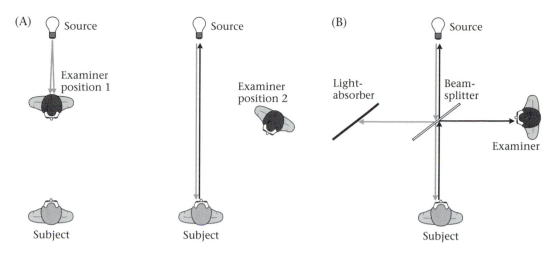

2.2   MEASURING LIGHT REFLECTED FROM THE EYE. (A) If an examiner looks directly into a subject's eye, he blocks the light path from the source and casts a shadow, making it impossible to see a reflected image. If the examiner moves out of the light path, the image is reflected back toward the source (solid line). (B) The beam-splitter permits the examiner to see some of the light reflected from the interior of the eye.

Flamant (1955) first measured the retinal image using a modified ophthalmoscope[2] in which a light-sensitive recording device, a **photodetector**, was placed at the position normally reserved for the ophthalmologist's eye. In this way, she measured the intensity pattern of the light reflected from the back of the subject's eye. Campbell and Gubisch (1966) used Flamant's method to build their apparatus, which is sketched in Figure 2.3. Campbell and Gubisch measured the reflection of a single bright line, which served as the input stimulus in their experiment. As shown in the figure, a beam-splitter placed between the input light and the subject's eye divides the input stimulus into two parts. The beam-splitter causes some of the light to be turned away from the subject and lost; this stray light is absorbed by a light baffle. The rest of the light continues toward the subject. When the light travels in this direction, the beam-splitter is an annoyance, serving only to lose some of the light; it will accomplish its function on the return trip.

The light that enters the subject's eye is brought to a focus on the retina by a lens. A small fraction of the light incident on the retina is reflected and passes through the optics of the eye a second time. On the return path, the beam-splitter now plays its functional role. The

---

[2] The great nineteenth-century scientist Hermann von Helmholtz built the first ophthalmoscope, a device for seeing light reflected from the interior of the eye. The design shown in Figure 2.2B is unconventional, though it does satisfy the basic need to arrange a light path so that the examiner's eye does not cast a shadow. A bright source light is required since the back of the human eye is not very reflective. A more conventional design is found in Appendix III of *Visual Perception* by Cornsweet (1970).

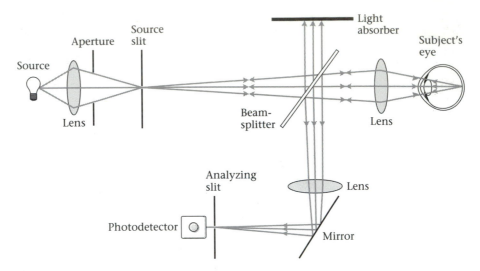

2.3   A MODIFIED OPHTHALMOSCOPE can measure the human retinal image. Light from a bright source passes through a slit and beam-splitter and into the eye. A fraction of the light is reflected from the retina and is measured by a photodetector. The intensity of the reflected light is measured at different spatial positions by varying the location of the analyzing slit. After Campbell and Gubisch, 1966.

reflected image would normally return to a focus at the light source. But the beam-splitter divides the returning beam so that a portion of it is brought to focus in a measurement plane to one side of the apparatus. Using a very fine slit in the measurement plane, with a photodetector behind it, Campbell and Gubisch measured the reflected light and used the measurements of the reflected light to infer the shape of the image on the retinal surface.

What part of the eye reflects the image? Figure 2.4 shows a cross section of the peripheral human retina. In normal vision, the image is focused on the retina at the level of the photoreceptors. The light measured by Campbell and Gubisch probably contains components from several different planes at the back of the eye. Thus, their measurements probably underestimate the quality of the image at the level of the photoreceptors.

Figure 2.5 shows several examples of Campbell and Gubisch's measurements of the light reflected from the eye when the observer is looking at a very fine line. The different curves show measurements for different pupil sizes. When the pupil is wide open (top, 6.6 mm diameter) the reflected light is more blurred than when the pupil is closed (1.0 mm). Notice that the measurements made with a large pupil opening are less noisy; when the pupil is wide open more light passes into the eye and more light is reflected, improving the quality of the measurements.

The light measured by Campbell and Gubisch passed through the optical elements of the eye twice, while the retinal image normally

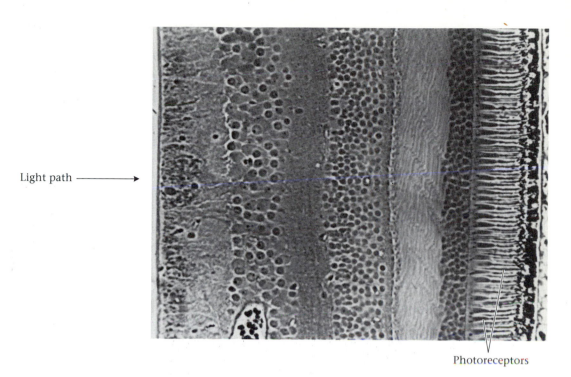

Light path ——————→

Photoreceptors

2.4 THE RETINA contains the light sensitive photoreceptors where light is focused. This cross section of a human retina outside the fovea shows that there are several layers of neurons in the optical path between the lens and the photoreceptors. As we will see later, in the central fovea these neurons are displaced to leave a clear optical path from the lens to the photoreceptors. From Boycott and Dowling, 1969.

passes through the optics only once. It follows that the spread in these curves is wider than the spread we would observe if we measured at the retina. How can we use these **double-pass** measurements to estimate the blur at the retina? To solve this problem, we must understand the general features of Campbell and Gubisch's experiment. It is time for some theory.

Linear-Systems Methods

When we study transformations, we must specify their inputs and outputs. As an example, we will consider how simple one-dimensional intensity patterns displayed on a video display monitor are imaged onto the retina (Figure 2.6A). In this case, the input is the light signal incident at the cornea. One-dimensional patterns have a constant intensity along one dimension (say, the horizontal dimension) and vary along the perpendicular (vertical) dimension. We will call the pattern of light intensity we measure at the monitor screen the **monitor image**. We can measure the intensity of the one-dimensional

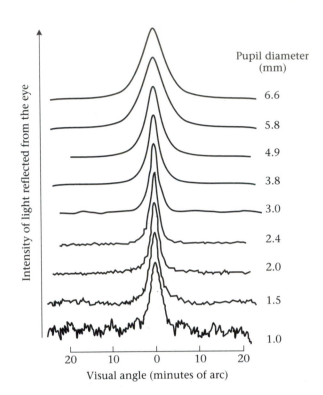

Pupil diameter
(mm)

6.6

5.8

4.9

3.8

3.0

2.4

2.0

1.5

1.0

Intensity of light reflected from the eye

2.5 EXPERIMENTAL MEASUREMENTS of light that has been reflected from a human eye looking at a fine line. The reflected light has been blurred by double passage through the optics of the eye. Source: Campbell and Gubisch, 1966.

20   10   0   10   20

Visual angle (minutes of arc)

image by placing a light-sensitive device called a **photodetector** at different positions on the screen. The vertical graph in Figure 2.6B shows a measurement of the intensity of the monitor image at all screen locations.

The output of the optical transformation is the image formed at the retina. When the input image is one-dimensional, the retinal image will be one-dimensional, too. Hence, we can represent it using a curve as in the bottom of Figure 2.6B. We will discuss the optical components of the visual system in more detail later in this chapter, but from simply looking at Figures 2.1 and 2.4 we can see that the monitor image passes through a lot of biological material before arriving at the retina. Because the optics of the eye are not perfect, the retinal image is not an exact copy of the monitor image: the retinal image is a blurred copy of the input image.

A good theoretical account of a transformation, such as the mapping from monitor image to retinal image, should have two important features. First, the theoretical account should suggest *which* measurements we should make to characterize the transformation fully. Second, the theoretical account should describe *how* to use these measurements to predict the retinal image distribution for all other monitor images.

(A)

(B)

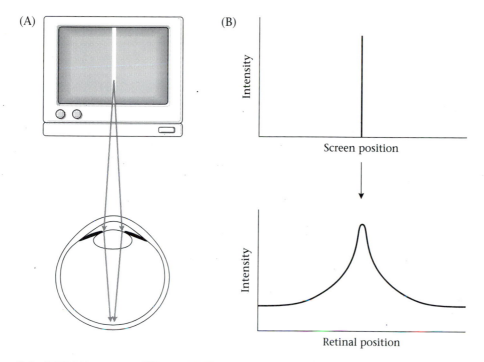

2.6   **RETINAL IMAGE FORMATION,** illustrated with a single-line input image. (A) A one-dimensional monitor image consists of a set of lines at different intensities. The image is brought to focus on the retina by the cornea and lens. (B) We can represent the intensity of a one-dimensional image using a simple graph (top) that shows the light as a function of horizontal screen position. Only a single value is plotted, since the one-dimensional image is constant along the vertical dimension. The retinal image (bottom) is a blurred version of the one-dimensional input image. The retinal image is also one-dimensional and is represented by a single curve.

    The monitor image described in Figure 2.6 is but one example of an infinite array of possible input images. Since there is no hope of measuring the response to every possible input, in order to characterize optical blurring completely we must build a model that specifies how any input image is transformed into a retinal image. We will use a set of general tools referred to as **linear-systems methods** to develop a method of predicting the retinal image from any input image. These tools will permit us to solve the problem of estimating the optical transformation from the monitor to the retinal image. The tools are sufficiently general, however, that we will be able to use them repeatedly throughout this book.

    There is no single theory that applies to all measurement situations. But linear-systems theory does apply to many important experiments. Best of all, we have a simple experimental test that permits us to decide whether linear-systems theory is appropriate to our measurements. To see whether linear-systems theory is appropriate, we must check to

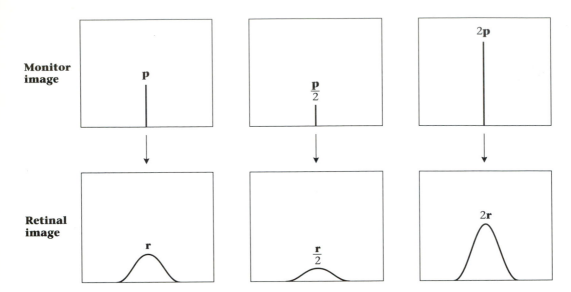

2.7   THE PRINCIPLE OF HOMOGENEITY. Input stimuli (top) and corresponding retinal images (bottom) are shown in each part of the figure. The three input stimuli are the same except for a scale factor. Homogeneity is satisfied when the corresponding retinal images are scaled by the same factor. The top left panel shows an input image at unit intensity, while the top middle and top right panels show the image scaled by 0.5 and 2.0, respectively.

see that our data satisfy the two properties of **homogeneity** and **superposition**.

Homogeneity

A test of homogeneity is illustrated in Figure 2.7. The top three panels show a series of monitor images, and the bottom three panels show the corresponding measurements of reflected light.[3] Suppose we represent the intensities of the lines in the one-dimensional monitor image using the vector **p** and we represent the retinal image measurements by the vector **r**. Now, suppose we scale the input signal by a factor a, so that the new input is $a\mathbf{p}$. We say that the system satisfies homogeneity if the output signal is also scaled by the same factor of a, and thus the new output is $a\mathbf{r}$. For example, if we halve the input intensity, then the reflected light measured at the photodetector should be one-half the intensity (middle panel). If we double the light intensity, the response

---

[3] I will use vectors and matrices in calculations to eliminate burdensome notation. Matrices will be denoted by boldface, uppercase roman letters (for example, $\mathbf{M}$). Column vectors will be denoted using lowercase boldface roman letters (for example, $\mathbf{v}$). The transpose operation will be denoted by a superscript T, $\mathbf{v}^T$. Scalar variables will be in italic typeface, and they will usually be denoted using the English alphabet (for example, a), except when tradition demands the use of Greek symbols (for example, α). The ith entry of a vector, $\mathbf{v}$, is a scalar and will be denoted as v_i. The ith column of a matrix, $\mathbf{M}$, is a vector, denoted $\mathbf{m}_i$. The scalar entry in the ith row and jth column of the matrix $\mathbf{M}$ will be denoted m_{ij}.

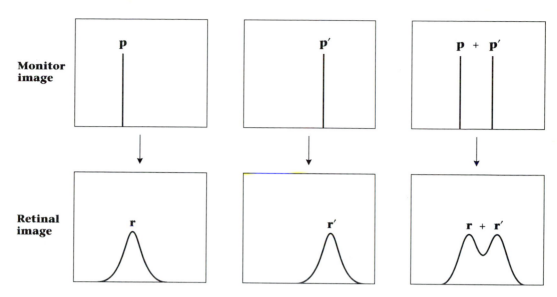

2.8 THE PRINCIPLE OF SUPERPOSITION. Each of the three parts of the picture shows an input stimulus and the corresponding retinal image. The stimulus shown in the left panel is a single-line image; in the middle panel the stimulus is a second line displaced from the first; the stimulus shown in the right panel is the sum of the first two lines. Superposition holds if the retinal image in the right panel is the sum of the retinal images in the middle and left panels.

should double (right panel). Campbell and Gubisch's measurements of light reflected from the human eye satisfy homogeneity.

Superposition

Suppose we measure the response to two different input stimuli. For example, suppose we find that input pattern **p** generates the response **r**, and input pattern **p′** generates response **r′**. Now we measure the response to a new input stimulus equal to the sum of **p** and **p′**. If the response to the new stimulus is the sum of the responses measured singly, **r** + **r′**, then the system is a linear system (Figure 2.8). By measuring the responses stimuli individually and then the response to the sum of the stimuli, we test superposition. When the response to the sum of the stimuli equals the sum of the individual responses, then we say the system satisfies superposition. Campbell and Gubisch's measurements of light reflected from the eye satisfy this principle.

Superposition, used as both an experimental procedure and a theoretical tool, is probably the single most important idea in this book. You will see it again and again in many forms.

We can summarize homogeneity and superposition succinctly using two equations. Write the linear optical transformation that maps the input image to the light intensity at each of the receptors as

$$\mathbf{r} = L(\mathbf{p}) \qquad (2.1)$$

Homogeneity and superposition are respectively defined by the following pair of equations:[4]

$$L(a\mathbf{p}) = aL(\mathbf{p}) \tag{2.2}$$

$$L(\mathbf{p} + \mathbf{p}') = L(\mathbf{p}) + L(\mathbf{p}') \tag{2.3}$$

Implications of Homogeneity and Superposition

Figure 2.9 illustrates how we will use linear-systems methods to characterize the relationship between the input signal from a monitor and light reflected from the eye.[5] First, we make an initial set of measurements of the light reflected from the eye for each single-line monitor image, with the monitor image set to unit intensity. If we know the measurements of reflections from single-line images, and we know that the system is linear, then we can calculate the light reflected from the eye for any monitor image: any one-dimensional image is the sum of a collection of lines.

Consider an arbitrary one-dimensional image, as illustrated at the top of Figure 2.9. We can conceive of this image as the sum of a set of single-line monitor images, each at its own intensity, p_i. We have measured the reflected light from each single-line image alone, call this $\mathbf{r}_i$ for the ith line. By homogeneity it follows that the reflected light from ith line will be a scaled version of this response, namely $p_i\mathbf{r}_i$. Next, we combine the light reflected from the single-line images. By superposition, we know that the light reflected from the original monitor image, $\mathbf{r}$, is the sum of the light reflected from the single-line images,

$$\mathbf{r} = \sum_i^N p_i\mathbf{r}_i \tag{2.4}$$

Equation 2.4 defines a transformation that maps the input stimulus, $\mathbf{p}$, into the measurement, $\mathbf{r}$. Because of the properties of homogeneity and superposition, the transformation is the weighted sum of a fixed collection of vectors: when the monitor image varies, only the weights (p_i) in the formula vary, but the vectors ($\mathbf{r}_i$; the reflections from single-line stimuli) remain the same. Hence, the reflected light will always be the weighted sum of these reflections.

---

[4] Notice that the superposition leads us to expect homogeneity for integer scalars since
$$L(2\mathbf{p}) = L(\mathbf{p} + \mathbf{p}) = L(2\mathbf{p}) = 2L(\mathbf{p})$$
and in general if we sum n copies of $\mathbf{p}$
$$L(n\mathbf{p}) = nL(\mathbf{p})$$
I consider homogeneity separately from superposition to avoid the tedium of treating the case of irrational numbers in certain proofs.
[5] I analyze a one-dimensional monitor images to simplify the notation. The principles remain the same, but the notation becomes cumbersome, when we consider two-dimensional images.

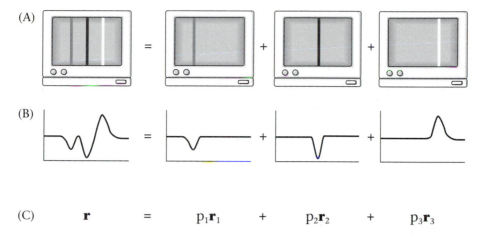

(C) $\mathbf{r}$ = $p_1\mathbf{r}_1$ + $p_2\mathbf{r}_2$ + $p_3\mathbf{r}_3$

2.9 APPLICATION OF HOMOGENEITY AND SUPERPOSITION. (A) A one-dimensional monitor image is the weighted sum of a set of lines. An example of a one-dimensional image is shown on the left and the individual monitor lines comprising the monitor image are shown separately on the right. (B) Each line in the component monitor image contributes to the retinal image. (C) The retinal image generated by the ith monitor line at unit intensity is represented by the vector $\mathbf{r}_i$. The intensity of the ith monitor line is p_i. By homogeneity, the retinal image of the ith monitor line is $p_i\mathbf{r}_i$. By superposition, the retinal image of the collection of monitor lines is sum of the individual retinal images, $\sum p_i\mathbf{r}_i$.

To represent the weighted sum of a set of vectors, we use the mathematical notation of **matrix multiplication**. Multiplying a matrix times a vector computes the weighted sum of the matrix columns; the entries of the vector define the weights. Matrix multiplication and linear-systems methods are closely linked. In fact, the set of all possible matrices define the set of all possible linear transformations of the input vectors.

Matrix multiplication has a shorthand notation to replace the explicit sum of vectors in Equation 2.4. In the example here, we define a matrix, **R**, whose columns are the responses to individual monitor lines at unit intensity, $\mathbf{r}_i$. The matrix **R** is called the **system matrix**. Matrix multiplication of the input vector, **p**, times the system matrix **R**, transforms the input vector into the output vector. Matrix multiplication is written using the notation

$$\mathbf{r} = \mathbf{R}\mathbf{p} \qquad (2.5)$$

Matrix multiplication follows naturally from the properties of homogeneity and superposition. Hence, if a system satisfies homogeneity and superposition, we can describe the system response by creating a system matrix that transforms the input to the output.

A NUMERICAL EXAMPLE OF A SYSTEM MATRIX. Suppose we measure a monitor that displays only three lines. We can describe the monitor image using a column vector with three entries, $\mathbf{p} = (p_1, p_2, p_3)^{\mathrm{T}}$. The lines of unit intensity are $(1,0,0)^T$, $(0,1,0)^T$ and $(0,0,1)^T$. We measure the response to these input vectors to build the system matrix. Suppose the measurements for these three lines are $(0.1,0.2,0.5,0.3,0,0)^T$, $(0,0.1,0.2,0.5,0.1,0)^T$, and $(0,0,0.2,0.5,0.3,0)^T$, respectively. We place these responses into the columns of the system matrix:

$$\mathbf{R} = \begin{pmatrix} 0.1 & 0 & 0 \\ 0.2 & 0.1 & 0 \\ 0.5 & 0.2 & 0.2 \\ 0.3 & 0.5 & 0.5 \\ 0 & 0.1 & 0.3 \\ 0 & 0 & 0 \end{pmatrix} \tag{2.6}$$

We can predict the response to any monitor image using the system matrix. For example, if the monitor image is $\mathbf{p} = (0.5, 1.0, 0.2)^T$ we multiply the input vector and the system matrix to obtain the response, on the left side of Equation 2.7.

$$\begin{pmatrix} 0.05 \\ 0.20 \\ 0.49 \\ 0.75 \\ 0.16 \\ 0 \end{pmatrix} = \begin{pmatrix} 0.1 & 0 & 0 \\ 0.2 & 0.1 & 0 \\ 0.5 & 0.2 & 0.2 \\ 0.3 & 0.5 & 0.5 \\ 0 & 0.1 & 0.3 \\ 0 & 0 & 0 \end{pmatrix} \begin{pmatrix} 0.5 \\ 1.0 \\ 0.2 \end{pmatrix} \tag{2.7}$$

Why Linear Methods Are Useful

Linear systems methods are a good starting point for answering an essential scientific question: how can we generalize from the results of measurements using a few stimuli to predict the results we will obtain when we measure using novel stimuli? Linear-systems methods tell us to examine homogeneity and superposition. If these empirical properties hold in our experiment, then we will be able to measure responses to a few stimuli and predict responses to many other stimuli.

This is very important advice. Quantitative scientific theories are attempts to *characterize* and then *explain* systems with many possible input stimuli. Linear-systems methods tell us how to organize experiments to characterize our system: measure the responses to a few individual stimuli, and then measure the responses to mixtures of these stimuli. If superposition holds, then we can obtain a good characterization of the system we are studying. If superposition fails, the work will not be wasted since we will need to explain the results of superposition experiments to obtain a complete characterization of the measurements.

To explain a system, we need to understand the general organizational principles concerning the system parts and how the system works in relationship to other systems. Achieving such an explanation is a creative act that goes beyond simple characterization of the input and output relationships. But any explanation must begin with a good characterization of the processing the system performs.

Shift-Invariant Linear Transformations

Shift-Invariant Systems: Definition

Since homogeneity and superposition are well satisfied by Campbell and Gubisch's experimental data, we can predict the result of any input stimulus by measuring the system matrix that describes the mapping from the input signal to the measurements at the photodetector. But recall that the experimental data are measurements of light that has passed through the optical elements of the eye *twice*, and we want to know the transformation that takes place when light passes through the optics *once*. To correct for the effects of double passage, we will take advantage of a special property of optics of the eye, **shift-invariance**. Shift-invariant linear systems are an important class of linear systems, and they have several properties that make them simpler than general linear systems. The following section briefly describes these properties and how we take advantage of them. The mathematics underlying these properties is not hard; I sketch proofs of these properties in Appendix A.

Suppose we start to measure the system matrix for the Campbell and Gubisch experiment by measuring responses to different lines near the center of the monitor. Because the quality of the optics of the human eye is fairly uniform near the fovea, we will find that our measurements, and by implication the retinal images, are nearly the same for all single-line monitor images. The only way they will differ is that, as the position of the input shifts, the position of the output will shift by a corresponding amount. The shape of the output, however, will not change. An example of two measurements we might find when we measure using two lines on the monitor is illustrated in the left and middle panels of Figure 2.8. As we shift the input line, the measured output shifts. This is a good feature for a lens to have, because as an object's position changes, the recorded image should remain the same (except for a shift). When we shift the input and the form of the output is invariant, we call the system shift-invariant.

Shift-Invariant Systems: Properties

Shift-invariant systems have two important properties for our purposes:

1. *We can define the system matrix of a shift-invariant system from the response to a single stimulus.* Ordinarily, we need to build the system matrix by combining the responses to many individual

lines. The system matrix of a linear shift-invariant system is simple to estimate since these responses are all the same except for a shift. Hence, if we measure a single column of the matrix, we can fill in the rest of the matrix. For a shift-invariant system, there is only one response to a line. This response is called the **linespread** of the system. We can use the linespread function to fill in the entire system matrix.

2. *The response to a harmonic function at frequency f is a harmonic function at the same frequency.* Sinusoids and cosinusoids are called **harmonics** or **harmonic functions**. When the input to a shift-invariant system is a harmonic at frequency f, the output will be a harmonic at the same frequency. The output may be scaled in amplitude and shifted in position, but it still will be a harmonic at the input frequency.

For example, when a sinusoidal input stimulus is defined at locations $i = 1, \ldots, N$ then its values are $\sin(2\pi f i/N)$, and the response of a shift-invariant system will be a scaled and shifted copy of the sinusoid, $s_f \sin(2\pi f i/N + \phi_f)$. There is some uncertainty concerning the output because there are two unknown values, the scale factor, s_f, and the phase shift, ϕ_f. However, for each sinusoidal input we know a lot about the output; the output will be a harmonic of the same frequency as the input.

We can express this same result another useful way. Expanding the sinusoidal output using the summation rule we have

$$s_f \sin\left(\tfrac{2\pi f i}{N} + \phi_f\right) = a_f \cos\left(\tfrac{2\pi f i}{N}\right) + b_f \sin\left(\tfrac{2\pi f i}{N}\right) \qquad (2.8)$$

where

$$a_f = s_f \sin(\phi_f)$$

$$b_f = s_f \cos(\phi_f) \qquad (2.9)$$

In words, when the input is a sinusoid at frequency f, the output is the weighted sum of a sinusoid and a cosinusoid, both at the same frequency as the input. In this representation, the two unknown values are the weights of the sinusoid and the cosinusoid.

For many optical systems, the relationship between harmonic inputs and the output is even simpler. When the input is a harmonic function at frequency f, the output is a scaled copy of the function, and there is no shift in spatial phase. For example, when the input is $\sin(2\pi f i/N)$, the output will be $s_f \sin(2\pi f i/N)$, and only the scale factor, which depends on frequency, is unknown.

The Optical Quality of the Eye

We are now ready to correct the measurements for the effects of double passage through the optics of the eye. To make the method easy to understand, I will analyze how to do the correction by first making the assumption that the optics introduce no phase shift into the retinal image; this means, for example, that a cosinusoidal stimulus creates a cosinusoidal retinal image, scaled in amplitude. It is not necessary to assume that there is no phase shift, but the assumption is reasonable, and the main principles of the analysis are easier to see if we assume there is no phase shift.

To understand how to correct for double passage, consider a hypothetical alternative experiment Campbell and Gubisch might have done (Figure 2.10). Suppose Campbell and Gubisch had used input stimuli equal to cosinusoids at various spatial frequencies, f. Because the optics are shift-invariant and there is no frequency-dependent phase shift, the retinal image of a cosinusoid at frequency f is a cosinusoid scaled by a factor s_f. The retinal image passes back through the optics and is scaled again, so that the measurement would be a cosinusoid

(A)

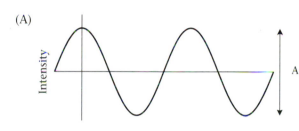

(B)

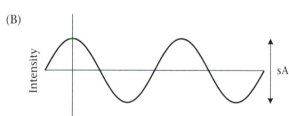

(C)

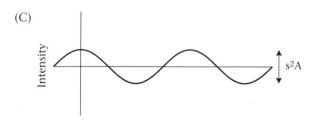

Spatial position

2.10 SINUSOIDS AND DOUBLE PASSAGE. The amplitude, A, of an input cosinusoidal stimulus (A) is scaled by a factor, s, after passing through the eye's optics (B). (C) Passage through the optics a second time scales the amplitude again, resulting in a signal with amplitude s^2A.

scaled by the factor $s_f{}^2$. Hence, had Campbell and Gubisch used a co-sinusoidal input stimulus, we could deduce the retinal image from the measured image easily: the retinal image would be a cosinusoid with an amplitude equal to the square root of the amplitude of the measurement.

Campbell and Gubisch used a single line, not a set of cosinusoidal stimuli. But we can still apply the basic idea of the hypothetical experiment to their measurements. Their input stimulus, defined over N locations, is

$$p_i = \begin{cases} N & \text{if } i = 0 \\ 0 & \text{if } 1 \le i < N \end{cases} \tag{2.10}$$

Appendix A explains how one can express the stimulus as the weighted sum of harmonic functions by using the **discrete Fourier series**. The representation of a single line is equal to the sum of cosinusoidal functions

$$\hat{p}_i = 0.5 + \sum_{f=1}^{N-1} \cos(2\pi f i/N) \tag{2.11}$$

Because the system is shift-invariant, the retinal image of each cosinusoid is a scaled cosinusoid, say, with scale factor s_f. The retinal image is scaled again during the second pass through the optics to form the cosinusoidal term they measured.

Using the discrete Fourier series, we also can express the measurement as the sum of cosinusoidal functions,

$$\text{Measurement} = 0.5 + \sum_{f=1}^{N-1} (s_f)^2 \cos(2\pi f i/N) \tag{2.12}$$

We know the values of $s_f{}^2$, since this was Campbell and Gubisch's measurement. The image of the line at the retina, then, must have been

$$l_i = 0.5 + \sum_{f=1}^{N-1} s_f \cos(2\pi f i/N) \tag{2.13}$$

The values l_i define the linespread function of the eye's optics. We can correct for the double passage and estimate the linespread because the system is linear and shift-invariant.

As you read further about experimental and computational methods in vision science, remember that there is nothing inherently important about sinusoids as visual stimuli; we must not confuse the stimulus with the system or with the theory we use to analyze the system. When the system is a shift-invariant linear system, sinusoids can be helpful in simplifying our calculations and reasoning, as we have just seen. The sinusoidal stimuli are important only insofar as they help us to measure or clarify the properties of the system. If the system is not shift-invariant, the sinusoids may not be important at all.

The Linespread Function

Figure 2.11 contains Campbell and Gubisch's estimates of the linespread functions of the eye. Notice that as the pupil size increases, the width of the linespread function increases, which indicates that the focus is worse for larger pupil sizes. As the pupil size increases, light reaches the retina through larger and larger sections of the lens. As the area of the lens affecting the passage of light increases, the amount of blurring increases.

The measured linespread functions, l_i, along with our belief that we are studying a shift-invariant linear system that introduces no phase

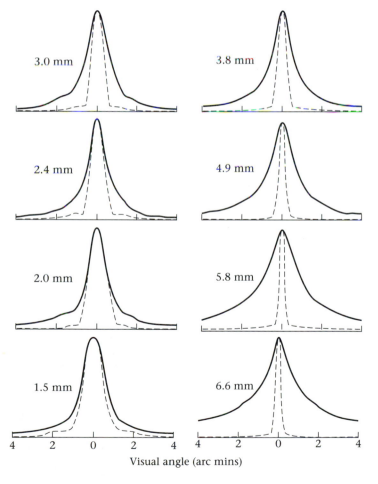

2.11 THE LINESPREAD FUNCTION OF THE HUMAN EYE. The panels show measurements for a variety of pupil diameters. The solid line in each panel is a measurement of the linespread. The dotted lines are the diffraction-limited linespread for a pupil of that diameter. (Diffraction is explained below). Source: Campbell and Gubisch, 1966.

3.0 mm

3.8 mm

2.4 mm

4.9 mm

2.0 mm

5.8 mm

1.5 mm

6.6 mm

4   2   0   2   4   4   2   0   2   4

Visual angle (arc mins)

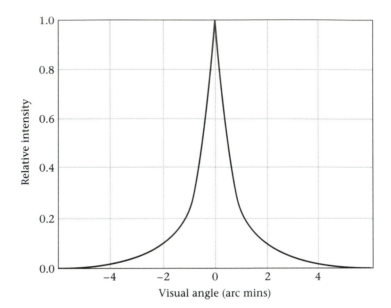

2.12 THE HUMAN LINE-SPREAD FUNCTION. An analytic approximation for an eye with a pupil diameter of 3.0 mm. Source: Westheimer, 1986.

shift, permit us to predict the retinal image for any one-dimensional input image. To calculate these predictions, it is convenient to have a function that describes the linespread of the human eye. Westheimer (1986) suggested the following formula to describe an even-symmetric linespread function that is consistent with the measurements of the human eye, when in good focus and when the pupil diameter is near 3 mm:

$$l_i = 0.47e^{-3.3i^2} + 0.53e^{-0.93|i|} \qquad (2.14)$$

where the variable i refers to position on the retina specified in terms of minutes of visual angle. A graph of this linespread function is shown in Figure 2.12.

We can use Westheimer's linespread function to predict the retinal image of any one-dimensional input stimulus.[6] Some examples of the predicted retinal image are shown in Figure 2.13. Because the optics blur the image, even the light from a very fine line is spread across several photoreceptors. I will discuss the relationship between the optical defocus and the positions of the photoreceptors in Chapter 3.

The Modulation Transfer Function

In correcting for double passage, we thought about the measurements in two separate ways. Since our main objective was to derive the line-

[6] Westheimer's linespread function is for an average observer under one set of viewing conditions. As the pupil changes size and as observers age, the linespread function can vary. Consult IJspeert et al. (1993) and Williams et al. (1994) for alternatives to Westheimer's formula.

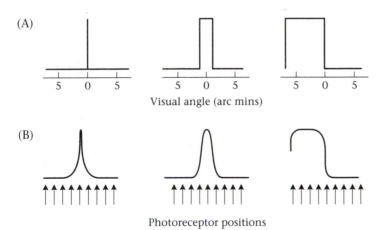

(A)

Visual angle (arc mins)

(B)

Photoreceptor positions

2.13 EXAMPLES OF THE EFFECT OF OPTICAL BLURRING. (A) Images of a line, an edge, and a bar pattern. (B) The estimated retinal image after blurring by Westheimer's linespread function. The spacing of the photoreceptors in the retina is shown by the stylized arrows.

spread function (a function of spatial position), we considered the measurements in terms of light intensity as a function of spatial position. When we corrected for double passage through the optics, however, we also considered a hypothetical experiment in which the stimuli were harmonic functions (cosinusoids). To perform this calculation, we found that it was easier to correct for double passage by thinking of the stimuli as the sums of harmonic functions, rather than as functions of spatial position.

These two ways of looking at the system, in terms of spatial functions or as sums of harmonic functions, are equivalent. To see this, notice that we can use the linespread function to derive the retinal image to any input image. Hence, we can use the linespread to compute the scale factors of the harmonic functions. Conversely, we already saw that by measuring how the system responds to the harmonic functions, we can derive the linespread function. It is convenient to be able to reason about system performance in both ways.

The **optical transfer function** defines the system's complete response to harmonic functions. The optical transfer function is a complex-valued function of spatial frequency. The complex values code both the scale factor and the phase shift the system induces in each harmonic function.

When the linespread function of the eye is an even-symmetric function, there is no phase shift of the harmonic functions. In this case, we can describe the system completely using a real-valued function, the **modulation transfer function**. This function defines the scale factors applied to each spatial frequency. The data points in Figure 2.14 show measurements by Williams et al. (1994) of the modulation transfer function of the human eye. These data points were obtained using a method called visual interferometry, which is described in Chapter 3. Along with the data points, I have plotted the predicted modulation transfer function using Westheimer's (1986) linespread function and a

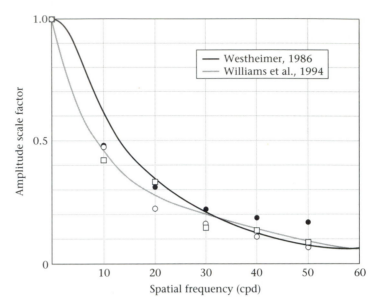

**2.14 MODULATION TRANS-
FER FUNCTION** measurements
of the optical quality of the
eyes of three different observers
made by Williams et al. (1994)
using visual interferometry (see
Chapter 3). The data are compared with the predictions from
the linespread suggested by
Westheimer (1986) and a curve
fit through the Williams et al.
data.

curve fit to the data reported by Williams et al. The curve derived by
Westheimer using completely different data sets differs from the measurements by Williams et al. by no more than about 20 percent. This
should tell you something about the relative precision of these descriptions of the optical quality of the lens.

The linespread function and the modulation transfer function offer us two different ways to think about the optical quality of the lens.
The linespread function in Figure 2.12 describes defocus as the spread of
light from a fine slit across the photoreceptors: the light is spread across
3–5 photoreceptors. The modulation transfer function in Figure 2.14 describes defocus as an amplitude reduction of harmonic stimuli: beyond
12 cycles per degree (cpd) the amplitude is reduced by more than a factor of 2.

Lenses, Diffraction, and Aberrations

Lenses and Accommodation

What prevents the optics of the eye from focusing the image perfectly?
To answer this question we should consider why a lens is useful in
bringing objects to focus at all.

As a ray of light is reflected from an object, it will travel along along
a straight line until it reaches a new material boundary. At that point,
the ray may be absorbed by the new medium, reflected, or refracted.
The latter two possibilities are illustrated in Figure 2.15A. We call the
angle between the incident ray of light and the perpendicular to the
surface the **angle of incidence**. The angle between the reflected ray and

the perpendicular to the surface is called the **angle of reflection**, and it equals the angle of incidence. Of course, reflected light is not useful for image formation at all. The useful rays for imaging must pass from the first medium into the second. As they pass between the two media, the rays may change direction, in which case we say that the light is refracted. The angle between the refracted ray and the perpendicular to the surface is called the **angle of refraction**.

The relationship between the angle of incidence and the angle of refraction was first discovered by a Dutch astronomer and mathematician, Willebrord Snell, in 1621. He observed that when ϕ is the angle of incidence, and ϕ' is the angle of refraction, then

$$\frac{\sin \phi}{\sin \phi'} = \frac{v'}{v} \tag{2.15}$$

where v' and v are the **refractive indices** of the two media. The relationship in Equation 2.15 is known as **Snell's law**. The refractive index of an optical medium is the ratio of the speed of light in a vacuum to the speed of light in the optical medium. The refractive index of glass is 1.520; for water the refractive index is 1.333; and for air it is nearly

(A)

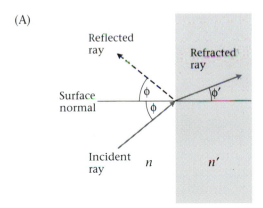

(B)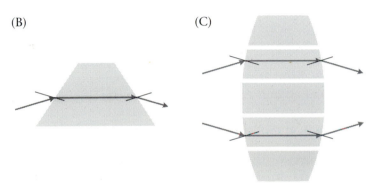

(C)

2.15 SNELL'S LAW. (A) When a light ray passes from one medium to another, the ray can be refracted so that the angle of incidence (ϕ) does not equal the angle of refraction (ϕ'). Instead, the angle of refraction depends on the refractive indices of the two media (n and n') a relationship called Snell's law, which is defined in Equation 2.15. (B) A prism causes two refractions of the light ray and can reverse the ray's direction from upward to downward. (C) A lens combines the effect of many prisms in order to converge the rays diverging from a point source.

1.000. The refractive index of the human cornea is 1.376, quite similar to that of water (which is the main content of our eyes).

Now, consider the consequence of applying Snell's law twice, as light passes into and then out of a prism, as illustrated in Figure 2.15B. We can draw the path of a ray of light as it enters the prism using Snell's law. The symmetry of the prism and the reversibility of the light path make it easy to draw the exit path. Passage through the prism bends the ray's path downward. The prism causes the light to deviate significantly from a straight path; the amount of the deviation depends upon the angle of incidence and the angle between the two sides of the prism.

We can build a lens by smoothly combining many infintesimally small prisms to form a convex lens, as illustrated in Figure 2.15C. In constructing such a lens, any deviations from the smooth shape, or imperfections in the material used to build the lens, will cause the individual rays to be brought to focus at slightly different points in the image plane. These small deviations of shape or materials are a source of the imperfections in the image.

Objects at different depths are focused at different distances behind the lens. The **lensmaker's equation** relates the distance between the source and the lens to the distance between the image and the lens. The lensmaker's equation depends on **focal length** of the lens. Call the distance from the center of the lens to the source d_s, the distance to the image d_i, and the focal length of the lens f. Then the lensmaker's equation is

$$\frac{1}{d_s} + \frac{1}{d_i} = \frac{1}{f} \tag{2.16}$$

From this equation, notice that we can measure the focal length of a convex thin lens by using it to image a very distant object. In that case, the term $1/d_s$ is zero so that the image distance is equal to the focal length. When I first moved to California, I spent a lot of time measuring the focal length of the lenses in my laboratory by going outside and imaging the sun on a piece of paper behind the lens; the sun was a convenient and reliable source at optical infinity. (It had been a less reliable source in my previous home of Pennsylvania.)

The **optical power** of a lens is a measure of how strongly the lens bends the incoming rays. Since a lens with a short focal length bends the incident ray more than a long-focal-length lens, the optical power is the inversely related to focal length. The optical power is defined as the reciprocal of the focal length measured in meters and is specified in units of **diopters**. When we view faraway objects, the distance from the middle of the cornea and the flexible lens to the retina is 0.017 m. Hence, the optical power of the human eye is $1/0.017 = 58.8$, or roughly 60 diopters.

From the optical power of the eye $(1/f)$ and the lensmaker's equation, we can calculate the image distance of a source at a known distance. For example, the top curve in Figure 2.16 shows the relationship between image distance (d_i) and source distance (d_s) for a 60-diopter lens. Sources beyond 1.0 m are imaged at essentially the same distance behind the optics. Sources closer than 1.0 m are imaged at a longer distance, so that the retinal image is blurred.

To bring nearby sources into focus on the retina, muscles attached to the lens change its shape and thus change the power of the lens. The bottom two curves in Figure 2.16 illustrate that sources closer than 1.0 m can be focused onto the retina by increasing the power of the lens. The process of adjusting the focal length of the lens is called **accommodation**. You can see the effect of accommodation by first focusing on your finger placed near your noise and noticing that objects in the distance appear blurred. Then, while leaving your finger in place, focus on the distant objects. You will notice that your finger now appears blurred.

Pinhole Optics and Diffraction

The only way to remove lens imperfections completely is to remove the lens. It is possible to focus images without any lens at all by using **pinhole optics**, as illustrated in Figure 2.17. A pinhole serves as a useful focusing element because only the rays passing within a narrow angle are used to form the image. As the pinhole is made smaller, the angular deviation is reduced. Reducing the size of the pinhole serves to reduce the amount of blurriness due to the deviation among the rays. Another advantage of using pinhole optics is that, no matter how distant the source point is from the pinhole, the source is rendered in sharp focus.

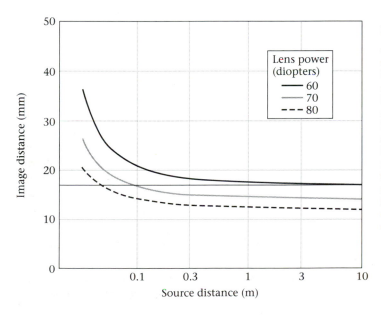

2.16 DEPTH OF FIELD OF THE HUMAN EYE. Image distance is shown as a function of source distance. The solid horizontal line shows the distance of the retina from the lens center. A lens power of 60 diopters brings distant objects into focus, but not nearby objects; to bring nearby objects into focus the power of the lens must increase. The depth of field (the distance over which objects will continue to be in reasonable focus) can be estimated from the slope of the curve.

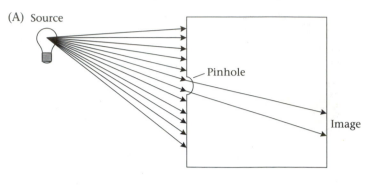

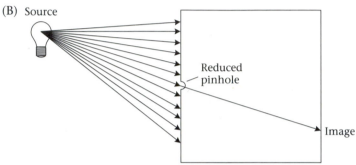

2.17 PINHOLE OPTICS. Using ray-tracing, we see that only a small pencil of rays passes through a pinhole. (A) If we use a wide pinhole, light from the source spreads across the image, making it blurry. (B) If we narrow the pinhole, only a small amount of light is let in. The image is sharp; the sharpness is limited by diffraction.

Since the focusing is due to selecting out a thin pencil of rays, the distance of the point from the pinhole is irrelevant, and accommodation is unnecessary.

The pinhole design has two disadvantages, however. First, as the pinhole aperture is reduced, less and less of the light emitted from the source is used to form the image. The reduction of signal has many disadvantages for sensitivity and acuity. There is a second fundamental limit to the pinhole design that we must consider. When light passes through a small aperture, or near the edge of an aperture, the rays do not travel in a single straight line. Instead, the light from a single ray is scattered into many directions and produces a blurry image. The dispersion of light rays that pass by an edge or narrow aperture is called **diffraction**. Diffraction scatters the rays coming from a small source across the retinal image and therefore serves to defocus the image. The effect of diffraction when one makes an image using pinhole optics is shown in Figure 2.18.

Diffraction can be explained in two different ways. First, diffraction can be explained by thinking of light as a wave phenomenon. A wave exiting from a small aperture expands in all directions; a pair of coherent waves from adjacent apertures creates an interference pattern. Second, diffraction can be understood in terms of quantum mechanics; indeed, the explanation of diffraction is one of the important achievements of quantum mechanics. Quantum mechanics supposes that there are limits to how well one may know both the position and direction of

(A)   (B)   (C)

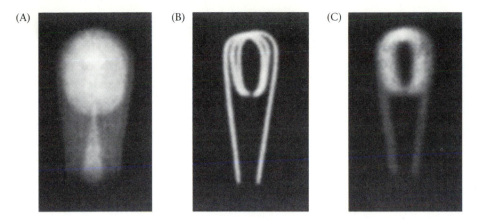

2.18   DIFFRACTION LIMITS THE QUALITY OF PINHOLE OPTICS. These three images of a bulb filament were made using pinholes with decreasing size. (A) When the pinhole is relatively large, the image rays are not properly converged, and the image is blurred. (B) Reducing the size of the pinhole improves the focus. (C) Reducing the size of the pinhole further worsens the focus, due to diffraction. From Ruechardt, 1958.

travel of a photon of light.[7] The more we know about a photon's position, the less we can know about its direction. If we know that a photon has passed through a small aperture, then we know something about the photon's position, and we must pay a price in terms of uncertainty concerning its direction of travel. As the aperture becomes smaller, our certainty concerning the position of the photon becomes greater; this uncertainty takes the form of the scattering of the direction of travel of the photons as they pass through the aperture. For very small apertures, for which our position certainty is high, the photon's direction of travel is very broad, producing a very blurry image.

There is a close relationship between the uncertainty in a photon's direction of travel and the shape of the aperture (Figure 2.19). In all cases, however, when the aperture is relatively large, our knowledge of the spatial position of the photons is insignificant, and diffraction does not contribute to defocus. As the pupil size decreases, and we know more about the position of the photons, the diffraction pattern becomes broader and spoils the focus.

In the human eye, diffraction takes place because light must pass through the circular aperture defined by the pupil. When the ambient light intensity is high, the pupil may become as small 2 mm in diameter. For a pupil opening this small, the optical blurring in the human eye is due only to the small region of the cornea and lens near the center of our visual field. With this small an opening of the pupil, the quality of the cornea and lens is rather good, and the main source of image blur is diffraction. At low light intensities, the pupil diameter is as

---

[7] Light may be described in two complementary ways. For certain calculations, we describe light as being composed of discrete packets of energy called *photons* or *quanta*. For other calculations, we describe light as a continuous wavefront traveling through space.

(A)

(B)

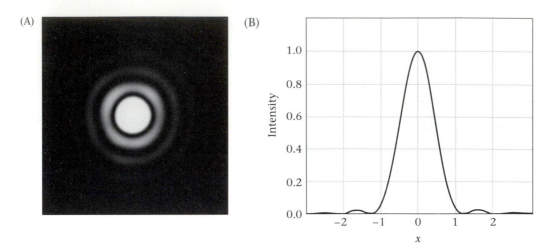

2.19 DIFFRACTION PATTERN CAUSED BY A CIRCULAR APERTURE. (A) The image of a diffraction pattern measured through a circular aperture. (B) A graph of the cross-sectional intensity of the diffraction pattern. After Goodman, 1968.

large as 8 mm. When the pupil is open quite wide, the distortion due to cornea and lens imperfections is large compared to the defocus due to diffraction.

One way to evaluate the quality of the optics is to compare the blurring in the eye to the blurring from diffraction alone. The dashed lines in Figure 2.11 plot the blurring expected from diffraction for different pupil widths. Notice that when the pupil diameter is 2.0 mm, the observed linespread is about equal to the amount expected by diffraction alone; the lens causes no further distortion. As the pupil opens, the observed linespread is worse than the blurring expected by diffraction alone. For these pupil sizes the defocus is due mainly to imperfections in the optics.[8]

The Pointspread Function and Astigmatism

Most images, of course, are not composed of weighted sums of lines. The set of images that can be formed from sums of lines oriented in the same direction are all one-dimensional patterns. To create more complex images, we must either use lines with different orientations or use a different fundamental stimulus: the point.

Any two-dimensional image can be described as the sum of a set of points. If the system we are studying is linear and shift-invariant, we can use the response to a point and the principle of superposition

---

[8] Helmholtz (1909) calculated that this was the case long before any precise measurements of the optical quality of the eye were possible. He wrote, "The limit of the visual capacity of the eye as imposed by diffraction, as far as it can be calculated, is attained by the visual acuity of the normal eye with a pupil of the size corresponding to a good illumination" (p. 442).

(A)

(B)

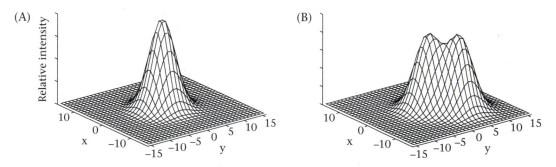

2.20   THE POINTSPREAD FUNCTION. (A) A pointspread function and (B) the sum of two pointspreads. The pointspread function is the image created by a source consisting of a small point of light. When the optics are shift-invariant, the image to any stimulus can be predicted from the pointspread function.

to predict the response of a system to any two-dimensional image. The measured response to a point input is called the **pointspread function**. A pointspread function and the superposition of two nearby pointspreads are illustrated in Figure 2.20.

Since lines can be formed by adding together many different points, we can compute the system's linespread function from the pointspread. In general, we cannot deduce the pointspread function from the linespread because there is no way to add a set of lines, all oriented in the same direction, to form a point. If it is known that a pointspread function is circularly symmetric, however, a unique pointspread function can be deduced from the linespread function. The calculation is described in Goodman (1968) and in Yellott et al. (1984).

When the pointspread function is not circularly symmetric (Figure 2.21), measurements of the linespread function will vary with the orientation of the test line. It may be possible to adjust the accommodation of this type of system so that any single orientation is in good focus,

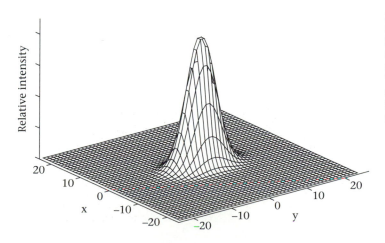

2.21   ASTIGMATISM implies an asymmetric pointspread function. The pointspread shown here is narrow in one direction and wide in another. The spatial resolution of an astigmatic system is better in the narrow direction than the wide direction.

but it will be impossible to bring all orientations into good focus at the same time. For the human eye, astigmatism can usually be modeled by describing the defocus as being derived from the contributions of two one-dimensional systems at right angles to one another. The defocus in intermediate angles can be predicted from the defocus of these two systems.

Chromatic Aberration

The light incident at the eye is usually a mixture of different wavelengths. When we measure the system response, there is no guarantee that the linespread or pointspread function we measure with different wavelengths will be the same. Indeed, for most biological eyes the pointspread function is very different with different wavelengths of light. When the pointspread functions of different wavelengths of light are quite different, then the lens is said to exhibit **chromatic aberration**.

When the incident light is a mixture of many different wavelengths (as for white light), then we can see a chromatic fringe at edges. The fringe occurs because the different wavelength components of the white light are focused more or less sharply. Figure 2.22 plots one measure of the chromatic aberration. The smooth curve plots the lens power (mea-

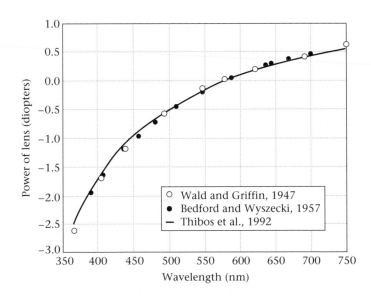

2.22 CHROMATIC ABERRATION OF THE HUMAN EYE. The data points measure the optical power one must add to the human eye in order to bring different wavelengths into a common focus with a 578-nm light. The smooth curve plots a formula created by Thibos et al. (1992) that predicts the measurements and interpolates smoothly between them. The formula is $D(\lambda) = p - q/(\lambda - c)$, where λ is wavelength in micrometers, $D(\lambda)$ is the defocus in diopters, $p = 1.7312$, $q = 0.63346$, and $c = 0.21410$. After Marimont and Wandell, 1993.

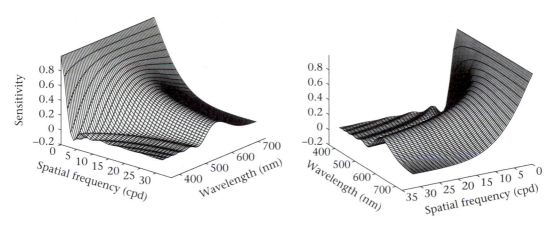

2.23   TWO VIEWS OF THE MODULATION TRANSFER FUNCTION OF A MODEL EYE at various wavelengths. The model eye has the same chromatic aberration as the human eye (see Figure 2.22) and a 3-mm pupil diameter. The eye is in focus at 580 nm; the curve at 580 nm is diffraction-limited. The retinal image has no significant contrast beyond 4 cpd at short wavelengths. After Marimont and Wandell, 1993.

sured in units of diopters) needed to bring each wavelength into focus along with a 578-nm light. When the various wavelengths pass through the correcting lens, the optics will have the same power as the eye's optics at 578 nm. The two sets of measurements agree well with one another and are similar to what would be expected if the eye were simply a bowl of water. The smooth curve through the data is a curve used by Thibos et al. (1992) to predict the data.

An alternative method of representing the axial chromatic aberration of the eye is to plot the modulation transfer function at different wavelengths. The two surface plots in Figure 2.23 show the modulation transfer function at a series of wavelengths. The plots show the same data, but seen from different points of view (so that you can see around the "hill"). The calculation in the figure is based on an eye with a pupil diameter of 3 mm, the same chromatic aberration as the human eye, and in focus at 580 nm.

The retinal image contains very poor spatial information at wavelengths that are far from the best plane of focus. By accommodation, the human eye can place any wavelength into good focus, but it is impossible to focus all wavelengths simultaneously.[9]

---

[9] A possible method of improving the spatial resolution of the eye to different wavelengths of light is to place the different classes of photoreceptors in slightly different image planes. Ahnelt et al. (1987) and Curcio et al. (1991) have observed that the short-wavelength photoreceptors have a slightly different shape and length from the middle- and long-wavelength photoreceptors. In principle, this difference could play a role to compensate for the chromatic aberration of the eye; however, the difference is very small, and it is unlikely that it plays any significant role in correcting for axial chromatic aberration.

Exercises

1. Matrix calculations:

   (a) Consider the matrix

   $$A = \begin{pmatrix} 1 & 2 \\ 2 & -4 \\ 4 & 6 \end{pmatrix}$$

   Write the transpose of A, the matrix A^T.

   (b) Compute the result of multiplying A with the column vector

   $$v = \begin{pmatrix} 1 \\ 0 \end{pmatrix}$$

   (That is, compute Av).

   (c) Compute the result of multiplying A with the column vector

   $$\begin{pmatrix} 1 \\ 1 \end{pmatrix}$$

   (d) Compute the result of multiplying A with the column vector

   $$\begin{pmatrix} 1 \\ -1 \end{pmatrix}$$

   (e) Compute the result of multiplying A by the matrix

   $$B = \begin{pmatrix} 1 & 1 & 1 \\ 0 & 1 & -1 \end{pmatrix}$$

   (f) How do the results of multiplying by the matrix compare with the results of multiplying by the individual vectors?

2. Answer the following questions about lens specifications:

   (a) When your eye doctor prescribes lenses for you, she tells you the visual correction you require in terms of diopters. What does it mean to require a 6-diopter optical correction?

   (b) What does visual astigmatism mean?

   (c) Do you think it is likely that different people vary greatly in the extent of chromatic aberration in their eyes? Why or why not?

   (d) Suppose one individual needs a 6-diopter correction and another individual needs a 3-diopter correction. Give your best guess about the relative linespread functions of the two individuals. Give your best guess about the relative modulation transfer functions of the two individuals.

3. Answer these questions with respect to experimental estimates of the linespread function of the eye's optics:

   (a) What instrumentation might Campbell and Gubisch have used to measure the pointspread function of the eye? What additional problems would they have had if they had measured the pointspread? (See Artal et al. [1989] for such measurements.)

(b) Can the linespread function be determined from the pointspread function? If so, how?

(c) Can the pointspread function be determined from a single linespread function? If so, how? (See the appendix in Yellott et al. [1984].)

(d) Do you think it is possible that Campbell and Gubisch measured the light reflected precisely from the photoreceptor plane? Why or why not? If not, how should one evaluate their estimated linespread function, compared to the linespread function in the plane of the photoreceptors?

(e) IJspeert et al. (1993) recently described a new set of equations to characterize the optical linespread of the eye. These equations are intended to generalize Westheimer's function described in the text. Read their paper and compare their new curves with Westheimer's formula.

4. In the text we reviewed how to derive the linespread function from double-pass measurements. In that derivation, I assumed that the linespread function introduces no phase shift into the retinal image, so that the true linespread is an even-symmetric function. Artal et al. (1995) have shown that, in fact, measurements made using the double-pass method do not capture accurately the phase-shifts that are present in the true linespread function: the double-pass measurements always produce an even-symmetric linespread function no matter what the true shape of the linespread. Read their article to understand why this is so. Then explain why, even with the loss of phase information, the double-pass measurements still yield an accurate estimate of the modulation transfer function.

3

The Photoreceptor Mosaic

In Chapter 2 we reviewed Campbell and Gubisch's (1966) measurements of the optical linespread function. Their data are presented in Figure 2.11 as smooth curves, but the actual measurements must have taken place at a series of finely spaced intervals, or **sample points**. In designing their experiment, Campbell and Gubisch must have considered carefully how to space their sample points because they wanted to space their measurement samples only finely enough to capture the intensity variations in the measurement plane. Had they positioned their samples too widely, they would have missed significant variations in the data. On the other hand, spacing the sample positions too closely would have made the measurement process wasteful of time and resources.

Just as Campbell and Gubisch sampled their linespread measurements, so too the retinal image is sampled by the nervous system. Since only those portions of the retinal image that stimulate the visual photoreceptors can influence vision, the sample positions are determined by the positions of the photoreceptors. If the photoreceptors are spaced too widely, the image encoding will miss significant variation present in the retinal image. On the other hand, if the photoreceptors are spaced very close to one another compared to the spatial variation that is possible given the inevitable optical blurring, then the image encoding will be redundant, using more neurons than necessary to do the job. In this chapter we will consider how the spatial arrangement of the photoreceptors, called the **photoreceptor mosaic**, limits our ability to infer the spatial pattern of light intensity present in the retinal image.

The Photoreceptor Types

We will consider separately the photoreceptor mosaics of each of the different types of photoreceptors. There are two fundamentally different types of photoreceptors in the human eye: the **rods** and the **cones**. There are approximately 5 million cones and 100 million rods in each eye. The positions of these two types of photoreceptors differ in many ways across the retina. Figure 3.1 shows how the relative densities of cone photoreceptors and rod photoreceptors vary across the retina.

The rods initiate vision under low illumination levels, called **scotopic** light levels, while the cones initiate vision under higher, **photopic** light levels. The intensities under which both rods and cones can initiate vision are called **mesopic** intensity levels. At most wavelengths of light, the cones are less sensitive to light than the rods. Rods are very sensitive light detectors: they generate a detectable photocurrent response when they absorb a single photon of light (Hecht et al., 1942; Schwartz, 1977; Baylor et al., 1987).

The region of highest visual acuity in the human retina is the **fovea**. As Figure 3.1 shows, the central fovea contains no rods, but it does contain the highest concentration of cones. There are approximately 50,000 cones in the central human fovea. This explains why we cannot see very dim sources, such as weak starlight, when we look straight at them. These sources are too dim to be visible through the all-cone fovea. The dim source only becomes visible when it is placed in the

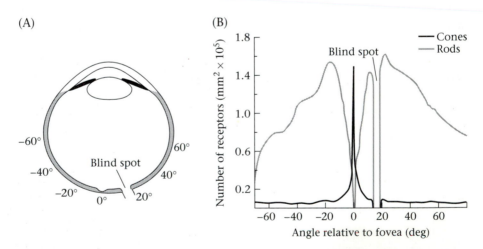

3.1 THE DISTRIBUTION OF ROD AND CONE PHOTORECEPTORS across the human retina. (A) Degrees of visual angle relative to the position of the fovea for the left eye; the position of the blind spot is also shown. (B) The cone receptors are concentrated in the fovea. The rod photoreceptors are absent from the fovea and reach their highest density between 10 and 20 degrees peripheral to the fovea. No photoreceptors are present in the blind spot.

periphery and can be detected by the rods. Since there are no photoreceptors at the optic disk, where the ganglion cell axons exit the retina, there is a **blind spot** in that region of the retina (see Chapter 5).

Figure 3.2 contains schematic diagrams of mammalian rod and cone photoreceptors. Light imaged by the cornea and lens is shown entering the receptors through the **inner segment**. The light passes into the **outer segment**, which contains light-absorbing **photopigments**. As light passes from the inner to the outer segment of the photoreceptor, it will either be absorbed by one of the photopigment molecules in the outer segment or it will simply continue through the photoreceptor and exit out the other side. Some light imaged by the optics will pass between the photoreceptors. Overall, less than 10 percent of the light entering the eye is absorbed by the photoreceptor photopigments (Baylor, 1987).

The rod photoreceptors contain a photopigment called **rhodopsin**. The rods are small, there are many of them, and they sample the retinal image very finely. Yet visual acuity under scotopic viewing conditions is very poor compared to visual acuity under photopic conditions. The reason for this is that the signals from many rods converge onto a single neuron within the retina, so that there is a many-to-one relationship between rod receptors and neurons in the optic tract. The density of rods and the convergence of their signals onto single neurons improve the sensitivity of rod-initiated vision, but rod-initiated vision does not resolve fine spatial detail.

The foveal cone signals do not converge onto single neurons. Instead, several neurons encode the signal from each cone, so that there is a one-to-many relationship between the foveal cones and optic-tract neurons. The dense representation of the foveal cones suggests that the spatial sampling of the cones must be an important aspect of the visual encoding.

There are three types of cone photoreceptors within the human retina. Each cone can be classified based on the wavelength sensitivity of the photopigment in its outer segment. Estimates of the spectral sensitivity of the three types of cone photoreceptors are shown in Figure 3.3. These curves are measured from the cornea, so they include

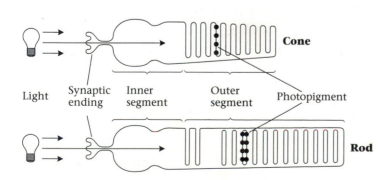

3.2 MAMMALIAN ROD AND CONE PHOTORECEPTORS contain the light-absorbing pigments that initiate vision. Light enters the photoreceptors through the inner segment and is funneled to the outer segment, which contains the photopigment.

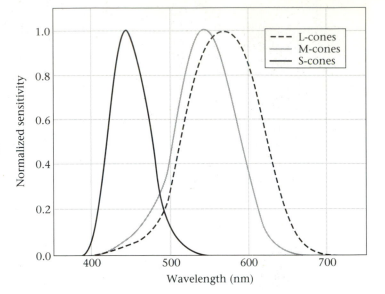

3.3 SPECTRAL SENSITIVITIES OF THE L-, M-, AND S-CONES in the human eye. The measurements are based on a light source at the cornea, so that the wavelength loss due to the cornea, lens, and other inert pigments of the eye plays a role in determining the sensitivity. Source: Stockman and MacLeod, 1993.

light loss due to the cornea, lens, and inert materials of the eye. In the next chapter we will study how color vision depends upon the differences in wavelength selectivity of the three types of cones. Throughout this book I will refer to the three types of photoreceptors as the **L-cones**, **M-cones**, and **S-cones**.[1]

Because light is absorbed after passing through the inner segment, the position of the inner segment determines the spatial sampling position of the photoreceptor. Figure 3.4 shows cross sections of the human cone photoreceptors at the level of the inner segment in the human fovea (Figure 3.4A) and just outside the fovea (Figure 3.4B). In the fovea, the cross section shows that the inner segments are very tightly packed and form a regular sampling array. A cross section just outside the fovea shows that the rod photoreceptors fill the spaces between the cones and disrupt the regular packing arrangement. The scale bar represents 10 μm; the cone photoreceptor inner segments in the fovea are approximately 2.3 μm wide with a minimum center-to-center spacing of about 2.5 μm. Figure 3.4C shows plots of the cone densities from several different human retinas as a function of the distance from the foveal center. The cone density varies across individuals.

Units of Visual Angle

We can convert cone sizes and separations into degrees of visual angle as follows. The distance from the effective center of of the eye's optics to the retina is 1.7×10^{-2} m (17 mm). We compute the visual angle spanned by one cone, ϕ, from the trigonometric relationship in Figure 3.5: the tangent of an angle in a right triangle is equal to the ratio of

[1] The letters refer to long-, **middle**-, and short-wavelength peak sensitivity, respectively.

(A)

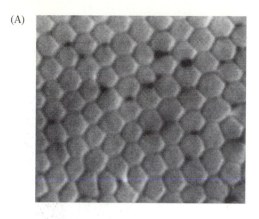

(B)

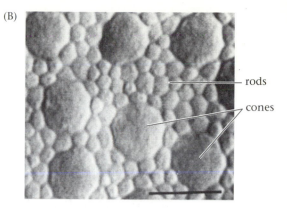

rods

cones

(C)

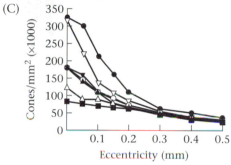

3.4 THE SPATIAL MOSAIC OF THE HUMAN CONES. Cross sections of the human retina at the level of the inner segments showing (A) cones in the fovea, and (B) cones in the periphery. Note the size difference (scale bar = 10 μm), and that, as the separation between cones grows, the rod receptors fill in the spaces. (C) Cone density plotted as a function of distance from the center of the fovea for seven human retinas; cone density decreases with distance from the fovea. Source: Curcio et al., 1990.

the lengths of the sides opposite and adjacent to the angle. This leads to the following equation:

$$\tan(\phi) = (2.5 \times 10^{-6}\ m)/(1.7 \times 10^{-2}\ m)$$

$$= 1.47 \times 10^{-4} \tag{3.1}$$

The width of a cone in degrees of visual angle, ϕ, is approximately 0.0084 degrees, or roughly 0.5 minutes of visual angle. In the center of

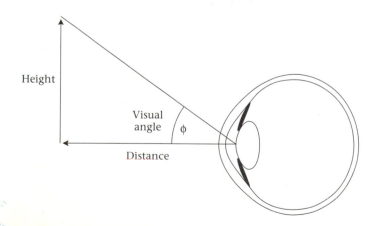

3.5 CALCULATING THE VIEWING ANGLE. By trigonometry, the tangent of the viewing angle, ϕ, is equal to the ratio of height to distance in the right triangle shown. Therefore, ϕ is the inverse tangent of that ratio (see Equation 3.1).

the eye, then, where the cone photoreceptors are packed densely, their centers are separated by about half of a minute of visual angle.

The S-Cone Mosaic

Behavioral Measurements

Just as the rods and cones have different spatial sampling distributions, so too the three types of cone photoreceptors have different spatial sampling distributions. The sampling distribution of the short-wavelength cones was the first to be measured empirically, and it has been measured both with behavioral and physiological methods. Behavioral experiments by Williams et al. (1981) took advantage of several features of the short-wavelength photoreceptors. As background to their work, I shall first describe these features.

The photopigment in the short-wavelength photoreceptors is significantly different from the photopigment in the other two types of photoreceptors. Notice that the wavelength sensitivity of the L and M photopigments are very nearly the same (see Figure 3.3). The sensitivity of the S photopigment is significantly higher than that of the other two photopigments in the short-wavelength part of the spectrum. As a result, if we present the visual system with a very weak light, containing energy only in the short-wavelength portion of the spectrum, the S-cones will absorb relatively more quanta than the other two classes. Indeed, the discrepancy in the absorptions is so large that it is reasonable to suppose that when short-wavelength light is barely visible, at detection threshold, perception is initiated uniquely from a signal that originates in the short-wavelength receptors.

We can give the short-wavelength receptors an even greater sensitivity advantage by presenting a blue test target on a steady yellow background. As I will discuss in later chapters, steady backgrounds suppress visual sensitivity. By using a yellow background, we can suppress the sensitivity of the L- and M-cones and the rods and yet keep the sensitivity of the S-cones. This improves the relative sensitivity advantage of the short-wavelength receptors in detecting the short-wavelength test light.

A second special feature of the S-cones is that they are very rare in the retina. Based on other experiments which will be described in Chapter 4, it has been suspected for many years that no cones containing short-wavelength photopigment are present in the central fovea. It has also been suspected for some time that the number of cones containing the short-wavelength photopigment is quite small compared to the other two classes. If the S-cones are widely spaced, and if we can isolate them with these choices of test stimulus and background, then we can measure the mosaic of short-wavelength photoreceptors.

During the experiment, the subjects visually fixated on a small mark. After the eye was perfectly fixated, the subject pressed a button and initiated a stimulus presentation, and indicated whether or not the stimulus was visible. If light from the short-wavelength test light fell upon a region that contained S-cones, sensitivity should be relatively high. On the other hand, if that region of the retina contained no S-cones, sensitivity should be rather low. Hence, from the spatial pattern of visual sensitivity, Williams et al. inferred the spacing of the S-cones.

The sensitivity measurements are shown in Figure 3.6. First, notice that in the very center of the visual field, in the central fovea, there is a large valley of low sensitivity. In this region, there appear to be no short-wavelength cones at all. Second, beginning about half a degree from the center of the visual field there are small, punctate spatial regions of high sensitivity. We interpret these results by assuming that these peaks correspond to the positions of this observer's S-cones. The gaps in between, where the observer has rather low sensitivity, are likely to be patches of L- and M-cones. Around the central fovea, the typical separation between the inferred S-cones is about 8–12 minutes of visual angle. Thus, there are 5–7 S-cones per degree of visual angle.

Biological Measurements

There have been many biological measurements of the S-cone mosaic, and we can compare some of these these with the behavioral measurements. Marc and Sperling (1977) used a stain that is taken up by cones when they are active. They applied this stain to a baboon retina and

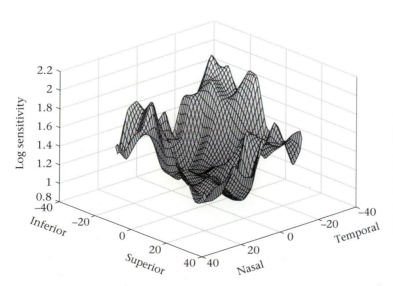

3.6 PSYCHOPHYSICAL ESTIMATE OF THE SPATIAL MOSAIC OF THE S-CONES. The height of the surface represents the observer's threshold sensitivity to a short-wavelength test light presented on a yellow background. The test was presented at a series of locations spanning a grid around the fovea. The local peaks in sensitivity probably correspond to the positions of the S-cones. From Williams et al., 1981.

then stimulated the retina with short-wavelength light in the hopes of staining only the short-wavelength receptors. They found that only a few cones were stained when the stimulus was a short-wavelength light. The typical separation between the stained cones was about 6 minutes of arc, a smaller value than the separation that Williams et al. observed, which may reflect a species-related difference.

DeMonasterio et al. (1985) discovered that when the procion-yellow dye is applied to the retina, it stains only a small subset of the photoreceptors' inner segments completely. Figure 3.7 shows a spatial mosaic of these stained cones in a tangential section of the retina at the inner segment level just outside the fovea. The inner segments that take up this dye fully appear as light disks; the dark disks are also cone inner segments; the small disks in between are rods. By studying many such images across the retina, DeMonasterio et al. found that these cones are absent from the central fovea, they have their peak density 1 degree from the central fovea, and they are spaced widely compared to the other cones. These factors are consistent with the psychophysical observations concerning the positions of the S-cones, and thus it seems likely that the stained inner segments are the S-cones.

Why would the S-cones stain more strongly than the other cone types? The S-cones are generally more susceptible to disease than the other two cone types. Hence, it is possible that when they react to the procion-yellow dye, their membranes break apart more readily than the L- and M-cone membranes, and the stain is absorbed more completely.

In the above experiments, the arguments identifying these special cones as S-cones are rather indirect. A more certain procedure was developed by Curcio and her colleagues. They used a biological marker that had been developed using knowledge of the genetic code for the S-cone photopigment to label selectively the S-cones in the human retina (Curcio et al., 1991). Their measurements agree well quantitatively with

3.7 A BIOLOGICAL ESTIMATE OF THE S-CONE SPATIAL MOSAIC as revealed by procion-yellow dye in the macaque retina. This image is a cross-section of the retina at the cone inner segment layer. Cone inner segments that absorbed the procion-yellow dye strongly appear as lightly colored large spots; the dark spots show the positions of cone inner segments that did not absorb the stain strongly. The small circles in between the cones show the positions of the rods. From DeMonasterio et al., 1985; courtesy of Stan Schein.

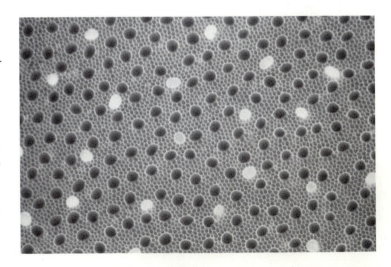

Williams's psychophysical measurements and show that the average spacing between the S-cones is 10 minutes of visual angle. Curcio and her colleagues could also confirm some early anatomical observations that the S-cones differ slightly in size and shape from the L- and M-cones. The S-cones have a wider inner segment, and they appear to be inserted within an orderly sampling arrangement of their own between the sampling mosaics of the other two cone types (Ahnelt et al., 1987).

Why Are the S-Cones Widely Spaced?

The spacing between the S-cones is much larger than the spacing between the L- and M-cones. Why should this be? The large spacing between the S-cones is consistent with the strong blurring of the short-wavelength component of the image due to the axial chromatic aberration of the lens. Recall that axial chromatic aberration of the lens blurs the short-wavelength portion of the retinal image, the part S-cones are particularly sensitive to, more than the middle- and long-wavelength portion of the image (see Figure 2.22). In fact, under normal viewing conditions the retinal image of a fine line at 450 nm falls to one half its peak intensity nearly 10 minutes of visual angle away from the location of its peak intensity. At that wavelength, the retinal image only contains significant contrast at spatial frequency components below 3 cpd of visual angle, and the retinal image encoded by the S cones contains no rapid spatial variation. Because the image changes smoothly over space, it can be represented using few spatial samples. For reasons I will describe later in this chapter, when the highest spatial frequency in the image is 3 cpd we can represent the retinal pattern using the responses of only 6 S-cones per degree of visual angle. Thus, the theoretical expectations and empirical observations concerning the S cone sampling mosaic are in good agreement.

Interestingly, the *spatial* defocus of the short-wavelength component of the image also implies that signals initiated by the S-cones will vary slowly over *time*. In natural scenes, temporal variation occurs mainly because of movement of the observer or an object. When a sharp boundary moves across a cone position, the light intensity changes rapidly at that point. However, if the boundary is blurred, changing gradually over space, then the light intensity changes more slowly. Since the short-wavelength signal is blurred by the optics, and temporal variation is mainly due to motion of objects, the S-cones will generally be coding slower temporal variations than the L- and M-cones.

At the very earliest stages of vision, we see that the properties of different components of the visual pathway fit smoothly together. The optics set an important limit on visual acuity, and the S-cone sampling mosaic can be understood as a consequence of the optical limitations.

As we shall see, the L- and M-cone mosaic densities also make sense in terms of the optical quality of the eye.

This explanation of the S-cone mosaic flows from our assumption that visual acuity is the main factor governing the photoreceptor mosaic. For the visual streams initiated by the cones, this is a reasonable assumption. However, there are other important factors that can play a role in the design of a visual pathway. For example, acuity is not the dominant factor in the visual stream initiated by rod vision. In principle the resolution available in the rod encoding is comparable to the acuity available in the cone responses; but visual acuity using rod-initiated signals is very poor compared to acuity using cone-initiated signals. The high density of the rods and their convergence onto individual neurons suggest that we think of rod-initiated vision in terms of improving the signal-to-noise ratio under low light levels. In the rod-initiated signals, the visual system trades visual acuity for an increase in the signal-to-noise ratio.

When we ask why the visual system has a particular property, we need to relate observations from the different disciplines that make up vision science. Questions about anatomy require us to think about the behavior the anatomical structure serves. Similarly, behavior must be explained in terms of algorithms and the anatomical and physiological responses of the visual pathway. By considering the visual pathways from multiple points of view, we piece together a complete picture of how the system functions.

Visual Interferometry

We would like to use behavioral experiments to measure threshold repeatedly through individual L- and M-cones using small points of light, as we did with the S-cones. However, this method cannot succeed for the L- and M-cones because the pointspread function distributes light over a region containing about 20 cones, so that the visibility of even a small point of light may involve any of the cones from a large pool (see Figures 2.11 and 2.12). We can, however, use a method introduced by LeGrand in 1935 to defeat the optical blurring. The technique is called **visual interferometry**, and it is based upon the principle of diffraction.

Thomas Young, the brilliant scientist, physician, and classicist, demonstrated that it is possible to use the interference of light waves emanating from a pair of **mutually coherent sources** to create a pattern of light (Young, 1802). A pair of light sources is mutually coherent when the wavefront of the two sources is the same except for a constant shift of the wavefront. Young demonstrated this effect to the Royal Society of England by means of an apparatus like the one shown in Figure 3.8. He passed light from an ordinary source through a single slit, and then

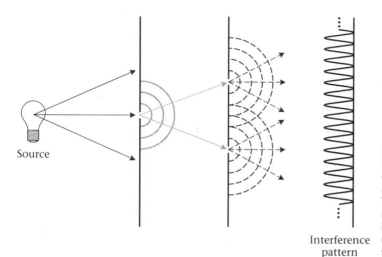

Source

Interference
pattern

3.8 YOUNG'S DOUBLE-SLIT EXPERIMENT uses a pair of coherent light sources to create an interference pattern of light. The intensity of the resulting image is nearly sinusoidal, and its spatial frequency depends upon the spacing between the two slits.

through a pair of slits.[2] Because the light from the double slits originates from a common source, these two sources are mutually coherent. Young showed that the waves from the double slits interfere with one another and create a nearly sinusoidal interference pattern.

We can also achieve this interference effect by using a laser as the original source. The key elements of a visual interferometer used by MacLeod et al. (1992) are shown in Figure 3.9. Light from a laser enters the beam-splitter and is divided into one part that continues along a straight path (solid line) and a second part that is reflected along a path to the right (dashed line). These two beams, originating from a common source, will be the pair of sources to create the interference pattern on the retina. Light from each beam is reflected from a mirror toward a glass cube. By varying the orientation of the glass cube, the experimenter can vary the paths of the two beams. When the glass cube is at right angles to the light path, as is shown in Figure 3.9A, the beams continue in a straight path along opposite directions and emerge from the beam-splitter at the same position. When the glass cube is rotated, as is shown in Figure 3.9B, the refraction due to the glass cube symmetrically changes the beam paths; they emerge from the beam-splitter at slightly different locations and act as a pair of point sources. This configuration creates two coherent beams that act like the two slits in Thomas Young's experiment, creating an interference pattern; the amount of rotation of the glass cube controls the separation between the two beams.

Each beam passes through only a very small section of the cornea and lens. The usual optical blurring mechanisms do not interfere with the image formation, since the lens does not serve to converge the light

---

[2] Young used pinholes, not slits, in his original experiments. Slits are used commonly now to increase the intensity of the interference pattern.

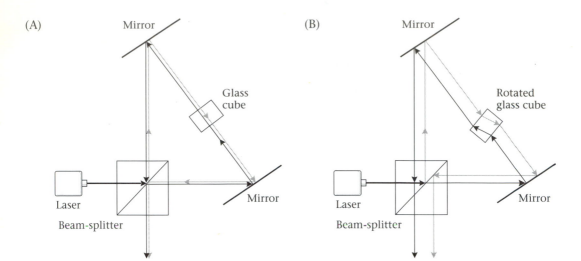

(A) Mirror Glass cube Laser Beam-splitter Mirror

(B) Mirror Rotated glass cube Laser Beam-splitter Mirror

3.9 A VISUAL INTERFEROMETER creates an interference pattern as in Young's double-slit experiment. In the device shown here, the original beam is split into two paths shown as the solid and dashed lines. (A) When the glass cube is at right angles to the light path, the two beams traverse an equal path and are imaged at the same point after exiting the interferometer. (B) When the glass is rotated, the two beams traverse slightly different paths, causing the images of the two coherent beams to be displaced and creating an interference pattern. After MacLeod et al., 1992.

(see the section on lenses in Chapter 2). Instead, the pattern that is formed depends upon the diffraction due to the restricted spatial region of the light source.

We can use diffraction to create retinal images with much higher spatial frequencies than are possible through ordinary optical imaging by the cornea and lens. Figure 3.10 is an image of a diffraction pattern created by a pair of slits. The intensity of the pattern is a nearly sinusoidal function of retinal position. The spatial frequency of the retinal image can be controlled by varying the separation between the focal points; the smaller the separation between the slits, the lower the spatial frequency in the interference pattern. Analogously, by rotating the glass cube in the interferometer and changing the separation of the two beams we can control the spatial frequency of the retinal image.

3.10 AN INTERFERENCE PATTERN. The image was created using a double-slit apparatus. The intensity of the pattern is nearly sinusoidal. From Jenkins and White, 1976.

Visual interferometry permits us to image fine spatial patterns at much higher contrast than when we image these patterns using ordinary optical methods. For example, Figure 2.14 shows that a 60-cpd sinusoid cannot exceed 10 percent contrast when imaged through the optics. Using a visual interferometer, we can present patterns at frequencies considerably higher than 60 cpd at 100 percent contrast.

However, a challenge remains: the interferometric patterns are not fine lines or points, but extended patterns (cosinusoids). Therefore, we cannot use the same logic as Williams et al. and map the receptors by carefully positioning the stimulus. We need to think a little bit more about how to use the cosinusoidal interferometric patterns to infer the structure of the cone mosaic.

Sampling and Aliasing

In this section we consider how the cone mosaic encodes the high-spatial-frequency patterns created by visual interferometers. The appearance of these high-frequency patterns will permit us to deduce the spatial arrangement of the combined L- and M-cone mosaics. The key concepts that we must understand to deduce the spatial arrangement of the mosaic are **sampling** and **aliasing**. These ideas are illustrated in Figure 3.11.

The most basic observation concerning sampling and aliasing is

(A)

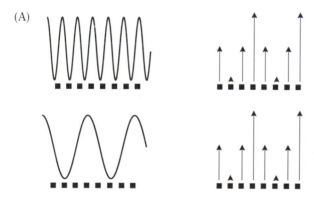

(B)

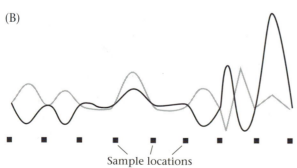

Sample locations

3.11 ALIASING of signals results when sampled values are the same but in-between values are not. (A) The continuous sinusoids on the left have the same values at the sample positions indicated by the black squares. The values of the two functions at the sample positions are shown by the height of the stylized arrows on the right. (B) Undersampling may cause us to confuse various functions, not just sinusoids. The two curves at the bottom have the same values at the sampled points, differing only in between the sample positions.

this: we can measure only that portion of the input signal that falls over the sample positions. Figure 3.11 shows one-dimensional examples of aliasing and sampling. Figure 3.11A depicts two different cosinusoidal signals (left), showing the locations of the sample points. The values of these two cosinusoids at the sample points are shown by the height of the arrows on the right. Although the two continuous cosinusoids are quite different, they have the same values at the sample positions. Hence, if cones are only present at the sample positions, the cone responses do not distinguish between these two inputs. We say that these two continuous signals are an aliased pair. Aliased pairs of signals are indistinguishable after sampling. Hence, sampling degrades our ability to discriminate between sinusoidal signals.

Figure 3.11B shows that sampling degrades our ability to discriminate between signals in general, not just between sinusoids. Whenever two signals agree at the sample points, their sampled representations agree. The basic phenomenon of aliasing is that signals which only differ between the sample points are indistinguishable after sampling.

Figure 3.12 shows an example of two square-wave patterns seen through a sampling grid. After sampling, the high-frequency pattern appears to be a rotated, low-frequency signal. Appendix F contains a computer program that can help you make sampling demonstrations like the one in Figure 3.12. If you print out square-wave patterns and various sampling arrays using the programs provided you can put the various patterns onto overhead transparencies and explore the effects of sampling.

3.12 SQUARE-WAVE ALIASING. The square wave on top is seen fairly accurately through the grid. The square wave on the bottom is at a higher spatial frequency than the grid sampling. When seen through the grid, the pattern appears at a lower spatial frequency and rotated.

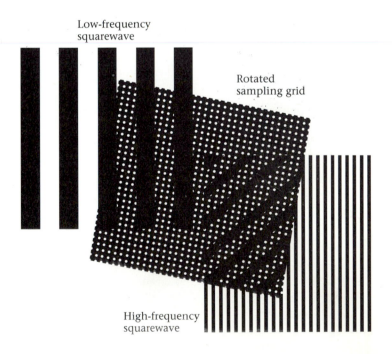

Low-frequency squarewave

Rotated sampling grid

High-frequency squarewave

Sampling Is a Linear Operation

The sampling transformation takes the retinal image as input and generates a portion of the retinal image as output. Sampling is a linear operation, as the following thought experiment reveals. Suppose we measure the sample values at the cone positions when we present image A; call the intensities at the sample positions $S(A)$. Now we measure the intensities at the sample positions for a second image, B; call the sample intensities $S(B)$. If we add together the two images, the new image, $A + B$, contains the sum of the intensities in the original images. The values picked out by sampling will be the sum of the two sample vectors, $S(A) + S(B)$.

Since sampling is a linear transformation, we can express it as a matrix multiplication. In our simple description, each position in the retinal image either falls within a cone inner segment or not. The sampling matrix consists of N rows representing the N sampled values. The entries in each row are all zeros except at the entry corresponding to that row's sampling position, where the value is 1.

Aliasing of Harmonic Functions

For uniform sampling arrays we have already observed that some pairs of sinusoidal stimuli are aliases of one another (see Figure 3.11A). We can analyze precisely which pairs of sinusoids form alias pairs using some algebra. Suppose that the continuous input signal is $\cos(2\pi f x)$. When we sample the stimulus at regular intervals, the output values will be the value of the cosinusoid at those regularly spaced sample points. Suppose further that within a single unit of distance there are N sample points, so that our measurements of the stimulus take place every $1/N$ units. Then the sampled values will be $S_f(k) = \cos(2\pi f k/N)$. A second cosinusoid, at frequency f' will be an alias if its sample values are equal, that is, if $S_{f'}(k) = S_f(k)$.

With a little trigonometry, we can prove that the sample values for any pair of cosinusoids with frequencies $N/2 - f$ and $N/2 + f$ will be equal. That is,

$$\cos\left(\frac{2\pi(N/2+f)k}{N}\right) = \cos\left(\frac{2\pi(N/2-f)k}{N}\right) \tag{3.2}$$

(To prove this, we must use the cosine addition law. The steps in the verification are left as Exercise 5 at the end of the chapter.)

The frequency $f = N/2$ is called the **Nyquist frequency** of the uniform sampling array; sometimes it is referred to as the **folding frequency**. Any cosinusoidal stimuli whose frequencies differ by equal amounts above and below the Nyquist frequency of a uniform sampling array will have identical sample responses.

Experimental Implications

The aliasing calculations suggest an experimental method to measure the spacing of the cones in the eye. If the cone spacing is uniform, then pairs of stimuli separated by equal amounts above and below the Nyquist frequency should appear indistinguishable. Specifically, a signal $\cos(2\pi(N/2 + f))$ that is above the Nyquist frequency will appear the same as the signal $\cos(2\pi(N/2 - f))$ that is an equal amount below the Nyquist frequency. Thus, as subjects view interferometric patterns of increasing frequency, as we cross the Nyquist frequency the perceived spatial frequency should begin to decrease even though the physical spatial frequency of the diffraction pattern increases.

Yellott (1982) examined the aliasing prediction for the primate retina using a nice graphical method (see Figure 3.12). He began with an image of the retina seen face-on that showed the spatial arrangement of the cones near the fovea. Then he made small holes in the paper at locations corresponding to each of the cone positions which served as a sampling mosaic through which he viewed other images. By restricting his view of other images with the sampling mosaic, he could see only those parts of the image that would be encoded by the cones. In this way, he could visualize the effects of spatial sampling by the cone mosaic. For example, by examining sine waves at different spatial frequencies, he could observe the Nyquist frequency at which aliasing begins through the cone mosaic.[3]

Williams and Collier (1983) used the properties of sampling and aliasing to estimate the spacing between the S-cones. Recall that by using small flashes of light Williams et al. (1981) had estimated the average S-cone separation to be 10 minutes of visual angle (six S-cones per degree of visual angle). Consequently, short-wavelength sinusoidal patterns seen only by the S-cones should appear as low frequency aliased patterns when the stimulus exceeds the Nyquist frequency of 3 cpd of visual angle. Experiments confirm this prediction (Williams and Collier, 1983).

The L- and M-Cone Mosaics

Experiments using a visual interferometer to image a high-frequency pattern at high contrast on the retina provide a powerful way to analyze the sampling mosaic of L- and M-cones. But, even before this was technical feat was possible, Helmholtz (1896) noticed that extremely fine patterns, looked at without any special apparatus, can appear wavy. He

---

[3] Yellott introduced the method and proper analysis, but he used Polyak's (1957) data on the outer segment positions rather than data on the inner segment positions. As a result, some of his conclusions were revised in later publications (Miller and Bernard, 1983).

attributed this observation to sampling by the cone mosaic. His perception of a fine pattern and his graphical explanation of the waviness in terms of sampling by the cone mosaic are shown in Figure 3.13A (boxed drawings).

Byram (1944) was the first to describe the appearance of high-frequency interference gratings. His drawings of the appearance of these patterns are shown in Figure 3.13B. The image on the left shows the appearance of a low-frequency diffraction pattern. The apparent spatial frequency of this pattern is faithful to the stimulus. Byram noted that as the spatial frequency increases toward 60 cpd, the pattern still appears to be a set of fine lines, but they are difficult to see (middle drawing). When the pattern significantly exceeds the Nyquist frequency, it becomes visible again but looks like the low-frequency pattern drawn on the right. Further, he reports that the pattern shimmers and is unstable, probably due to the motion of the pattern with respect to the cone mosaic.

Williams (1985b) used visual interferometry to measure the sampling density of the mosaic formed by the L- and M-cones together. These measurements were based both on the appearance and the visi-

(A)

(B)

(C)

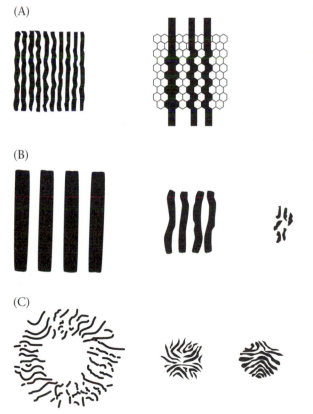

3.13 PERCEIVED ALIASING PATTERNS.
(A) Helmholtz (1896) observed aliasing of fine patterns, which he drew as depicted on the left. He offered an explanation of his observations in terms of cone sampling, as shown on the right. (B) Byram's (1944) drawings of three interference patterns at 40 (left), 85 (middle), and 150 cpd (right). (C) Drawings from Williams's laboratory (Williams, 1985b), of aliasing of patterns at 80 (left) and 110 cpd (middle and right).

bility of interference patterns seen mainly by the L- and M-cone mosaic. The two illustrations on the left of part Figure 3.13C are Williams's drawings of the appearance of 80-cpd and 110-cpd sinusoidal gratings created on the retina using a visual interferometer. The third drawing is by an artist who viewed a 110-cpd grating. The appearance of these patterns varies across the retina. The aliasing pattern for the 80-cpd stimulus appears to be a low-frequency pattern in the region surrounding the fovea and very little or no contrast in the fovea. At 110 cpd the alias pattern appears as high contrast stripes in the central fovea. These results, and many other related measurements, are consistent with a Nyquist sampling frequency of 60 cpd in the central fovea and decreasing with distance from the fovea. The variation in the Nyquist frequency is consistent with the coarser sampling density in the peripheral cone mosaic. The foveal Nyquist frequency is consistent with a center-to-center spacing between foveal cones of 30 seconds of visual angle.

Because the interferometric stimuli are one-dimensional, I have reported the sampling rate as if the mosaic were one-dimensional. In general, we should take into account the fact that the cones form a two-dimensional mosaic, not a one-dimensional array. Anatomical images of the cone mosaic (see Figure 3.4) show that in the central fovea the cones form a tightly packed triangular lattice, so that we do not expect any large effects at different orientations of the stimulus. Interferometric measurements have not shown any strong orientation dependencies. Some interesting visual effects occur when one varies the orientation of a stimulus seen only through its alias. As the images in Figure 3.12 show, the orientation of the low-frequency alias is not the same as the orientation of the input. Try the demonstration yourself and rotate the sampling grid.[4] You will see that the direction of motion of the alias is opposite to the motion of the input stimulus. These effects have been reported using visual stimuli presented by an interferometer (Coletta and Williams, 1987).

The cone sampling grid becomes more coarse and irregular outside the fovea. Just outside the fovea, rods push their way into the mosaic. The presence of the rods, coupled with the fact that the cones' widths increase with distance from the fovea, increases the spacing between the cones. Moreover, because the rods are interspersed in a random fashion, the cone mosaic is no longer a regular grid. As a result, we do not expect to see high-frequency interference patterns. Yellott (1982) has described this phenomenon, and he argues that it is a desirable and important feature of the cone mosaic. In the periphery, the sampling density of the cones is too low to capture the spatial variation of the retinal image. Were the cone mosaic regular, high spatial frequency

[4] You may use the PostScript program in Appendix F to print out a grid and a fine pattern.

patterns in the retinal image would be confused with regular low spatial frequency patterns that could easily be interpreted as significant objects. The disorder in the sampling mosaic prevents this confusion, causing the high spatial frequency patterns to alias with mottled noise that has no visual significance.

It has not been possible to draw firm experimental conclusions about the individual L- and M-cone mosaics using interferometric measurements. For the moment, we can only analyze the interferometric measurements in terms of a single mosaic formed from the combination of L- and M-cones. This is not too disturbing because, as we shall see in Chapter 9, there are several reasons to conceive of this combined mosaic as initiating a significant neural pathway that codes the intensity variation in the retinal image.

Visual Interferometry: Measurements of Human Optics

Using interferometry, we can estimate the quality of the optics of the eye. Suppose we ask an observer to set the contrast of a sinusoidal grating, imaged using an ordinary light source, such as a television monitor. The observer's sensitivity to the target will depend on the contrast reduction in the eye's optics and the observer's neural sensitivity to the target. Now, suppose that we create the same sinusoidal pattern using an interferometer. The interferometric stimulus bypasses the contrast reduction due to the optics. In this second experiment, then, the observer's sensitivity is limited only by the observer's neural sensitivity. Hence, the sensitivity difference between these two experiments is an estimate of the loss due to the optics.

The visual-interferometric method of measuring the quality of the optics has been used on several occasions. While the interferometric estimates are similar to estimates using reflections from the eye, they do differ somewhat. The difference is shown in Figure 2.14, which includes the Westheimer estimate of the modulation transfer function, created by fitting data from reflections, along with data and a modulation transfer function obtained from interferometric measurements. The current consensus is that the optical modulation transfer function is somewhat closer to the visual interferometric measurements than the reflection measurements. The reasons for the differences are discussed in several papers (e.g., Campbell and Green, 1965; Williams 1985; Williams et al., 1994).

Summary and Discussion

In this chapter we have reviewed the spatial arrangement of the photoreceptor mosaics, and have encountered several principles concerning image encoding. We have seen that the spatial properties of the photoreceptor mosaics may fulfill different visual goals. The rods are present in very high density, but many rod signals converge onto a single neuron so that we have very poor spatial resolution under scotopic visual conditions. The high spatial density of the rods, then, is probably to improve sensitivity, not spatial resolution. As we shall see in Chapter 4, signals from the foveal cones are carried on by single neurons. The spatial arrangement of the cone mosaics is probably organized to obtain high spatial resolution. In the central fovea, the L- and M-cones form a tightly packed mosaic with a sampling density that is high enough to capture all of the spatial variation present after the image has been blurred by the eye's optics. The cone sampling density in the peripheral retina is lower, and there the deleterious effects of aliasing are reduced by the disarray in the sampling mosaic.

We can image high spatial frequency patterns onto the cone mosaic by using a visual interferometer. From the appearance of these patterns and an understanding of aliasing, we can infer certain properties of the L-, M-, and S-cone mosaics. For stimuli seen through the S-cones just outside the fovea, aliasing begins at a spatial frequency near 3 cpd. This frequency is consistent with other estimates that predict a separation of 10 minutes of visual angle (36 S-cones/deg^2). For stimuli seen through the L- and M-cones in the fovea, the Nyquist frequency is consistent with a separation of 30 seconds of visual angle (1.4×10^4 cones/deg^2).

What are the limitations and theoretical assumptions of our current understanding? First, the spatial arrangement of the separate L- and M-cone mosaics are unknown (though data on this point should arrive shortly; see Mollon and Bowmaker, 1992), but current behavioral estimates of the relative number of L- and M-cones suggest that there are about twice as many L-cones as M-cones (Cicerone and Nerger, 1989). Second, we have not considered the effects of eye movements on the spatial resolution of the cone mosaics. With each eye movement, the photoreceptors receive new information about the scene. By integrating information obtained after such eye movements, spatial resolution could be improved.

In most experimental measurements, the effects of eye movements have been reduced by flashing the interference patterns briefly. So, we do not have many empirical studies of how information might be integrated over time to improve acuity. We do know that when one examines an interferometric pattern for substantial amounts of time, visual resolution for interferometric patterns does not improve. While information available across eye movements could be very useful, the analysis based on a static eye offers a good account of current empirical measurements. The nervous system plainly combines certain types of information across eye movements to see motion, yet it seems not to use information from different eye positions to improve visual resolution (Packer and Williams, 1992).

Exercises

1. Answer the following questions related to image properties on the retina:

    (a) Why does the retinal image not change size when the pupil changes size? Use a diagram to explain your answer.

    (b) What is the visual angle swept out by a building that is 200 meters tall seen from a distance of 400 meters?

    (c) Suppose a lens has a focal length of 100 mm. Where will the image plane of a line 1 m from the center of the lens be? Suppose the line is 5 mm high. Using a picture, show the size of the image.

    (d) Use the lensmaker's equation (from Chapter 2) to calculate the actual height on the retina of the image in part (c).

    (e) Good-quality printers generate output with 600 dots per inch. How many dots is that per degree of visual angle? (Assume that the usual reading distance is 12 inches.)

    (f) Good-quality monitors have approximately 1,000 pixels on a single line. How many pixels is that per degree of visual angle? (Assume that the usual monitor distance is 0.4 m and the width of a line is 0.2 m.)

    (g) Some monitors can only turn individual pixels on or off. It may be fair to compare such monitors with the printed page since most black-and-white printers can only place a dot or not place one at each location. However, it is not fair to compare printer output with monitors capable of generating different gray scale levels. How can gray scale levels improve the accuracy of reproduction without increasing the number of pixels? Justify your answer using a matrix-tableau argument.

2. A manufacturer is choosing between two blue phosphors in a display. The relative energy of the two phosphors at different wavelengths is shown in the figure. Ordinarily, users will be in focus for the red and green phosphors (not shown) around 580 nm.

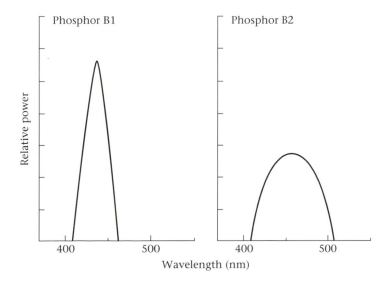

(a) Based on chromatic aberration, which of the two blue phosphors will yield a sharper retinal image? Why?

(b) If the peak phosphor values are 400 nm and 450 nm, what will be the highest spatial frequency imaged on the retina by each of the two phosphors? (Use the curves in Figure 2.23.)

(c) Given the highest frequency imaged at 450 nm, what is the Nyquist sampling rate required to estimate the blue phosphor image? What is the Nyquist sampling rate for a 400-nm light source?

(d) The eye's optics image light at wavelengths above 500 nm much better than wavelengths below that level. Using the curves in Figure 3.3, explain whether you think the S-cones will have a problem due to aliasing at those longer wavelengths.

(e) (Challenge) Suppose the eye is always in focus for 580-nm light. The quality of the image created by the blue phosphor will always be quite poor. How can you design a new layout for the blue phosphor mosaic on the screen to take advantage of the poor short-wavelength resolution of the eye? (Remember, you only need to match images after optical defocus.)

3. Reason from physiology to behavior and back to answer the following questions:

(a) Based purely on the physiological evidence from procion-yellow stains, is there any reason to believe that the cones in Figure 3.7 are the S-cones?

(b) What evidence do we have that the measurements of Williams et al. are due to the positions of the S-cones, rather than to the spacing of neural units in the visual pathways that are sensitive to short-wavelength light?

4. Answer the following questions about aliasing:

(a) Draw an example of aliasing for a set of sampling points that are evenly spaced, but do not use a sinusoidal input pattern.

(b) Consider the unevenly spaced sensor sample positions in the figure. Draw the response of this system to a constant-valued input signal.

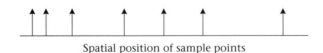

Spatial position of sample points

(c) Now, draw a picture of a stimulus that is nonuniform and that yields the same response as in the previous question.

(d) What rule do you use to make sure the stimuli yield equivalent responses?

(e) Suppose that we put a lens that strongly defocuses the stimuli prior to their arrival at the sensor positions. This defocus means that it will be impossible to generate patterns that vary rapidly across space. If this blur is introduced into the optical path, will you be able to deliver your stimulus to the sensor array? Explain.

5. Perform the following aliasing calculations:

   (a) In this chapter I asserted that $\cos(2\pi(N/2+f)/N) = \cos(2\pi(N/2-f)/N)$. Multiply out the arguments of the functions and write them both in the form of $\cos(i+j)$.

   (b) Use the trigonometric identity $\cos(i-j) = \cos(i)\cos(j) + \sin(i)\sin(j)$ to expand the two functions.

   (c) What is the value of $\sin(\pi)$? What is the value of $\cos(\pi)$? Use these values to obtain the final equality.

   (d) Suppose that we represent a signal using a vector with ten entries. Suppose that the signal is sampled at five locations and that we describe the sampling operation using a sampling matrix consisting of 0's and 1's. How many rows and columns would the sampling matrix have?

   (e) Write out the sampling matrix for a one-dimensional sampling pattern whose sample positions are at 1, 3, 5, 7, and 9.

   (f) Write out the sampling matrix for a nonuniform, one-dimensional pattern in which the sample positions are spaced at locations 1, 2, 4, and 8.

6. Answer each of the following questions about the relationship between the sampling mosaic and optics of the eye:

   (a) From time to time, some investigators have thought that the long-wavelength photopigment peak was near 620 nm, not 580 nm. Using Figure 2.23, discuss what implication such a peak wavelength would have for the Nyquist sampling rate required of these receptors.

   (b) In fact, as you can see from Figure 3.3, the L- and M-cones both have peak sensitivities in the range from 550 nm to 580 nm. What is required of their spacing in order to capture the retinal image accurately?

   (c) We have been assuming that the sensors in our array are equally sensitive to the incoming signal. Suppose that we have a sensor array that consists of alternating S- and L-cones. Draw the response of this array to a uniform field consisting of 450-nm light. Now, draw the intensity pattern that would have the same effect for 650-nm light.

4

Wavelength Encoding

Sir Isaac Newton's sketch in Figure 4.1 summarizes his investigations into the properties of light. In these experiments, Newton separated daylight into its fundamental components by passing it through a prism and creating a spectrum. Newton's demonstration that light can be decomposed into rays of different wavelength is at the foundation of our understanding of light and color.

To perform these experiments, Newton placed a shutter containing a small hole in the window in his room at Cambridge (Newton, *Opticks*). The light emerging from the hole in the window shutter served as a point source to illuminate his apparatus. The key elements of the apparatus are featured prominently in the center of the figure: the lens and prism. Newton's drawing shows that when the daylight passed through the prism, it formed an image of a "rainbow" on his wall. With two experimental manipulations, he showed that the components of the rainbow were fundamental constituents of light. In the upper-left portion of the sketch, we see a series of holes that Newton drilled in the wall permitting part of the rainbow to continue through to a second prism. This ray of light was cast upon a second surface, but the new image did not produce a second rainbow; rather, as Newton wrote in his *Opticks*,

> the color of the light was never changed in the least. If any part of the red light was refracted, it remained totally of the same red color as before. No orange, no yellow, no green or blue, nor other new color was produced by that refraction.

From this experiment, Newton concluded that the pass through the first prism had separated the daylight into its fundamental components.

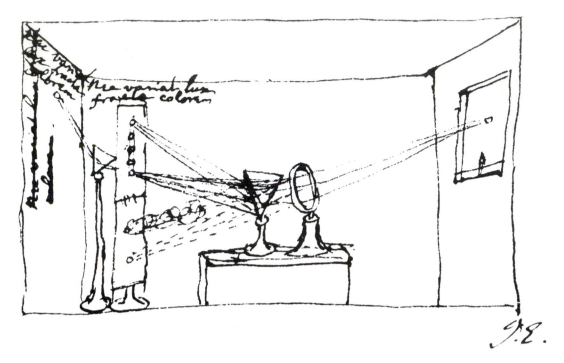

4.1 NEWTON'S SUMMARY DRAWING of his experiments with light. Using a point source of light and a prism, Newton separated sunlight into its fundamental components. By reconverging the rays, he also showed that the decomposition is reversible.

No further change was observed when the ray passed through a second prism.

At the bottom of the sketch Newton illustrated that the decomposition is reversible: passing light through the prism does not destroy the character of the light. To show this Newton converged the rays following their passage through the prism to form a new image; he found the color of the image to be the same as that of the source. Newton concluded that

> light being transmitted through the parallel surfaces of two prisms . . .
> if it suffered any change by the refraction by one surface, it lost that
> impression by the contrary refraction of the other surface.

From the second experiment, he concluded that passage through the prism had not destroyed, but merely revealed, the character of the light.

Measuring the Spectral Composition of Light

We now know that Newton succeeded in decomposing the sunlight into its **spectral components**, each with its own characteristic wavelength. The prism separates the rays because the prism bends each wavelength of light by a different amount (see the section on Snell's law in Chapter 3). When we see the spectral components separately, they each have a different color. Light with relatively long wavelengths appears red when viewed against a dark background. Light with relatively short wavelengths appears blue when viewed against a dark background. Shorter wavelengths of light are refracted more strongly than longer wavelengths. Spectral light, with energy only at a single wavelength, is also called **monochromatic light**.

Newton's apparatus suggests a simple device we might build to measure the amount of power a light has in each of the different wavelength bands. As illustrated in Figure 4.2A, by proper use of lenses and prisms, we can form a focused image of the spectral components in an image plane containing a movable slit. Behind the slit, we place a light sensor. To measure the energy at different wavelengths, we move the slit, passing only some of the spectral components at each position through to the sensor, and thus we measure the energy of the source at different wavelengths of light. In the visible region, the wavelength of light is on the order of a few hundred billionths of a meter, or **nanometers** (nm).

The **spectral power distribution** of a light is the function that defines the power in the light at each wavelength. In the modern theory of physics, the wavelength of light can be thought of in two different ways. We describe the light as if it were a continuous wave as it passes through a medium. When the light exchanges energy with some material, say by giving up its energy to be absorbed, we describe the light as if it were composed of discrete objects called **photons** or **quanta** (singular, *quantum*) of light. The amount of energy given up by the photon is predicted by the wavelength of the light.

The experimental aspect of light measurement that makes it useful and predictable is that the measurement satisfies the principle of superposition (see Chapter 2). We can demonstrate the superposition of light measurement as follows. First, measure the spectral power distri-

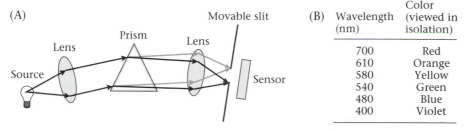

(A)

Lens   Prism   Lens   Movable slit

Source   Sensor

(B)

Wavelength (nm)	Color (viewed in isolation)
700	Red
610	Orange
580	Yellow
540	Green
480	Blue
400	Violet

4.2 A SPECTRORADIOMETER is used to measure the spectral power distribution of light. (A) A schematic design of a spectroradiometer includes a means for separating the input light into its different wavelengths and a detector for measuring the energy at each of the separate wavelengths. (B) The color names associated with the appearance of lights at a variety of wavelengths are shown. After Wyszecki and Stiles, 1982.

butions of two lights separately. Then, mix the two lights together and measure again. The spectral power distribution of the mixture will be the sum of the first two spectral power distributions. This property of light mixture is illustrated in Figure 4.3. Superposition is a crucial property of light measurement because it implies that we can measure the energy of a light at each wavelength separately and then predict the spectral power distribution when the spectral components are mixed together.

Suppose we wish to measure the spectral power distribution of a light source. How many wavelengths should we measure? Or, equivalently, how finely do we have to sample along the wavelength dimension? The answer to this question is important for both practical and theoretical reasons, because the number of samples can be quite large. For example, to sample the visible spectrum from 400 nm to 700 nm in 1-nm steps, we need about 300 measurements. To sample in 10 nm steps, we need about 30 measurements.

The answer to this sampling question depends on the same set of issues as the sampling questions we addressed in Chapter 3 on the spatial sampling of the retinal image by the photoreceptor mosaics. If the energy in the light varies rapidly as a function of wavelength, then we may have to sample quite finely to measure accurately; if the functions vary slowly, then only a few measurements are necessary. Also, the precision of the representation requires that we know how sensitive the photopigments in the receptors are to rapid changes in the energy as a function of wavelength. It is difficult to make accurate general-

4.3   THE MEASUREMENT OF LIGHT SPECTRAL POWER DISTRIBUTIONS satisfies the principle of superposition. The spectral power distributions of two lights measured separately are shown in (A) and (B) and together in (C). The spectral power distribution of the mixture is the sum of the individual measurements, thus demonstrating that superposition holds true.

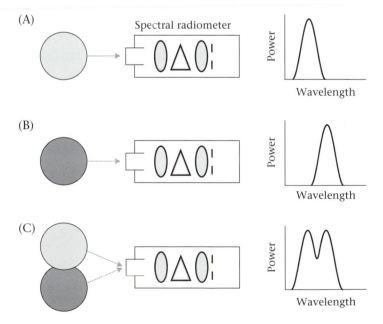

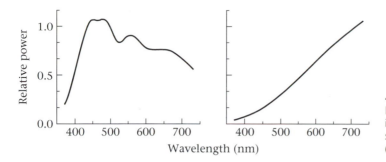

4.4 THE SPECTRAL POWER DISTRIBUTION of two important light sources are shown: (left) blue skylight and (right) a tungsten bulb.

izations about how spectral power distributions vary as a function of wavelength, but it is believed widely that for practical purposes one can approximate spectral power distributions using smooth, regular functions as shown in Figure 4.4. Also, it is known that the photopigments integrate broadly across the wavelength spectrum. Consequently, international standards organizations suggest making measurements every 5 nm to achieve an excellent representation of the signal. Practical measurements often rely on measurements spaced every 10 or 20 nm. We will consider this issue much more completely when we review color appearance, in Chapter 9.

Scotopic Wavelength Encoding

What information about the spectral power distribution is encoded when rods initiate vision, that is, under so-called scotopic conditions? We can answer this question by an experiment designed to measure how well people can discriminate different spectral power distributions. In the **scotopic matching experiment**, we present an observer with two lights, side by side in a bipartite field. One side of the field contains the **test light**; it may have any spectral power distribution whatsoever. The other side of the field contains the **primary light**; it has a fixed relative spectral power distribution and can vary only by an overall intensity factor. The observer's task in the scotopic matching experiment is to adjust the primary light intensity so that the primary light appears indistinguishable from the test light. The observer can adjust only the intensity of the primary light, so when the match is achieved the spectral power distributions of the test and primary lights that match are still different.

Under scotopic conditions, observers can adjust the primary light's intensity so that the primary light matches any test light. Since subjects can always make this match, we have a simple answer to our question: the rods encode nothing about the relative spectral density of a light. An observer can adjust the intensity of a primary light to match the appearance of a test light with any spectral power distribution. The relative spectral power distribution is immaterial; all that matters is the relative intensities of the two lights.

Matching: Homogeneity and Superposition

We can learn more about scotopic wavelength encoding by studying the quantitative properties of the matching experiment. To characterize the matching experiment completely, we must be able to predict how a subject will adjust the primary intensity to match any test light. We treat the experiment as a transformation by identifying the spectral power distribution of the test light as the input and the intensity of the primary light as the output. A quantitative description of the experiment tells us how to map the input to the output.

Naturally, we first ask whether we can characterize the matching-experiment transformation using linear-systems methods. Denote the spectral power distribution of the test and primary lights using the vectors $\mathbf{t}$ and $\mathbf{p}$ respectively. The n_λ entries of these vectors describe the power at each of the n_λ sample wavelengths. To test linearity, we evaluate whether the scotopic matching experiment satisfies the linear-systems properties of homogeneity and superposition. We can evaluate these properties from the following experimental tests:

- *Homogeneity:* If $\mathbf{t}$ matches $e\mathbf{p}$, will $a\mathbf{t}$ match $a(e\mathbf{p})$?

- *Superposition:* If $\mathbf{t}$ matches $e\mathbf{p}$ and $\mathbf{t}'$ matches $e'\mathbf{p}$, will $\mathbf{t} + \mathbf{t}'$ match $(e\mathbf{p}) + (e'\mathbf{p})$?

A hypothetical test of homogeneity is shown in Figure 4.5. The separate panels show the intensity of the test light on the horizontal axis and the intensity of the matching primary light on the vertical axis. Each panel plots the results using a spectral test light of a different wavelength along with a 510-nm primary light. In the scotopic

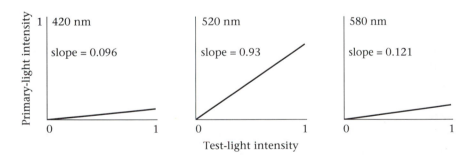

4.5 HYPOTHETICAL SCOTOPIC MATCHING EXPERIMENT. The horizontal scale measures the intensity of a monochromatic test light and the vertical scale measures the intensity a matching 510-nm primary light. Since the scotopic matching experiment satisfies homogeneity, the data will fall along a straight line. The slope of the line defines the relative scotopic sensitivity to each test wavelength.

matching experiment the data will fall on a straight line, consistent with the prediction from homogeneity. The slope of the line defines the relative scotopic sensitivity to the test and the primary lights. For example, in the right panel of Figure 4.5 the hypothetical results from an experiment with a 580-nm test light are shown. The slope of the line shows that we need $8.3 (= 1/0.121)$ units of energy at 580 nm to have the same effect as one unit of energy at 510 nm. Hence, the light at 510 nm is 8.3 times more effective, per unit energy, than the light at 580 nm.

Because the scotopic matching experiment is linear, there must be a system matrix, **R**, that maps the input (**t**, the test-light spectral power distribution), to the output (*e*, the primary-light intensity). The system matrix must have one row and n_λ columns. The test light, the system matrix, and the primary-light intensity are related by the product, $e = \mathbf{Rt}$.

We can write this matrix equation using a **matrix tableau** representation. This representation indicates the general shapes of the vectors and matrices and is often a helpful method for understanding their shapes and inter-relationships. The matrix tableau that represents the scotopic matrix is:

$$(e) = (r_1 \; r_2 \; \ldots \; r_{n_\lambda-1} \; r_{n_\lambda}) \begin{pmatrix} t_1 \\ t_2 \\ \vdots \\ t_{n_\lambda-1} \\ t_{n_\lambda} \end{pmatrix}$$

We can also write the matrix product **Rt** as a summation over the sample wavelengths:

$$e = \sum_{i=1}^{n_\lambda} r_i t_i \tag{4.1}$$

We can then relate the measurements in the scotopic matching experiment to the entries of the system matrix. Suppose we use a monochromatic test light of unit intensity, that is, an input **t** that has only a single nonzero wavelength, $(0, 0, \ldots, 0, 1, 0, \ldots, 0)^T$. Then Equation 4.1 becomes simply $e = r_i t_i$. This shows that the slope of the line relating the monochromatic test intensity, r_i, to the primary-light intensity, e, is the system matrix entry, r_i. Hence, we can estimate the system matrix from the slopes of the experimental lines measured in the test of homogeneity shown in Figure 4.5.

Figure 4.6 is a graphical method of representing the system matrix of the scotopic matching experiment. The curve shows the entries of **R**

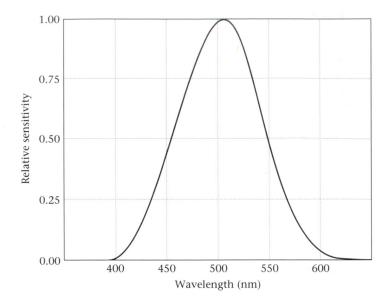

4.6 THE SCOTOPIC SPECTRAL SENSITIVITY FUNCTION defines the human wavelength sensitivity under scotopic viewing conditions. The curve is a plot of the entries of the scotopic system matrix.

as a function of wavelength, interpolated from experimental measurements at many sample wavelengths. The curve is called the **scotopic sensitivity function**.

Once we measure the system matrix, $\mathbf{R}$, we can predict whether any pair of lights will match under scotopic conditions. Suppose we have two test lights, $\mathbf{t}$ and $\mathbf{t}'$. Two lights will match when they are matched by the same intensity of the primary light, so these two lights will match when $\mathbf{Rt} = \mathbf{Rt}'$.

Uniqueness

The hypothetical experiment illustrated in Figure 4.5 assumed a 510-nm primary light. Suppose that we perform the scotopic matching experiment using a different primary light. How will this affect the system matrix, $\mathbf{R}$?

We can answer this question by a thought experiment. Call the second primary light $\mathbf{p}'$. We can set a match between the new primary light, $\mathbf{p}'$ and the first primary light $\mathbf{p}$. We will find that there is some scalar, k, such that $k\mathbf{p}'$ matches $\mathbf{p}$, and we expect that whenever $a\mathbf{p}$ matches a test light, $\mathbf{t}$, then $a[k\mathbf{p}']$ will match $\mathbf{t}$. In particular, since $R_i\mathbf{p}$ matches the ith monochromatic test light, we expect that $R_ik\mathbf{p}'$ will match the ith monochromatic test light as well. It follows that the entries of the new system matrix will be kR_i, equal to the original except for a constant scale factor, k. Hence, the new system matrix will be $k\mathbf{R}$, and we say that the estimate of $\mathbf{R}$ is unique up to an unknown scale factor.

The Biological Basis of Scotopic Matching

The scotopic matching experiment is remarkable in its simplicity. We can understand the biological basis of the experimental matches by studying the properties of the rod photopigment, rhodopsin. Rod photopigment is present in much higher density than any of the cone photopigments. Thus, researchers have been able to isolate and extract the rod photopigment for 50 years, whereas the cone photopigments have only become available recently through the methods of genetic engineering (Merbs and Nathans, 1992). Characteristically, when the rod photopigment is exposed to light, it undergoes a series of rapid changes in chemical state (Hubbard and Wald, 1951; Wald and Brown, 1956; Wald, 1968). Whenever a quantum of light is absorbed by the rhodopsin photopigment, it undergoes a specific sequence of events resulting in the decomposition of the rhodopsin molecule into opsin and vitamin A (Color Plate 1). It is the wavelength selectivity of the rhodopsin photopigment that provides the biological basis of scotopic matching. The relationship between the behavioral experiment and the properties of the rod photopigment is based on an important property called **univariance**.

Rushton (1965) emphasized that when a photopigment molecule absorbs light, the effect upon the photopigment is the same no matter what the wavelength of the absorbed light might be. Thus, even though quanta at 400 nm possess more energy than quanta at 700 nm, the sequence of rhodopsin reactions to absorption of a 400-nm quantum is the same as the sequence of reactions to a 700-nm quantum. Rushton used the word "univariance" for this principle to remind us that a single photopigment makes only a single-variable response to the incoming light. The photopigment maps all spectral lights into a single-variable output, the **rate of absorption**. The response of a single photopigment does not encode any information about the relative spectral composition of the light. This explains why we cannot discriminate between lights with different spectral power distributions under scotopic viewing conditions (Rushton, 1965; Naka and Rushton, 1966). Univariance does *not* mean, however, that the photopigment responds equally well to all spectral lights. The photopigment is much more likely to absorb some wavelengths of light than others. Univariance asserts that once absorbed, all quanta have same visual effect.

One can measure the probability of absorption using the experimental apparatus shown in Figure 4.7. A thin layer of photopigment is placed on a clear plate of glass. Monochromatic light is created by passing light from an ordinary source through a **monochromator**. The monochromator can be constructed using prisms or diffraction gratings to separate the incident light into its separate wavelengths, much as in Newton's original experiments. The amount of monochromatic light passed through the photopigment and the glass plate is measured by

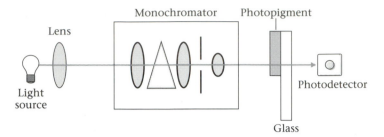

4.7   AN APPARATUS TO MEASURE THE SPECTRAL ABSORPTION OF A PHOTOPIGMENT. Using the monochromator, one can select light at one wavelength from the light source. To estimate the fraction of photons absorbed by the photopigment at that wavelength, we divide the number of photons detected through the glass and photopigment by the number detected after passing through the glass alone.

means of a light sensor at the rear of the apparatus. The glass plate is then moved upward, to remove the photopigment from the light path, and measurements are taken again. The difference in the photodetector signal measured in these two conditions is proportional to the amount of light absorbed by the photopigment.

If only a thin layer of photopigment is present, the experimental measurements of the absorptions will satisfy homogeneity and superposition. To test homogeneity, we increase the intensity of the test light. We will find that the number of absorptions will increase proportionately over a significant range (Figure 4.8). To test superposition, we measure the photopigment absorptions to a test light t to be a, and the number of absorptions to a second light t' to be a'. When we superimpose the two input lights, we will measure $a + a'$ absorptions. Since the measurement process is linear, we can estimate the system matrix of this absorption process, A, just as we measured the system matrix of the scotopic matching experiment, R.

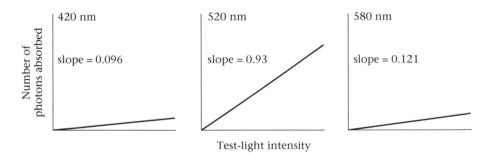

4.8   RHODOPSIN ABSORPTIONS AT DIFFERENT WAVELENGTHS. The number of absorptions in a thin layer of photopigment are proportional to the intensity of the input light and thus satisfy the principle of homogeneity. The slope of the linear relationship between the light intensity and the number of absorptions describes the fraction of photon absorptions. The slope varies with the wavelength of the test light, thus defining the photopigment wavelength sensitivity.

We can predict the matches in the scotopic matching experiment from the absorptions of the rhodopsin photopigment. A test light and primary light match in the scotopic matching experiment when the two lights create the same number of absorptions in the rhodopsin photopigment. We can demonstrate this by comparing the system matrices of the scotopic matching experiment and the rhodopsin absorption experiment. After we correct for the effects of the wavelength-sensitive elements of the eye, mainly the lens, we can plot the system matrices of the scotopic matching experiment R, and the rhodopsin absorption experiment, A, on the same graph. Wald and Brown (1956) made this comparison in the graph in shown Figure 4.9. The filled circles in the graph plot the measurements of the system matrix from the rhodopsin absorption experiment, A. The completely open circles plot estimates of the entries of R after correcting for the fact that the lens absorbs a significant amount of light in the short-wavelength part of the spectrum.

The agreement between the measurements of the rhodopsin photopigment and the scotopic matching experiment confirm a simple model of the observer's behavior. Under scotopic viewing conditions the observer's perception of the two halves of the bipartite field depends on a signal initiated by the rod photopigment absorptions. The two sides of the field appear identical when the rhodopsin absorption rates on the two sides of the bipartite field are equal. During the experiment,

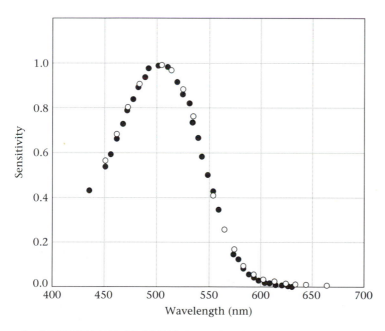

4.9 COMPARISONS OF SCOTOPIC MATCHING AND RHODOPSIN WAVELENGTH SENSITIVITY. The filled circles show human rhodopsin absorption measured as in Figure 4.7. The open circles show human scotopic sensitivity, corrected for light loss at the lens and optical media. Source: Wald and Brown, 1956.

then, the observer adjusts the intensity of the matching light to equalize the rod absorption rates on the two sides of the bipartite field. Since the absorption of the light is a linear process, the observer's behavior is linear, too.

The precise quantitative match between the scotopic matches and the rod photopigment make a very strong connection between performance and biological encoding of the light. This type of precise quantitative relationship between behavior and the biological encoding of light serves as a good standard to use when we consider the relationship between behavior and biology in other conditions.

Photopic Wavelength Encoding

When the cones initiate vision, that is, under photopic conditions, we do encode some information about the relative spectral power distribution of the incident light. Changes in the relative spectral power distributions result in changes of the color appearance of the light. Several of the important properties of color appearance can be traced to the way cone photoreceptors encode the relative spectral power distribution of light.[1]

The human ability to discriminate lights will be related to the properties of the cones just as was done with the rods. First, I will review the matching experiments that characterize how well people can discriminate between lights with different spectral power distributions. When we measure under photopic conditions, the experiment is called the **color-matching experiment**. The color-matching experiment is the foundation of color science and of direct significance to many color applications (see Appendix B). Second, I will relate the properties of the color-matching experiment to the properties of the cone photopigments. The analysis of photopic wavelength encoding parallels the analysis of scotopic wavelength encoding. The main differences are that (a) we must keep track of the photopigment absorptions in three cone photopigments rather than the single rod photopigment, and (b) until quite recently the cone photopigments were not available in sufficient quantity to define their properties with any certainty (Merbs and Nathans, 1992). Hence, the problem of relating color-matching and the cone photopigments was solved using other indirect biological measurements. We can learn a great deal from studying the logic of these methods.

Figure 4.10 shows a simple apparatus that can be used to perform the color-matching experiment. The observer views a bipartite visual field with a test light on one side. The test light may have any spectral power distribution. The second half of the bipartite field contains a

[1] Note that color appearance is not a simple consequence of the spectral power distribution of the incident light. We will discuss color appearance broadly in Chapter 9.

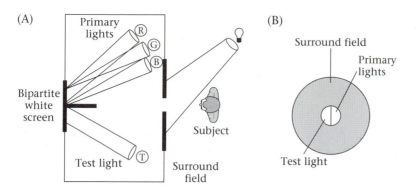

4.10   THE COLOR-MATCHING EXPERIMENT. The observer views a bipartite field and adjusts the intensities of the three primary lights to match the appearance of the test light. (A) A top view of the experimental apparatus. (B) The appearance of the stimuli to the observer. After Judd and Wyszecki, 1975.

mixture of *three* primary lights. Throughout the experiment, the relative spectral power distribution of each primary light is constant; only the absolute level of the primary lights can be adjusted. The observer's task is to adjust the intensities of the three primary lights so that the two sides of the bipartite field appear identical.

When the observer has completed setting an appearance match, the lights on the two sides of the bipartite field are not physically the same. The test light can have any spectral power distribution, while the mixture of primaries can only have a limited number of spectral power distributions determined by the possible weighted sums of the three primary-light spectral power distributions. Lights that are photopic appearance matches, but that are physically different, are called **metamers.** Figure 4.11 contains a pair of spectral power distributions that match visually but differ physically (i.e., a pair of metamers).

The metamers in Figure 4.11 illustrate that even under photopic viewing conditions we fail to discriminate between very different spectral power distributions. To understand the behavioral aspects of photopic wavelength encoding, we must try to predict which spectral power distributions we can discriminate. The first question we ask is whether we can predict performance in the photopic color-matching experiment using linear-systems methods.

We can define the measurements in the color-matching experiment in direct analogy with the definitions we used in the scotopic matching experiment. The input variable in the color-matching experiment is the light **t**, just as in scotopic matching. In the color-matching experiment, however, the subject's responses consist of three numbers, not just one. So, we record the responses using a three-dimensional vector, **e**. The entries of **e** are the intensities of the three primary lights (e_1, e_2, e_3). To test superposition in the color-matching experiment we follow the logic illustrated in Figure 4.12. We obtain a match to a **t** by adjusting the primary intensities to the levels in **e**. We then obtain a match to **t′** by ad-

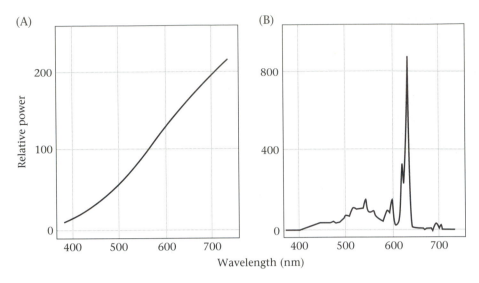

(A) (B)

Relative power

Wavelength (nm)

4.11 METAMERIC LIGHTS. Two lights with these spectral power distributions appear identical to most observers and are called metamers. (A) An approximation to the spectral power distribution of a tungsten bulb. (B) The spectral power distribution of light emitted from a conventional television monitor whose three phosphor intensities were set to match the light in panel A in appearance.

justing the three primary intensities to e'. We test additivity by verifying that the match to $t + t'$ is $e + e'$. Photopic color-matching satisfies homogeneity and superposition. We honor the person who first understood the importance of superposition in color-matching by calling this empirical property **Grassmann's additivity law**.

The photopic color-matching experiment defines a linear mapping from the test light spectral power distribution to the intensity of the three primary lights. Because the color-matching experiment linearly maps the physical stimulus to the primary intensities, there must be a $3 \times n_\lambda$ system matrix that maps the input to the output, $e = Ct$. We can express the whole relationship using a matrix tableau:

$$\begin{pmatrix} e_1 \\ e_2 \\ e_3 \end{pmatrix} = \begin{pmatrix} \text{Color-matching function of Primary 1} \\ \text{Color-matching function of Primary 2} \\ \text{Color-matching function of Primary 3} \end{pmatrix} \begin{pmatrix} t_1 \\ t_2 \\ \vdots \\ t_{n_{\lambda-1}} \\ t_{n_\lambda} \end{pmatrix}$$

We can estimate the system matrix C from the color matches in the same way as we estimated the scotopic system matrix: by setting matches to a collection of monochromatic test lights with unit intensity. Since the vector representing a monochromatic test light is zero at each entry but one, the product of the system matrix and the monochromatic test light vector equals a single column of the system

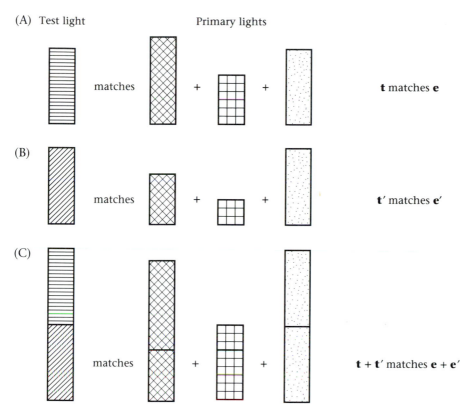

(A) Test light   Primary lights

matches   +   +   **t** matches **e**

(B)

matches   +   +   **t′** matches **e′**

(C)

matches   +   +   **t + t′** matches **e + e′**

4.12 THE COLOR-MATCHING EXPERIMENT SATISFIES THE PRINCIPLE OF SUPERPOSITION. In parts (A) and (B), test lights are matched by a mixture of three primary lights. In part (C) the sum of the test lights is matched by the additive mixture of the primaries, demonstrating superposition.

matrix. Thus, by matching a series of unit-intensity monochromatic lights, we can define each of the columns of the system matrix, C.

It is also useful to think of the system matrix in terms of its rows, which are called the **color-matching functions**. Each row of the matrix defines the intensity of a single primary light that was set to match the monochromatic test lights. We will relate the rows of the photopic system matrix to the properties of the cone photopigments just as we related the single row of the scotopic system matrix to the rhodopsin photopigment. However, to make the connection between the cone photopigments and the color-matching functions will require a little more work.

Measurements of the Color-Matching Functions

Two important caveats arise when we measure the color-matching functions. These are only a minor theoretical nuisance, but they have important implications for the laboratory experiment and for practical applications.

The first issue concerns the selection of primary lights. We should choose lights that are **visually independent**; that is, no additive mixture of two of the primary lights should be a visual match to the third primary. This is an obvious but important constraint: it would be unreasonable to choose a second primary light that looked the same as the first except for an intensity scale factor. This choice would be foolish since we could always replace the second light by an intensity-scaled version of the first primary light, adding nothing to the range of visual matches we can obtain. Similarly, a third primary light that can be matched by a mixture of the first two adds nothing. We must choose our primary lights so that they are independent of one another.

Even among collections of primary lights that are independent, some are more convenient than others. Empirically, it turns out that no matter which primary lights we choose, there will always be some test lights that cannot be matched by an additive mixture of the three primaries. To match these test lights, we must move one or even two of the primary lights from the matching side of the bipartite field to the test side of the bipartite field. Thus, ordinarily we obtain visual matches of the form

$$\mathbf{t} = e_1 \mathbf{p}_1 + e_2 \mathbf{p}_2 + e_3 \mathbf{p}_3 \qquad (4.2)$$

Shifting one of the primaries to the test side of the bipartite field means that our match has the form

$$\mathbf{t} + e_1 \mathbf{p}_1 = e_2 \mathbf{p}_2 + e_3 \mathbf{p}_3 \qquad (4.3)$$

To a mathematician Equation 4.3, is the same as

$$\mathbf{t} = -e_1 \mathbf{p}_1 + e_2 \mathbf{p}_2 + e_3 \mathbf{p}_3 \qquad (4.4)$$

Hence, when we encode the intensity of the primary light that has been shifted to the test side of the bipartite field we denote the match using a negative intensity value.[2]

Figure 4.13 plots color-matching functions measured by Stiles and Burch (1959) using three monochromatic primary lights at 645.2 nm, 525.3 nm, and 444.4 nm [denoted as $\bar{r}_{10}(\lambda)$, $\bar{g}_{10}(\lambda)$, and $\bar{b}_{10}(\lambda)$, respectively]. Each function describes the intensity of one of the primary lights used to match various monochromatic test lights. Notice that the intensity of the red primary, at 645.2 nm, is negative over a region of

---

[2] Changing the sign of the primary-light intensity is a trivial matter for the theorist. It is a nuisance in the laboratory, however, and usually impossible in applications such as color displays. Thus, the issue of selecting primary lights to minimize the number of times we must make this adjustment is of great practical interest.

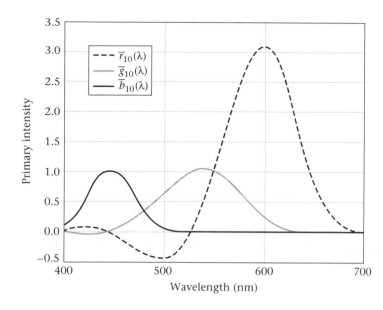

4.13 THE COLOR-MATCHING FUNCTIONS ARE THE ROWS OF THE COLOR-MATCHING SYSTEM MATRIX. The functions measured by Stiles and Burch (1959) using a 10-degree bipartite field and primary lights at the wavelengths 645.2 nm, 525.3 nm, and 444.4 nm with unit radiant power are shown. The three functions in this figure are called $\bar{r}_{10}(\lambda)$, $\bar{g}_{10}(\lambda)$, and $\bar{b}_{10}(\lambda)$.

test light wavelengths, indicating that over this range of test lights the 645.2 nm primary light was added to the test field.

The color-matching functions are extremely important in color technology, such as creating images on color monitors and color printers. I review the application of these methods to color monitors in Appendix B.

Uniqueness of the Color-Matching Functions

Suppose two research groups measure the color-matching functions using different sets of primary lights. One group measures the color-matching functions using three primary lights p_i, while the second group uses a different set of primary lights, p_i'. Because the groups use different primary lights, they will measure different sets of color-matching functions, C and C'. How will the two sets of color matching functions be related?

We can answer this question by the following thought experiment. First, create a matrix whose columns contain the spectral power distributions of the first group's primary lights, and call this matrix P. The spectral power distribution of a mixture of the primaries, with primary intensities e, is the weighted sum of the columns. We can express this mixture using the matrix product Pe. Now, we can use the color-matching functions to predict when a test light will match the mixture of three primaries. The test and primaries will match when

$$\mathbf{Ct} = \mathbf{CPe} \qquad (4.5)$$

Suppose the second group of researchers can also establish matches to this test light using their primaries. To describe their measurements, we create a second matrix whose columns contain the spectral power distributions of the second group's primary lights, $\mathbf{P}'$. Call the primary intensities used to match the test with the second primaries $\mathbf{e}'$. Since the light $\mathbf{P}'\mathbf{e}'$ is a visual match to the test light, we know that

$$\mathbf{Ct} = \mathbf{CP}'\mathbf{e}' \qquad (4.6)$$

By combining Equations 4.5 and 4.6, we find that the two vectors of primary intensities, $\mathbf{e}$ and $\mathbf{e}'$, are related by a linear transformation,

$$\mathbf{e} = (\mathbf{CP})^{-1}\mathbf{CP}'\mathbf{e}'$$

Finally, recall that the vectors in the columns of the color-matching functions are the primary-light intensity settings necessary to match the monochromatic lights. We have just shown that the primary-light intensities used to make matches with the two different sets of primaries are related by a linear transformation. Hence, the system matrices containing the color-matching functions $\mathbf{C}$ and $\mathbf{C}'$ must be related a linear transformation.

With a little more algebra, one can show that the color-matching functions are related by the following linear transformation:

$$\mathbf{C} = (\mathbf{CP}')\mathbf{C}' \qquad (4.7)$$

The 3×3 matrix relating the two sets of color-matching functions, $\mathbf{CP}'$, has a simple empirical interpretation; its columns contain the intensities of the new primary lights needed to match the original primaries. To see this, remember that each column of $\mathbf{P}'$ is the spectral power distribution of one of the primary lights, $\mathbf{p}_i'$. Thus, the first column of $\mathbf{CP}'$ is the vector of intensities of the first group of primaries needed to match $\mathbf{p}_1'$. Similarly the second and third columns of $\mathbf{CP}'$ contain the intensities of the first group of primary lights needed to match the corresponding primaries in $\mathbf{p}'$. The matrix $\mathbf{CP}'$ contains three columns equal to the primary-light intensities of $\mathbf{p}_i$ needed to match the new primary lights, $\mathbf{p}_i'$.

The photopic color-matching functions are not unique; when we measure using different sets of primaries we will obtain different color-matching functions. But, the color-matching functions are not completely free to vary either, since different pairs of color-matching functions will always be related by a linear transformation. We say that the color-matching functions are unique up to a free linear transformation.

A Standard Set of Color-Matching Functions

When the members of the Commisssion Internationale d'Eclairage (CIE; an international standards organization) met in 1931, they were fully aware that the color-matching functions were not unique. To facilitate communication about color, the CIE defined the standard system of color representation shown in Figure 4.14. This set of color-matching functions defines the **XYZ tristimulus coordinate system**; the color-matching functions in this system are called $\bar{x}(\lambda), \bar{y}(\lambda)$, and $\bar{z}(\lambda)$. They define one of the many possible system matrices of the color-matching experiment.

The standard color-matching functions were chosen for several reasons. First of all, $\bar{y}(\lambda)$ is a rough approximation to the brightness of monochromatic lights of equal size and duration. A second important reason is that the functions are nonnegative, which simplifies some aspects of the design of instruments to measure the tristimulus coordinates. But, as with any standards decision, there are some irritating aspects of the XYZ color-matching functions as well. One serious drawback is that there is no set of physically realizable primary lights that by direct measurement will yield the color-matching functions. Primary lights that would yield these functions would have to have negative energy at some wavelengths and cannot be instrumented. Another problem is that these early estimates have been improved upon. Specifically, Judd (1951) noted that the functions are inaccurate in the short-wavelength region, and he proposed a modified set of functions that are often used by scientists, although they have not displaced the industrial standard. Also, and perhaps most significantly, there is very little that

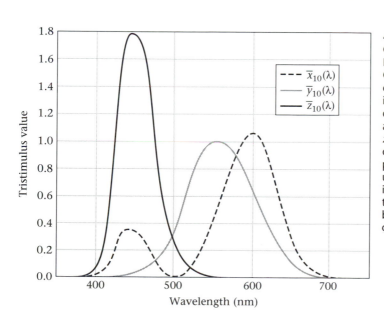

4.14 THE XYZ STANDARD COLOR-MATCHING FUNCTIONS. In 1931 the CIE standardized a set of color-matching functions for image interchange. These color-matching functions are called $\bar{x}(\lambda), \bar{y}(\lambda)$, and $\bar{z}(\lambda)$. Industrial applications commonly describe the color properties of a light source using the three primary intensities needed to match the light source that can be computed from the XYZ color-matching functions.

is intuitive about the XYZ color-matching functions. Although they have served quite well as a technical standard, and are understood by the mandarins of vision science, they have served quite poorly as tools for explaining the discipline to new students and colleagues outside the field.

The Biological Basis of Photopic Color-Matching

Just as we can explain the scotopic color-matching experiment in terms of the light-absorption properties of the rhodopsin photopigment, we also would like to explain the photopic color-matching experiment in terms of the light absorption properties of the cone photopigments. We related the rod photopigment to behavior by studying the system matrices of the scotopic matching experiment and light absorption by rhodopsin. We found that two lights were scotopic matches when $\mathbf{Rt} = \mathbf{Rt'}$, and we then showed that the entries in the $1 \times n_\lambda$ scotopic matching matrix, $\mathbf{R}$, was the same as the rhodopsin absorption function $\mathbf{A}$. For photopic vision, we use the same general approach. But there are two complications: there are three cone photopigments, instead of just one; and the photopic matching matrix is not unique.

Extending the analysis to account for three cone photopigments instead of one rod photopigment is straightforward. We measure the absorption properties of each of the three cone photopigments, and we create a $3 \times n_\lambda$ cone absorption system matrix, $\mathbf{B}$, whose three rows contain the three cone photopigment absorption functions. This matrix generalizes the rhodopsin system matrix $\mathbf{A}$, and we use it to predict the cone absorptions, $\mathbf{c} = (L, M, S)^{\mathrm{T}}$, by multiplying the test light times the cone absorption system matrix, namely $\mathbf{c} = \mathbf{Bt}$. Expressed in a matrix tableau this is:

$$\begin{pmatrix} L \\ M \\ S \end{pmatrix} = \begin{pmatrix} \text{Spectral sensitivity of L photopigment} \\ \text{Spectral sensitivity of M photopigment} \\ \text{Spectral sensitivity of S photopigment} \end{pmatrix} \begin{pmatrix} t_1 \\ t_2 \\ \vdots \\ t_{n_{\lambda-1}} \\ t_{n_\lambda} \end{pmatrix}$$

To verify that color-matching can be explained by the properties of the cone absorptions, we must compare the cone absorption system matrix, $\mathbf{B}$, with the color-matching experiment system matrix, $\mathbf{C}$. The cone absorptions can explain the color-matching results only if the two matrices are related by a linear transformation.

Based on our analysis of color-matching, it is clear that the color-matching system matrix is not unique; there is a collection of equivalent system matrices, all related by a linear transformation. Hence, to evaluate whether the cone absorption matrix can explain the color-matching experiment, we must evaluate whether the color-matching system matrix, **C**, is related to **B** by a linear transformation. Our next task, then, is to measure the cone absorption system matrix, **B**.

Measuring Cone Photocurrents

Currently, the best estimates of the cone photopigment absorptions are derived from measurements of the cone photocurrent, that is, the change in the current flow through the membrane of individual cones as they are stimulated by light. Relating the photocurrent to the photopigment absorptions requires some careful analysis because the photocurrent depends nonlinearly on the photopigment absorptions in the cone. In this section we will develop new theoretical methods to interpret the nonlinear cone photocurrent measurements and infer the linear absorption properties of the cone photopigments.

Baylor, Nunn, and Schnapf (1987; see also Baylor, 1987) were the first to measure cone photocurrents in the macaque retina. The macaque has three types of cones, and its behavior on most color tasks is quite similar to human behavior. Thus, the comparison between the properties of the macaque photoreceptors and human behavior is a good place to begin (DeValois et al., 1974).

To measure the cone photocurrents, Baylor, Nunn, and Schnapf removed the retina from the eye and chopped it into fine pieces about 100 μm across. The pieces were placed in a chamber containing special solutions that support the metabolism of the cells. Even though the retina had been dissected from the eye and chopped into pieces, the electrical response of the photoreceptors remained vigorous for several hours. Baylor and his colleagues recorded the photocurrent of individual cells using the experimental technique pictured in Figure 4.15. The figure shows a glass micropipette containing a single photoreceptor. The inner diameter of the micropipette is between 2 and 6 μm, only ten times as wide as the wavelength of visible light. A single photoreceptor outer segment is held inside the micropipette, and a thin ray of light is passed transversely through the photoreceptor to stimulate it.

Figure 4.16 shows the result of stimulating the photoreceptor with a brief impulse of light. The curves illustrate the membrane photocurrent following a brief light flash. The curves in Figure 4.16A plot the response to 500-nm light at a range of intensities. The curves in Figure 4.16B plot the response to 659-nm light at a range of intensities. Before the stimulus is presented, there is a steady inward flow of current consisting of a stream of positively charged sodium ions entering the photoreceptor through ion channels in the cell membrane. This steady level in the absence of light is called the **dark current**. It represents a baseline level and is denoted as zero in the graph. The plotted values are **biphasic**, varying both above and below the baseline.

When the photopigment absorbs light from the flash, the inward flow of sodium ions is slowed. The sodium current in darkness re-

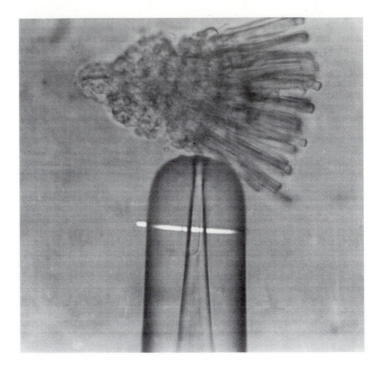

4.15 MEASURING CONE PHOTOCURRENTS. The image shows a portion of macaque retina suspended in solution. A single photoreceptor from this retinal section has been drawn into a micropipette and is being stimulated by a beam of light passing transversely through the photoreceptor and micropipette. Courtesy of Denis Baylor.

duces the negative electrical polarization of the cell interior. When light blocks the inward flow, the negative voltage difference between the inside and outside of the cell increases. Thus, the initial photoreceptor response to light is a **hyperpolarization**. After the initial blockage of inward flowing sodium current, the current flow is actively re-

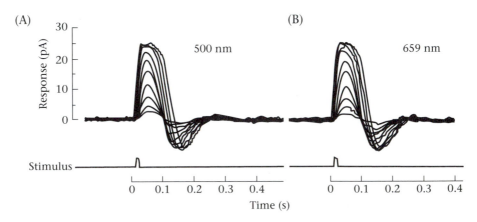

4.16 THE CONE PHOTOCURRENT in response to a brief test flash is biphasic. The amplitude of the photocurrent response increases with the stimulus intensity. The response functions are the same for different wavelengths of light: (A) stimulus wavelength = 500 nm; (B) stimulus intensity = 659 nm. The stimulus time course is shown below the photocurrent plots. Source: Baylor et al., 1987.

stored. The mechanism that restores balance overcompensates; during the second phase of the response, the total photocurrent flow reverses direction. Thus the photocurrent response first flows in one direction and then in the opposite direction, leading to the biphasic impulse response.

In this experiment the test light is the input, **t**, and the cone photocurrent response is the output. We can evaluate whether the input–output relationship satisfies the homogeneity requirement of a linear system from the graphs in Figure 4.16. Suppose the input signal is **t** and the photocurrent response is **i**, a vector representing the photocurrent as a function of time following the stimulus. To test homogeneity we should measure the response to the scaled input, k**t**. If the system is linear, then we expect that the photocurrent response will be k**i**. From a visual inspection of the curves in Figure 4.16 we can see that homogeneity fails. There are two features of the curves that should make this evident to you. First, notice that as the test intensity increases, the peak deviation is reached at about 25 pA (picoamps = amps $\times\ 10^{-12}$), after which the response levels off and then declines. This response is inconsistent with a strictly linear relationship between input intensity and output photocurrent. A second way to see that linearity fails is to consider the point of the biphasic response at which the output crosses the zero level at baseline. If the output photocurrent is proportional to the input intensity, points with a zero response level should always have a zero response level: multiplying zero by any intensity still yields zero. Hence, we expect that the zero-crossing should not change its position as we increase the test intensity. This prediction is true for lower test intensities, but as the input intensity increases to fairly high levels, the zero-crossing shifts its position in time.

How surprising! Human performance in the color-matching experiment satisfies the principles of a linear system, homogeneity and superposition, yet the cone photocurrent responses, a part of the chain of biological events that mediate the behavior, fail the simplest tests of linearity. How can the behavior be linear when the components mediating the behavior are nonlinear? We will answer this question in the following section. The answer is given specifically for color-matching, but the principles we will review are quite general. They will be helpful again when we consider the relationship between behavior and other neural responses throughout this book.

Static Nonlinearities: Photocurrents and Photopigments

By comparing the sets of photocurrent responses on the top and bottom of Figure 4.16, it appears that as we vary the level of the test signal we sweep out the same set of curves. The similarity of the measured photocurrent responses to the two test lights suggests that we can perform a color-matching experiment at the level of the photocurrent response.

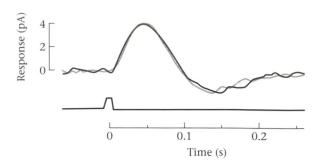

4.17 THE PRINCIPLE OF UNIVARIANCE states that absorption of a photon leads to the same neural response, no matter what the wavelength of the photon. The principle predicts that two stimuli at different wavelengths can be adjusted to equate the photocurrent response throughout its time course. This is shown here as the match between photocurrents in response to 550 nm (shaded line) and 659 nm (solid line) test lights set to a 9:1 intensity ratio. Source: Baylor et al., 1987.

We can perform such an experiment by choosing a test light and a primary light and adjusting the intensity of the primary light until the photocurrent responses of the test and primary lights are the same. The curves in Figure 4.17 show one example of such a match using a primary light at 500 nm and a test light at 659 nm.

The physiological preparation is very delicate, and it is difficult to keep the photoreceptors alive and functioning. This makes it impossible to get full photocurrent matches for arbitrary test and primary combinations. However, it is possible to carry out an efficient approximation of the full experiment. The two curves in Figure 4.18 summarize the photocurrent responses to a 659-nm test light and the 500-nm primary light at a series of different intensity levels. The data points show the peak value of the photocurrent response as a function of intensity; the peak value summarizes the full photocurrent time course. The smooth curves drawn through the points interpolate the peak response at any intensity level. From these interpolated measurements, we can estimate the intensity levels needed to obtain complete matches between the test and primary lights.

If the matching experiment performed at the level of the photocurrent satisfies homogeneity, the intensity of the test and primary lights that match should be proportional to one another. We can estimate the intensity of the test and primary lights that match at different response levels by drawing a horizontal line across the graph and noting the

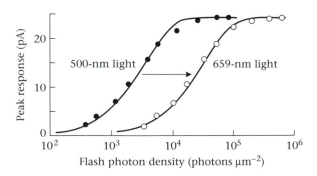

4.18 A MATCHING EXPERIMENT USING THE CONE PHOTOCURRENT AS RESPONSE. Lights at different wavelengths have equivalent effects on the cone photocurrent when the light intensity ratio is set properly. For this cone, the 659-nm light must be nine times more intense than the 500-nm light to have an equivalent effect. Source: Baylor et al., 1987.

intensity levels that produce the same peak photocurrent. The curves through the two sets of data points in Figure 4.18 are parallel on a logarithmic intensity axis, so that the intensities of pairs of points that match are separated by a constant amount. Since the axis is logarithmic, equal separation implies that, when the photocurrents match, the test and primary light intensities are in a particular ratio, precisely as required by homogeneity. Hence, the photocurrent-matching experiment satisfies homogeneity even though the photocurrent response itself is nonlinear.

From the separation between the two curves, we see that more 659-nm photons than 500-nm photons are needed to evoke the same response. For this pair of wavelengths, the curves are separated by 0.97 log units, which corresponds to a ratio of 9.3. It takes 9.3 times as many 659-nm quanta to equal the photocurrent produced by a given number of 500-nm quanta. By repeating this experiment using test lights at many different wavelengths, we can estimate the complete spectral responsivity curves for the cone photoreceptors. From a collection of such measurements we can estimate the wavelength sensitivity of a cone receptor. The wavelength sensitivity is due to the properties of the cone photopigment, so in this way we can derive the cone photopigment absorption function from the photocurrent measurements.

You will probably not be surprised to learn that Baylor, Nunn, and Schnapf (1987) found cones with three distinct spectral response functions: these measurements are plotted in Figure 4.19. Notice that the vertical axis spans six logarithmic units, so that they measured sensitivities varying over a factor of one million, an extraordinary technical measurement achievement.

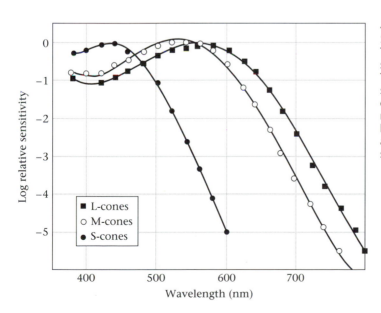

4.19 CONE PHOTOCURRENT SPECTRAL RESPONSIVITIES. The measurement range spans a factor of one million. The S-cone sensitivity at short wavelengths is high compared to behavioral measurements because in behavioral conditions the lens absorbs short-wavelength light strongly. After Baylor, 1987.

Static Nonlinearities: The Principle

We can analyze the photopigment sensitivity from the photocurrent response because the nonlinear relationship between the test light and the photocurrent signal is very simple. The photons are absorbed by a linear process; and the linear encoding is followed by a nonlinear process that converts the photopigment absorption rate into membrane photocurrent. The properties of the nonlinear process are independent of the linear encoding step, and thus we call this process a **static nonlinearity**. When a system is a linear process followed by a static nonlinearity, we can characterize the system performance completely.

It is worth spending a little time thinking about why we can characterize this type of nonlinear system. First, consider the linear process of light absorption by photopigments. There is a photopigment system matrix, say, A, that maps the test light into a photon absorption rate, At. Second, the static nonlinearity converts the photopigment absorption rate into a peak photocurrent response. Together, these two processes define the nonlinear system response, $F(At)$.

When we set a match between the peak photocurrent from the test light and the primary light, we establish an equation of the form

$$F(At) = F(aAp) \tag{4.8}$$

where a is the intensity of the primary light needed to match the test light. Since the nonlinear function F is monotonic, we can remove it from both sides of the equation and write

$$At = aAp \tag{4.9}$$

From this equation we see that there is a linear relationship between the primary- and test-light intensities, since if t matches ap, then kt will match kap. Thus, even if a system has a static nonlinearity, the system's performance in a matching experiment will satisfy the test of homogeneity. We can also show that in a matching experiment a system with a static nonlinearity will satisfy superposition.

Cone Photopigments and Color-Matching

How well do the spectral sensitivity of the cone photopigments predict performance in the photopic color-matching experiment? We predict that two lights are metamers when they have the same effect on the three types of cone photopigments. To answer how well the cone photopigments predict the color-matching results, we can perform the following calculation.

Create a matrix, B, whose three rows are the cone photopigment spectral sensitivities. We use this matrix to calculate the cone absorptions to a test light, so that Bt is a 3×1 vector containing the cone sensitivities to the test light. We predict that two lights t and t' will be a visual match when they have equivalent effects on the cone photopigments. Thus, two lights will be metamers when

$$\mathbf{Bt} = \mathbf{Bt}'$$

It follows that the cone absorption matrix **B** is a system matrix for the color-matching experiment. This is precisely what we mean when we say that the cone photopigments can explain the color-matching experiment. Earlier in this chapter, we saw that the color-matching functions are all related by a 3×3 linear transformation. Thus, there should be a linear transformation, say **Q**, that maps the cone absorption curves to the system matrix of the color-matching experiment, namely $\mathbf{C} = \mathbf{QB}$.

Baylor, Nunn, and Schnapf (1987) made this comparison.[3] They found a linear transformation to convert their cone photopigment measurements into the color-matching functions. Figure 4.20 shows the color-matching functions along with the linearly transformed cone photopigment sensitivity curves. From the agreement between the two data sets, we can conclude that the photopigment spectral responsivities provide a satisfactory biological basis to explain the photopic color-matching experiment.

Why This Is a Big Deal

The methods we have used to connect cone photopigments and color-matching are a wonderful example of how to relate physiological and behavioral data precisely. To make the connection between the behavioral and physiological data we have had to reason through some challenging issues. Still, we have obtained a close quantitative agreement between the behavioral and physiological measurements.

Notice that as we began our analysis, the properties of the neural measurements and the behavioral measurements appeared different. The linearity of the color-matching experiment contrasts with the non-linearity of the photocurrent response. But by comparing stimuli that cause equal performance responses, rather than comparing behavioral matches with raw photocurrent levels, we can see past the dissimilarities and understand their profound relationship. In this case, we know how to connect these two different measurements, and the simplicity and clarity of the relationship is easy to see. It makes sense, then, to ask what we can learn from this successful analysis that might help us when we move on to try to relate other behavioral and biological measurements.

We should remember that the relationship between behavior and biology may not always be found at the level of the measurements that

---

[3] After correcting for the absorptions by the lens and inert pigments in the eye.

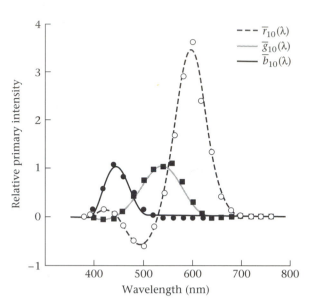

4.20 COMPARISON OF CONE PHOTOCURRENT RESPONSES AND THE COLOR-MATCHING FUNCTIONS. The cone photocurrent spectral responsivities are within a linear transformation of the color-matching functions, after a correction has been made for the optics and inert pigments in the eye. The smooth curves show the Stiles and Burch (1959) color-matching functions. The symbols show the matches predicted from the photocurrents of the three types of macaque cones. The predictions included a correction for absorption by the lens and other inert pigments in the eye. Source: Baylor, 1987.

are natural within each discipline. Direct comparisons between the intensity of the primary lights and the photocurrent signals do not help us to explain the relationship, even though each measure is natural within its own experiment. To make a deep connection, we needed to look at the structural properties of the experiment. When we perform the color-matching experiment, we learn about the equivalence of different stimuli. This equivalence is preserved under many transformations. Thus, we succeed at comparing the behavior and the biology when we compare the results at this level, although they seem different when we use other quantitative measures.

How do we know when we have the right set of biological and behavioral measures? There are many related physiological measures we might use to characterize the photoreceptors, and there are many variants of the behavioral color-matching experiment. For example, we could have asked the subject whether the brightness of the test light doubles when we double the intensity (the answer is no). Or we could have asked the subject to assess the change in redness or greenness. Just as the input–output relationship of the photocurrent may violate linearity for intense stimuli, so too many behavioral measures violate linearity. Finding the right measures to reveal the common properties of the two data sets is part science and part art. We learn about connections between these disciplines by trying to recast our experiments using different methods until the relationships become evident.

As we study the neural response in more central parts of the nervous system, you may be tempted to interpret a physiological measurement as a direct predictor of some percept. The rate at which a neuron responds and the stimulus that excites a neuron powerfully are natural biological measures. Remember, however, that there is no simple relationship between the photocurrent response and the intensity level of a primary light. We achieved a good link between the physiological and behavioral measures by structuring a theory of the information that is preserved in each set of experimental measurements. Understanding our measurements in terms of this level of abstraction—what information is present in the signal—is a harder but better way to forge links between different disciplines. Color science has been fortunate to have workers in both disciplines who seek to forge these links. We should take advantage of their experience when we relate behavior and biology in other domains.

Color Deficiencies

I have emphasized the fact that, for most observers, color-matching under the standard viewing conditions requires three primary lights to form a match, and thus we call color vision **trichromatic**. There are some viewing conditions in which only two different primary lights are necessary. Under these viewing conditions, color vision is **dichromatic**. Finally, when only a single primary is required, as under rod viewing conditions, performance is **monochromatic**.

Small-Field Dichromacy

Perhaps the most important of case of dichromacy occurs when we reduce the size of the bipartite field used in the color-matching experiment. If the field is greatly reduced in size, from 2 degrees to only 20 minutes of visual angle, then observers no longer need three independent primary lights; two primary lights suffice. Under these circumstances, observers act as if they have only two classes of photoreceptors, rather than three.

   Why should observers behave as if they had only two classes of receptors when the field is very small? If this observation surprises you, go back to Chapter 3 and read again the section on the S-cone mosaic. You will find that there are very few short-wavelength cones, and there are none in the central fovea. Oddly, we encode less about the spectral properties of the incident light in the central fovea than we record just slightly peripheral to the fovea. In the 20 minutes of the central fovea, people are dichromatic.

Dichromatic Observers

Some observers find that they can perform the color-matching experiment using only two primary lights throughout their entire visual field. Such observers are called **dichromats**. The vast majority of dichromats are male. By studying the family relationships of dichromats, it has been found that dichromacy is a sex-linked genetic trait

(Pokorny et al., 1979). Dichromatic observers can be missing the long-wavelength photopigment (**protanopes**), the middle-wavelength photopigment (**deuteranopes**), or the short-wavelength photopigment (**tritanopes**). Tritanopes are much more rare than either protanopes or deuteranopes. The difference in the probabilities arises because the gene responsible for the creation of the short-wavelength photopigment is on a different chromosome (Nathans et al., 1992).

It is possible to use the color-matching functions measured from dichromatic observers to estimate the photoreceptor spectral responsivities. Suppose we have two dichromatic observers: the first observer has only the L and M photoreceptors, and the second observer has only the L and S photoreceptors. Since the photoreceptor sensitivities are linearly related to the color-matching functions, a weighted sum of the first observer's color-matching functions will equal the L-cone absorption function, and a different weighted sum of the second observer's color-matching functions will equal the L-cone absorption function, too. This establishes a linear equation we can use to estimate the L-cone absorption function. Similarly, from a pair of dichromats who share only the M-cones, we can estimate the M-cone sensitivity, and so forth.

OTHER TESTS FOR COLOR DEFICIENCIES. For some purposes, we do not need the complete results of a color-matching experiment to learn about the observer's color vision. A much simpler test for dichromacy is to have a subject examine a set of colored images called the **Ishihara plates**. These plates were designed based on the results of the color-matching experiment and can be used to identify different types of dichromats based on a few simple judgments.

Each plate consists of a colored test pattern drawn against a colored background. The test and background are both made up of circles of random sizes; the test and background are distinguished only by their colors. The color difference on each plate is invisible to one of the three classes of dichromats. Hence, when a subject fails to see the test pattern, we conclude that the subject is missing that cone class.

The **Farnsworth–Munsell 100-hue test** is also commonly used to test for dichromacy. In this test, which is much more challenging than the Ishihara plates, the observer is presented with a collection of cylindrical objects, roughly the size of bottle caps and often called caps. The colors of the caps can be organized into a hue circle, from red, to orange, yellow, green, blue-green, blue, purple, and back to red. Despite the name of the test, there are a total of 85 caps, each numbered according to its position around the hue circle. The color of the caps differ by roughly equal perceptual steps.

The observer's task is to take a random arrangement of the caps and place them in order around the color circle. At the beginning of the task, four of the caps (1, 23, 43, and 64) are used to establish anchor points for the color circle. The subject is asked to arrange the remaining color caps "to form a continuous series of colors."

The hue steps separating the colors of the caps are fairly small; subjects with normal color vision often make mistakes. After the subject finishes sorting the caps, the experimenter computes an error score for each of the 85 positions along the hue circle. The error score is equal to the sum of the differences between the number on the cap and its neighbors. For example, in a correct series, the caps are ordered, say 1-2-3. In that case, the difference between the cap in the middle and the one on the left is −1, and the one on the right is +1. The error score is 0 in this case. If the caps are ordered 1-3-2, the two differences are +2 and +1 and the error is 3. Normal observers do not produce an error greater than 2 or 3 at any location.

The subject's error scores are plotted at 85 positions on a circular chart as in Figure 4.21. An error score of zero corresponds to the innermost circle, and increasing error scores correspond to points farther away from the center. Subjects missing the L-cones (protanopes), M-cones (deuteranopes), and S-cones (tritanopes) show characteristically different error patterns that cluster along different portions of the hue circle.

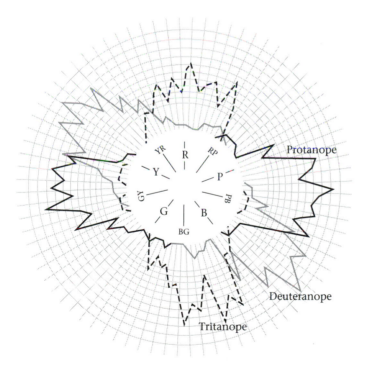

4.21 REPRESENTING ERRORS IN THE FARNSWORTH-MUNSELL 100-HUE TEST. Each of the test objects, called "caps," is assigned a position around the circle. The error score is indicated by the radial distance of the line from the center of the circle. Observers with normal color vision rarely have an error score greater than 2. Errors characteristic of an observer missing the L-cone photopigment (protanope), the M-cone photopigment (deuteranope), and the S-cone photopigment (tritanope) are shown. Source: Kalmus, 1965.

Anomalous Observers

Dichromatic observers have only two types of cones. A slightly larger population of observers who are called **anomalous observers**, have three types of cones and require three primaries in the color-matching experiment. The matches that they set are stable, but they are well outside of the range set by most of the population. These observers have cone photopigments that are slightly different in structure from most of the population, which is why they are called anomalous. The color-matching functions for anomalous observers are not within a linear transformation of the normal color-matching functions. This is equivalent to the experimental observation that lights that visually match for these observers do not match for normal observers, and vice versa.

Neitz, Neitz, and Jacobs (1993) have argued on genetic grounds that the eyes of many people contain small amounts of the anomalous photopigments so that there are more than three cone photopigments present in the normal eye. Because the anomalous photopigments are not very different from the normal ones, it is hard to discern their presence in all but the most sensitive experimental tasks. They attribute the trichromatic behavior in the color-matching experiment to a neural bottleneck, rather than to a limit on the number of photopigment types. Since the differences between the normal and anomalous photopigments are very small, however, this hypothesis will be difficult to prove or disprove, and it will have very little impact on color technologies.

The relationship between anomalous observers and normal observers parallels the relationship between color cameras and normal observers. The spectral responsivities of the color sensors in most color cameras differ from the spectral responsivity of the human cone photoreceptors. Worse yet, the camera sensors are not within a linear transformation of the cone photopigments. As a result, lights that cause the same effect on the camera, that is, lights that are visual matches when measured at the camera sensors, may be discriminable to the human observer. Conversely, there will be pairs of lights that are visual matches but that cause different responses in the camera sensors. I will return to this topic in Chapter 9.

Color Appearance

Color-matching provides a standard of precision to strive for when we analyze the relationship between behavior and physiology. The work in color-matching is also important because it has had an impact well beyond basic science, into engineering and technology.

The success of color-matching and its explanation is so impressive that there is a tendency to believe that color-matching explains more than it does. The theory and data of photopic color-matching provide a remarkably complete explanation of when two lights will match; but the theory is silent about what the lights look like.

Often, students who are introduced to color-matching for the first time are surprised that the words "brightness," "saturation," and "hue" never enter the discussion. The logic of the color-matching experiment, and what the color-matching experiment tells us about human vision, does not speak to color appearance. What we learn from color-matching is fundamental, but it is not everything we want to know (Color Plate 2).

To build theories of color appearance we will need to incorporate experimental factors, such as the viewing context, that are not included in either the theory or experimental manipulations of the color-matching experiment. It is precisely because the important discoveries recounted in this chapter do not solve the problem of color appearance that the chapter is so oddly titled. We will review the topic of color in Chapter 9.

Exercises

1. Our analysis of color encoding begins with the color-matching experiment. Make sure you can explain the highlights of this experiment.

    (a) Describe a procedure to measure the color-matching functions for an observer who is using three primary lights.

    (b) What constraints apply to your selection of primary lights?

    (c) What restrictions must you be aware of when you select the primary lights in a color-matching experiment?

    (d) Suppose you and a friend measure a color match to a test light, but you use different sets of primary lights. What will be the relationship between the color-matching intensities you find and those that your friend finds?

2. When the eye is adapted to a steady light, the nervous system readjusts its visual sensitivity in a variety of ways. For example, when you walk into a dark theater from the outdoors, at first you cannot see well. But after some time, your visual system adjusts, and it becomes easy to see dim lights. Similarly, a light presented on a bright background is difficult to see, but the same light presented on a weak background may be easy to see.

    In the following questions, think about the difference between a pair of lights that match one another versus what the lights look like—color-matching versus color appearance.

    (a) Suppose that we establish a pair of foveal lights as metamers by adjusting them to match on a zero (black) background. (Since the lights are viewed purely in the fovea, they are matched by the cones.) Now, suppose we view the metamers on an intense red background. Based on the theory that color matches are photopigment matches, will the two lights continue to be metamers?

(b) Neitz et al. (1991) claimed that some color-normal males change their matches when test lights are superimposed on red fields. In a related article, they argue that there are more than three types of cones in the human eye (Neitz et al., 1993). Read their articles and evaluate their claims.

(c) Suppose that, in fact, lights continue to match when they are superimposed upon various backgrounds. Seen on the bright background, the two lights are only barely visible. Will the lights still match when they are presented in the dark, against no background? What if we present the lights in the periphery, where there are many rods?

(d) When the two lights are seen on the bright background and on the dim background, will their *appearance* be unchanged?

3. Suppose we represent two lights by the three-dimensional vectors that represent each light's cone photopigment sensitivities, **a** and **b**. The vector difference between the two representation of the two lights is **d** = **a** − **b**. Finally, consider two lights **m** and **n** that also differ by this same vector, **d** = **m** − **n**.

(a) Suppose that we double the intensity of **a** and **b**. What happens to the vector representing each of the lights? What happens to the vector representing the difference between the scaled lights?

(b) Suppose that we express the coordinates of these lights in another color space obtained by applying a linear transformation, T. What will be the vector difference between **a** and **b** in the new color space? What will be the vector difference between **m** and **n** in the new color space?

(c) Do you think the two lights represented by **a** and **b** will be as discriminable as the lights **m** and **n**? Why or why not? Do you know of any experimental data to support your claim? What relevant data might be collected?

4. For many practical applications, people wish to use only two dimensions to describe colored lights. Specifically, they wish to compare the direction of the three-dimensional vectors and ignore the length of the vectors. The reduction in dimension of the representation is usually done by introducing *chromaticity coordinates* via the following formula. Suppose the entries of the three-dimensional color vector are L, M, S. Then we define two chromaticity coordinates, l and m as

$$l = \frac{L}{L + M + S}$$

$$m = \frac{M}{L + M + S}$$

(a) Show that two vectors with color representations that differ by a scale factor have the same chromaticity coordinates.

(b) Consider the following four lights:

$$(1, 1, 0), (0.7, 1.0, 0.3), (0.3, 1.0, 0.7), (0, 1, 1)$$

These lights are weighted mixtures of the two components, $(1, 1, 0)$ and $(0, 1, 1)$. Compute the chromaticity coordinates of lights that are formed as weighted sums of the lights. Plot them on a graph whose axes are l and m.

(c) Compute the general formula for the chromaticity of a pair of lights formed as the mixture

$$a(L, M, S) + b(L', M', S')$$

(d) (Challenge) The chromaticity coordinates of a mixture of two lights as given in (c) describe a set of points on the chromaticity diagram that depend on the weights, a and b. Call these points, $(l(a, b), m(a, b))$, and prove that they always fall on a straight line.

5. The table lists estimates of the proportion of photons absorbed per second for unit-intensity lights in the human eye. The table begins at 400 nm and increments by 10-nm steps.

Photopigment Absorption Sensitivities

L-Cones	M-Cones	S-Cones
0.004249	0.004602	0.174419
0.008655	0.009716	0.364341
0.015893	0.018921	0.662791
0.023446	0.031705	0.906977
0.030212	0.047814	1.000000
0.034461	0.063667	0.918605
0.041385	0.086167	0.802326
0.062785	0.130657	0.693798
0.102282	0.189210	0.468992
0.162392	0.267706	0.279070
0.263572	0.397597	0.166667
0.424233	0.596778	0.096899
0.618411	0.810534	0.046512
0.775138	0.944515	0.023256
0.885759	1.000000	0.011628
0.956412	0.989772	0.003876
0.995909	0.925850	0.003876
1.000000	0.809000	0.000000
0.967113	0.653030	0.000000
0.896459	0.478650	0.000000
0.796696	0.318844	0.000000
0.672069	0.194068	0.000000
0.531393	0.110458	0.000000
0.380960	0.058553	0.000000
0.257120	0.029660	0.000000
0.159559	0.014319	0.000000
0.091581	0.007159	0.000000
0.048308	0.003324	0.000000
0.025806	0.001534	0.000000
0.012431	0.000767	0.000000
0.006294	0.000256	0.000000

After Boynton, 1979, based on Smith and Pokorny, 1975.

(a) How many photons will be absorbed during one second from a light at 500 nm and 5 units of intensity? What about a light at 600 nm and 10 units of intensity? Answer for both receptor classes.

(b) How many photons will be absorbed in each receptor class when we present the superposition of the two lights? Again, answer for both receptor classes.

(c) How would you set the intensities of the 500-nm and 600-nm lights so that the absorptions to these lights equal the absorptions to a unit-intensity 550-nm light?

(d) Can you set the intensities of the 500-nm and 600-nm lights so that the absorption rate matches a 400-nm light at 10 units of intensity?

6. Now, suppose you are studying the color-matching performance of a dichromat, a person with only the L- and M-cones. We can summarize the properties of the two-receptor system using some simple drawings.

(a) Make a graph whose x-axis is the rate of absorptions by the first photoreceptor and whose y-axis is the rate of absorption by the second photoreceptor. Plot the rate of absorptions to each of the unit-intensity monochromatic lights.

(b) On the same graph, plot the number of absorptions during one second to a 500-nm light at 0.5 units of intensity and 2 units of intensity. Plot the number of absorptions during one second to a 600-nm light at 0.5 units of intensity.

(c) On the same graph, plot the number of absorptions in one second to mixtures of 500-nm and 600-nm lights when their respective intensities are (0.2, 0.8), (0.5, 0.5), and (0.8, 0.2).

7. Answer the following questions about scotopic sensitivity:

(a) Suppose you study the wavelength sensitivity of an observer under scotopic viewing conditions. At the end of the experiment, you discover that the observer was wearing tinted contact lenses. The observer has to go on an extended holiday tomorrow, but is willing to leave his contact lenses behind. What measurements do you need to make to correct your estimate of the observer's wavelength sensitivity?

(b) There are some intensity ranges in which both rods and cones actively respond to lights. At those intensity levels, human observers are still trichromatic, even though there are four active receptor classes. How can this be?

(c) Suppose we adjust a pair of lights so that they are metamers under scotopic vision. Will they be metamers under photopic vision?

(d) Suppose we adjust a pair of lights so that they are metamers under photopic vision. Will they be metamers under scotopic vision?

(e) A yellow daisy and a blue lilac may be perceived to be equally bright under scotopic conditions. Purkinje noticed that this does not occur under photopic conditions; the yellow flower is perceived to be much brighter. This phenomenon is called the Purkinje shift. Explain the phenomenon.

8. Answer the following questions on the limits of color-matching:

(a) Use a computer drawing program to make a pattern of fine yellow and blue lines. Make sure that the colors in the lines look blue and yellow when you are close to the monitor. Step away from the monitor three or four meters. What happens to the color appearance of the lines? Try the same with white and black lines. What happens to their appearance?

(b) What optical effects could be playing a role in the experiment in part (a)?

(c) Given what you know about the optics of the eye, do you think we will obtain the same color-matching functions if we repeat our experiments using a 10-cpd sinusoidal pattern rather than a uniform 2-degree spot? What qualitative expectations do you have about the experiments with a 10-cpd sinusoidal pattern?

(d) Suppose you establish a metameric match. Then you put on a pair of sunglasses. Will the metameric match be preserved? Describe why or why not.

(e) As we age, the wavelength transmissivity of our cornea and lens changes. What effect will this have on the color-matching functions?

9. In an abstract for a meeting, Knoblauch and McMahon (1993) described a test of a cure for dichromacy. The idea, which is also found in Cornsweet (1970), is simple: dichromats should wear a tinted lens over one eye. This changes the spectral absorption of the photopigments in that eye, providing enough information in the photopigment absorptions to permit discrimination of lights that were previously perceived as identical.

Now consider a dichromatic subject, Mr. X, as described by James Clerk Maxwell (1855, pp. 275–298):

> By furnishing Mr X. with a red and a green glass, which he could distinguish only by their shape, I enabled him to make judgements in previously doubtful cases of a colour with perfect certainty. I have since had a pair of spectacles constructed with one eye-glass red and the other green. These Mr X. intends to use for a length of time, and he hopes to acquire the habit of discriminating red from green tints by their different effects on his two eyes. Though he can never acquire our sensation of red, he may then discern for himself what things are red, and the mental process may become so familiar to him as to act unconsciously like a new sense.

Do you agree with Maxwell that Mr. X's experience of color would be the same if he were to wear the tinted-lens glasses? Knoblauch and McMahon, who are protanopes, thought that the ability to perform discriminations did change when wearing the glasses. Even if you are not a dichromat, try this idea for yourself. Do you agree with their conclusions?

OUR UNDERSTANDING OF how the visual pathways represent images is based upon a diverse collection of methods, drawn from several different fields. Four broad principles emerge from the studies in these different disciplines.

First, anatomical studies show that the neurons in the visual pathway are segregated into different visual streams. The functional role of the visual streams must be inferred from the anatomical properties along with the way the neurons in these separate streams respond to light stimulation.

Second, the most important information represented by the visual pathways is the image contrast, not the absolute light level. The image contrast is the ratio of the local intensity and the average image intensity. To represent the image contrast, neurons in the visual pathway change their sensitivity to compensate for changes in the mean illumination level. This process, called visual adaptation, permits the visual system to represent information in terms of the relative intensity of different portions of the visual field.

Third, behavioral and electrophysiological measurements suggest that contrast information is represented at different spatial scales and orientations.

Finally, as we try to integrate information from these diverse areas, we will consider the question of what standards we can apply to merge measurements from these different fields of study.

PART TWO

Representation

Visual Streams

The visual system consists of a collection of pathways, each responsible for analyzing different aspects of the retinal image. The specialization of the visual pathways begins at the peripheral stages of the visual encoding, with the segregation into rods and cones. The specialization is elaborated in the retina and continues into the cortical areas.

The distinction between rod and cone vision is clear: the division of labor between rods and cones permits us to extend the range of illumination conditions under which we can see. It seems likely that the visual streams throughout the visual pathways exist to meet various functional requirements. How can we establish their roles?

One visual stream in the retina contains the signals communicated to control eye movements. This visual stream can be identified based in part on its anatomical connections and in part from the fact that the neurons in this stream respond to light differently from the neurons that signal pattern and shape information. The spatiotemporal image information needed to control eye movements differs from the information needed to analyze fine detail and color in spatial patterns.

In the primate retina, two other visual streams, whose signals are kept separate up to the primary visual cortex, have been studied extensively. One of these streams represents contrast information that varies slowly over space but rapidly over time, while the other represents information that varies rapidly over space but slowly over time. The specialization of these visual streams, too, must serve a purpose in extending visual performance.

Separate visual areas exist within the visual cortex as well. These cortical areas can be identified from their unique patterns of interconnection. The functional significance of these areas is an important question in modern vision science, and I will review some of the hypotheses about these areas in the later chapters.

Adaptation and Contrast

It would be impractical to create a new visual stream to meet every visual challenge. Neurons within individual pathways must be able to adjust their sensitivity to light stimulation in response to changes in the imaging conditions.

The most salient adjustment of the image representation is the compensation in response to variation in the illumination level, visual adaptation. As the mean illumination level increases, the light sensitivity of individual neurons in the visual pathway, and of the whole observer, decreases.

Under many conditions the change in sensitivity achieves a constant representation of image contrast, rather than image light level. Image contrast is the ratio of the light at a point compared to the light at nearby points. Since for reflective objects this ratio is preserved as the level of ambient illumination decreases, preserving image contrast enhances our ability to distinguish and recognize objects in the image.

Multiresolution Representations

Behavioral studies of contrast sensitivity suggest that image contrast is represented within separate visual streams that each specialize in coding the information within a certain range of spatial frequencies and orientations. This multiresolution representation is qualitatively consistent with measurements of receptive-field properties in the primary visual cortex.

Multiresolution image representations have become a standard tool in computational applications, including image compression, segmentation, and analysis. To understand the implications of multiresolution for the visual pathways, we will spend some time thinking about how these computational applications can be designed to work with multiresolution representations.

Linking Hypotheses

Within vision science, biological and behavioral measurements are frequently compared. G. S. Brindley called hypotheses that relate measurements between these fields "linking hypotheses." He advised that we adopt a very conservative position in drawing connections between biological and behavioral measurements. This conservatism is far from universally accepted. For example, Zeki argues that a fearless attitude in speculating about linking hypothesis is to be admired and emulated. Begin by formulating guesses about the brain and perception, he argues.

The next few chapters contain many examples in which behavior and physiology are compared. What standard should we adopt before we accept a neural phenomenon as corresponding to a behavioral phenomenon?

A necessary condition for accepting a neural measurement as an explanation of a behavioral measurement is that the logic of the separate experiments must stand alone. An analogy between a few behavioral measurements and the receptive field properties of a neuron may be suggestive, but it should only serve as an inspiration for more perspiration.

Use the relationship between color-matching behavior and photopigment sensitivities as your model of a complete story. The linking hypothesis for color-matching is built by connecting a quantitative set of behavioral measurements and a quantitative set of physiological measurements. For each type of measurement, we can derive a clear set of rules that define how the system will respond to a wide range of stimuli. When each analysis stands on its own, the link between behavior and physiology is strongest.

5

The Retinal Representation

The retina is a thin layer of neural tissue that lines the eye. In this chapter we will review the structure of the retina and its role in organizing visual information. The retina is important to scientists and clinicians for a variety of reasons. Retinal neurons develop from the same cells that give rise to the brain; hence, the retina is part of the central nervous system. Indeed, the retina, which can be examined using an ophthalmoscope, is the only part of the central nervous system that can be examined without surgery. For this reason it is a convenient site to look for early signs of diseases of the central nervous system. Also, the retina performs many different visual functions. In Chapters 3 and 4 we reviewed some of the ways in which photoreceptors in the retina encode the light signal. In this chapter we will review how other retinal neurons convert the photoreceptor signals into neural activity that is sent to the brain. The anatomical connections and neural specializations within the retina combine to create a set of parallel neural pathways that communicate different types of information about the image to the brain. Finally, the sensitivity of photoreceptors and other retinal neurons varies with the intensity of the ambient viewing conditions. Because individual neurons adjust their sensitivity in response to changes in ambient light levels, the retina effectively communicates image information across conditions ranging from a moonless night to a bright sunny day, more than six orders of magnitude. By studying the way the retina organizes image information and responds to changes in the ambient viewing conditions, we obtain many insights about how the brain organizes and interprets images.

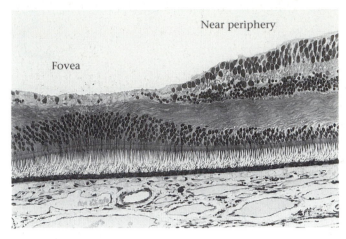

Near periphery

Fovea

Ganglion cell layer

Inner plexiform layer

Inner nuclear layer

Outer plexiform layer

Photoreceptors

5.1   THE HUMAN RETINA, seen here in cross-section, is a thin sheet of neural tissue that lines the back of the eye. In the periphery and near periphery, the retina is a multilayered structure. The cornea and lens would be at the top of this picture, so in the periphery light must pass through the several retinal layers before being absorbed by the photoreceptors. In the fovea, the retina consists of only a single layer of photoreceptors, as the neurons responsible for carrying the responses of the foveal cones are displaced to the side, out of the light path. Micrograph courtesy of Anita Hendrickson.

An Overview of the Retina

Retinal Structure

Over most of its extent, the primate retina is approximately 0.5 mm thick and consists of three layers of cell bodies and two layers containing the synaptic interconnections between the neurons. Near the optical axis of the eye, however, the primate retina contains a specialized region, the fovea, consisting of only a single layer of neurons, the cone photoreceptors. Both of these structural properties of the retina can be seen in the anatomical cross section of a human retina shown in Figure 5.1.

Figure 5.2 shows two types of retinal neurons and identifies some of their parts, including the **dendrites, cell bodies,** and **axons**. The dendritic fields receive input from other neurons; the axon, which may branch, carries the neuron's output to its destination.[1] The shape of a neuron's dendritic field and its axonal branches are generally important features for distinguishing broad classes of neurons. In order to classify and understand retinal neurons, we will use many features, including the locations of cell bodies, dendrites, and axons; the size and shape of their cell bodies and dendritic fields; and their interconnections with other neurons.

---

[1] Some neurons have no axon, exerting their influence only at local interconnections via synapses within the dendritic field.

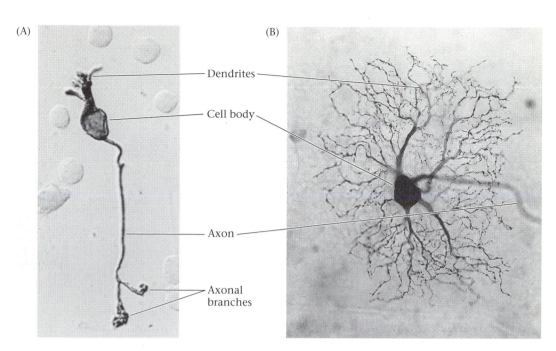

(A)

(B)

Dendrites

Cell body

Axon

Axonal branches

5.2 RETINAL NEURONS have many different shapes and sizes. (A) The cell body of a bipolar cell resides in the outer nuclear layer. Its dendrites make contact with the photoreceptors and horizontal cells and its axon carries the output of the bipolar cell to the inner plexiform layer (see Figure 5.1), where it contacts the dendritic field of a ganglion cell. (B) The retinal ganglion cell bodies reside in the ganglion cell layer of the retina (see Figure 5.1). The axons of the retinal ganglion cells comprise the optic nerve. Several types of retinal ganglion cells can be distinguished based on the properties of their dendritic fields, their interconnections, and their cell bodies. The cell shown here was called a parasol cell by Stephen Polyak (1941, 1957). Sources: A from Yamashita and Wässle, 1991; B from Dacey and Petersen, 1992.

There are five basic categories of retinal neurons, although each category has several subclassifications. The major categories of retinal neurons are distinguished by the location of their cell bodies, dendritic fields, and axon terminals. The photoreceptors' cell bodies are located in the **outer nuclear layer** of the retina. The synaptic terminals of the photoreceptors make contact with the dendritic fields of the **bipolar cells** and **horizontal cells** in the **outer plexiform layer**. The cell bodies of the bipolar and horizontal cells are located in the **inner nuclear layer**. Both the dendrites and the branching axon terminals of the horizontal cells make connections with cells in the outer nuclear layer. The bipolar cells, however, make connections onto the the dendrites of the **ganglion cells** within the **inner plexiform layer**. Since only the bipolar cells link the signals in the outer and inner plexiform layers, all visual signals must pass through the bipolar cells.

The **amacrine cell** bodies are also located in the inner nuclear layer. Santiago Ramón y Cajal gave these cells their name to indicate that they have no identifiable axons, but only dendrites. The dendritic fields of the amacrine cells make connections with the dendritic fields of the ganglion cells in the inner plexiform layer. The retinal ganglion cell bodies are located in the **ganglion cell layer**, and their dendritic fields connect with the axon terminals of the bipolars and the dendritic fields of the amacrine cells.

The axons of the retinal ganglion cells provide the only retinal output signal. The ganglion cell axons comprise the optic nerve, and they exit from the retina at a single location in the retina called the **optic disk**. There are no photoreceptors at the optic disk, so we do not encode or perceive the light that falls there. Consequently, the optic disk is also called the "blind spot." We are not aware of the blind spot in our eyes ordinarily, since the portion of the visual field falling in the blind spot of one eye falls on a functional portion of the retina in the other eye. You can perceive your blind spot by doing the demonstration in Figure 5.3.

Retinal Function: Specialization

The retina segregates visual information into parallel neural pathways specialized for different visual tasks. In earlier chapters, we reviewed one example of neural specialization in the retina: there are two different types of photoreceptors, the rods and the cones, which both sample the image. These two photoreceptors types are responsible for encoding the visual image in different intensity ranges.

The segregation of rod and cone signals continues through several synaptic connections within the retina. Kolb (1994) and her collaborators have shown that the signals initiated within the rods follow a

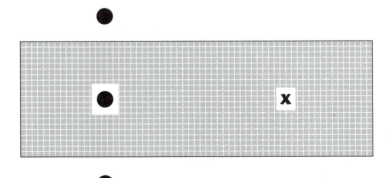

5.3   A DEMONSTRATION OF THE BLIND SPOT. Place the page about 10 cm from your eye. Then close your right eye and fixate on the X; the white square containing the black spot will disappear. If it does not, then slowly move the book back and forth, carefully maintaining fixation on the X until the spot does disappear. The two spots above and below become hard to see in the periphery, but they do not disappear. This demonstrates that the disappearance of the central square is not merely due to a general loss of visibility at this eccentricity.

separate **rod pathway** within the retina until the signals arrive at the retinal ganglion cells (Figure 5.4). The rods make connections with a class of bipolar cells, the **rod bipolars**, which integrate the responses of many different rod photoreceptors. Presumably, pooling the signals from many rods enhances the sensitivity of this rod pathway. The rod bipolars synapse directly onto **type-AII amacrine cells**, but unlike other bipolars the rod bipolars do not synapse directly onto ganglion cells. The rod bipolars synapse on the AII amacrine cells within a narrow level of the inner plexiform layer. Finally, the AII amacrines synapse onto retinal ganglion cells both within the same level of the inner plexiform layer and also at a second level of the inner plexiform layer. The ganglion cells that connect with the AII amacrine cells also receive signals via a cone-initiated pathway. Hence, the rod pathway merges with a cone-initiated pathway and disappears as a unique entity at this point.

By examining the properties of the rod pathway, we can see certain general features that might also be true of the organization of other visual pathways. First, the rod pathway only exists over a few synapses, serving its function and then merging with the main visual signal. As a

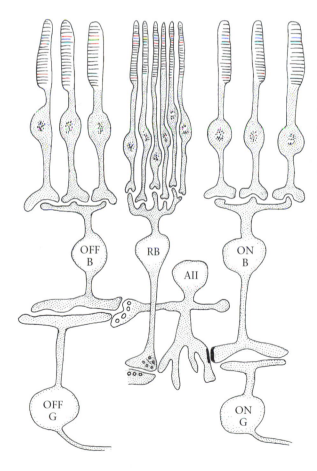

5.4 A ROD-INITIATED PATHWAY in the vertebrate retina. Axons from more than 1000 rods converge upon a single rod bipolar cell (RB). The rod bipolars send their outputs to a specialized amacrine cell (AII) located in the inner plexiform layer. The AII amacrine cell communicates the rod-initiated signal to two types of ganglion cells, one whose dendritic field is in the upper layers of the inner plexiform layer and another whose dendritic field is in the lower layers. Ganglion cells with dendritic fields in the upper layer (OFF G) also receive input from bipolar cells whose response is inhibited by light (OFF B); ganglion cells whose dendritic fields are in the lower layer (ON G) also receive input from bipolar cells that are excited by light (ON B). Source: Boycott and Wässle, 1991.

result, central processing elements that define shape, form, and so forth can analyze both the rod and cone signals and need not be duplicated. Thus, a visual pathway may serve its purpose within a few synapses and then disappear.

Second, we see that visual pathways may be created to serve fairly rudimentary functions, such as enhancing some aspect of the information in the image. The strong convergence of signals within the rod pathway—a single rod bipolar may integrate the signal from 1,500 rods—makes the rod pathway well-suited to capturing information at low light levels while paying a penalty in terms of visual acuity. This example shows that the anatomical connections of individual visual pathways may serve specialized computational goals. In this case, the converging anatomical connections within the rod pathway integrate light energy that is spread across the retina and improve absolute sensitivity to light.

The visual system is comprised of pathways whose anatomical connections and specialized neurons serve a variety of different computational goals. For example, some types of behaviors may require precise visual information of one sort, say, to track a moving object. To improve this type of performance, one may require a pathway with excellent temporal resolution. Other behaviors may require precise visual information of another sort, say, to identify a texture pattern. This might require a pathway with very high spatial sampling resolution. Rodieck et al. (1993) estimate that there may be as many as 20 pathways originating within the retina and that each of these pathways communicates its signal to a different location in the central nervous system. Like the rods and cones, each subcategory of retinal ganglion cell obtains a fairly complete copy of the retinal image. We may presume that each subcategory of ganglion cell type specializes in communicating about certain types of visual information.

We will refer to the connected series of neurons carrying information in parallel as visual pathways or **visual streams**. The precise site where information is segregated into different visual streams within the retina is not certain, but it seems likely that the segregation begins immediately at the output of the rods and cones. In fact, there appear to be about 15–20 different bipolar cells that make contact with each cone. The information encoded by each of the bipolars may serve as the starting point for the visual streams that have been identified at points further along the visual pathway (Rodieck et al., 1993; Boycott and Wässle, 1991).

Evidently, one of the important functions of the retina is to organize the information encoded by the photoreceptors into a collection of visual streams. Presumably, the purpose of these separate visual streams is to communicate relevant image information efficiently to brain areas engaged in specialized types of visual processing. This observation reinforces the view that the existence of these visual streams can be an important clue about the functional organization of the visual pathways. We presume that each visual stream carries an efficient representation of the spatiotemporal component of the image that is most relevant for tasks carried out in the visual area where the ganglion cell output is sent. Hence, by studying the response sensitivity of the neurons within a visual stream to different kinds of stimuli, we learn something about the functional role of that stream.

Retinal Function: Image Contrast and Adaptation

There are some visual challenges that are common to all of the specialized visual streams. It makes sense to meet these challenges at the initial encoding of the visual signal in the retina, before the visual signals are sent to widely separated destinations within the brain. One such challenge is that retinal neurons must remain sensitive to image pattterns despite the fact that the ambient light intensity, from a dim evening to a sunny day, can vary over six orders of magnitude. Encoding the light image across this dynamic range is a difficult challenge because individual neurons have a much smaller response range of only two or three orders of magnitude.

Neurons in the peripheral visual system solve this problem, in part, by signaling the **local contrast** in the image rather than the absolute stimulus level. The local contrast is the percentage change in the image intensity relative to the local average. The range of contrasts in a typical image remains constant as the ambient illumination level changes and typically spans no more than two orders of magnitude. By coding contrast, rather than the absolute stimulus level, neurons with small dynamic range can convey essential information about the retinal image despite enormous variation in the absolute level of light. In later chapters we will review computational issues, and we will find that contrast is an important signal in its own right. The contrast signal is closely coupled to the properties of surfaces, and surfaces are often the visual entity we want to identify or recognize.[2]

Visual Streams

I will begin by reviewing the kinds of methods we can use to classify retinal neurons. Then I will review the principal features of the information carried within two specific visual streams, the parvocellular

---

[2] In some books, the dynamic-range problem is treated by explaining that the photoreceptors respond to light intensity using a compressive function of intensity, such as a logarithmic or power function. A compressive function maps a light stimulus ranging over six orders of magnitude into neural responses of one to two orders of magnitude above their intrinsic variability. In the modern literature, this view has been substantially replaced by a formulation based on stimulus and response contrast.

pathway and the magnocellular pathway. I focus on these two streams because we know most about them and because their output represents a very large fraction of the total output of the retina.

Methods of Classifying Neurons

The form and structure of a neuron, including its dendritic field, cell body, and axonal projections, are called the neuron's morphology. The most fundamental method of distinguishing categories of neurons is simply to study their morphology. A second type of data we can use is the neuron's electrical responsiveness to different signals, that is, its electrophysiology. A third approach is to study the chemical substances used to build the neuron, that is, the neuron's biochemistry. A fourth approach is to study the anatomical pattern of interconnections a neuron makes with other neurons. The most satisfying classification of neurons occurs when the evidence from these different sources converge.

Recall that we used all of these methods in Chapter 3 to distinguish the photoreceptors into rods and cones. The rods and cones can be classified based on their cell morphology (rod-like shape versus cone-like shape), their electrical response to light, the type of photopigment they contain, and their interconnections (rods make no connections in the fovea). Taken together, the classification of rods and cones also suggests a difference in function, namely, that cones carry visual information used for high-acuity tasks and rods are specialized for low-illumination conditions.

It is natural to use our successes at peripheral levels to guide our next analysis of cellular function. So, we begin the analysis of the retinal ganglion cells by considering how we can use these methods to categorize the retinal ganglion cells into groups serving various visual functions.

Morphology of Parasol and Midget Ganglion Cells

When examining the retinal ganglion cell layer using a light microscope, one sees ganglion cells of many different sizes and shapes and with many different patterns of dendritic fields. In an extraordinary set of studies, Ramón y Cajal (1892, 1972) examined the retinal cell types in many mammalian eyes (but no primates) and identified the basic anatomical structure of the retina (Figure 5.5). To classify neurons, Cajal used several morphological properties, relying mainly on the location of the dendritic arbor terminations.

The modern era of anatomical studies in the primate retina began with the work of Stephen Polyak (1941, 1957), who wrote a remarkable pair of books describing his investigations into the primate visual system. Polyak described many aspects of the anatomical structure of the

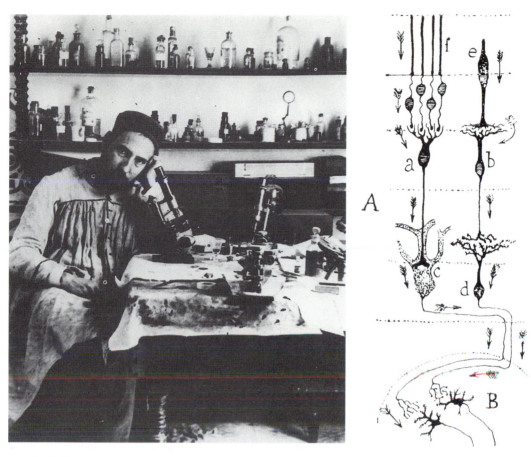

5.5 RAMÓN Y CAJAL. (Left) Cajal is shown at work at his lab bench along with
a drawing he made (right) of the direction of visual signals in a mammalian retina.
The labeled cells in part A of Cajal's drawing are (a) rod bipolar, (b) cone bipolar,
(c, d) ganglion cells, and (e, f) cone and rod photoreceptors. The connections with a
subcortical visual center are shown in part B. From Rodieck, 1973.

retina specifically and the primate vertebrate visual system generally. In
his work on the retinal ganglion cells, Polyak identified five different
categories of cells using the size of their cell bodies and the properties of
their dendritic fields. One of the principal classifications he made, and
the one that will concern us here, was based on the size and spread of
the dendritic arborizations of the retinal ganglion cells. At most locations within the retina one can identify some neurons whose dendritic
fields are relatively dense and compact compared to other retinal ganglion cells. Near the fovea these neurons are particularly conspicuous
since they make contact with only a single bipolar cell which in turn
makes contact with only a single cone. Polyak was the first to identify
these retinal ganglion cells which are abundant in primates but absent

in other mammals. Polyak named these ganglion cells **midget cells**. Several midget ganglion cells at different positions within the retina are illustrated in Figure 5.6A.

The morphology of the midget ganglion cells contrasts with a second class of ganglion cells shown in Figure 5.6B and called **parasol cells** by Polyak. The parasol cells have a sparse dendritic tree and medium-size to large cell bodies.

Variation with Retinal Eccentricity

As Polyak noted, the size of many types of retinal neurons increases with distance from the fovea. For example, a cell body or dendritic field that is relatively small in the fovea will be relatively large in the periphery. While Polyak showed that the midget ganglion cells are present throughout the retina, due to retinal inhomogeneity the midget ganglion cells in the periphery are larger than the parasol cells near the

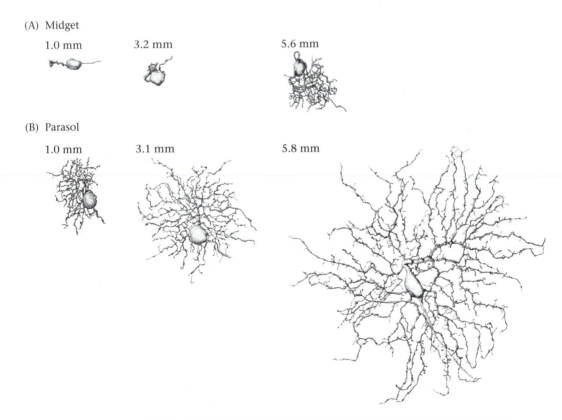

(A) Midget

1.0 mm   3.2 mm   5.6 mm

(B) Parasol

1.0 mm   3.1 mm   5.8 mm

5.6 A COMPARISON OF MIDGET AND PARASOL RETINAL GANGLION CELL MORPHOLOGY at various distances from the fovea. Camera lucida drawings of (A) midget ganglion cells and (B) parasol ganglion cells from a series of positions within the retina. At comparable positions within the retina, the dendritic tree of the midget ganglion cell is smaller and denser than that of the parasol cell. For both types of cells, however, the absolute size of the dendritic field increases with distance from the fovea. Source: Watanabe and Rodieck, 1989.

fovea. If absolute size is not a reliable indicator, what can we use to decide whether neurons at different distances from the fovea, that is, different **visual eccentricities**, are of the same type? In a seminal paper, Boycott and Wässle (1974) showed how to make such a determination in the retina of the domestic cat. The idea is simple and elegant: make measurements that span a wide range of retinal eccentricities and compare the trends within the neural population that defines one cell type. Boycott and Wässle's methods and observations have been extended from the cat to the primate and human (Leventhal et al., 1981; Perry and Cowey 1981, 1984; Rodieck et al., 1985; Watanabe and Rodieck, 1989; Dacey and Petersen, 1992).

Figure 5.7 shows that the size of dendritic fields of the midget and parasol ganglion cells increases with eccentricity in the human retina. Although both cell types increase in size, within each cell type the dendritic field size varies smoothly, and at each retinal eccentricity the sizes of the two populations remain distinct. The graph in Figure 5.7 suggests that the signals from the midget cells form one unified visual stream and the parasol cells form a second visual stream. Further evidence that these two classes of neurons form independent visual streams comes from their coverage of the retinal image. Both midget and parasol cells are present at every location within the retina. Thus, each class of neuron encodes a complete copy of the retinal image (Figure 5.8).

Although the two populations both receive a complete copy of the image, they do not encode the image at the same spatial resolution. In the fovea, midget ganglion cells receive input from a single cone. (Note that this does not mean that a cone sends its output to a single bipolar or ganglion cell!) From the spread of their dendritic fields, we see that the parasol cells receive convergent input from a much wider area of the retina. The fine resolution achieved by the midget ganglion cells means that more of them are needed to encode the entire retinal image. There appear to be 7–9 times as many midget cells as parasol cells (Perry et

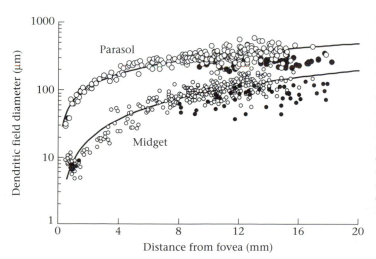

5.7 DENDRITIC FIELD SIZE AS A FUNCTION OF ECCENTRICITY in the human retina. The graph shows the dendritic field size of midget and parasol neurons. Filled symbols represent neurons in the nasal retina and open symbols represent neurons in the temporal retina. The dendritic field size increases with eccentricity for both types of neurons, but at each eccentricity the cells are easily classified. Source: Dacey and Petersen, 1992.

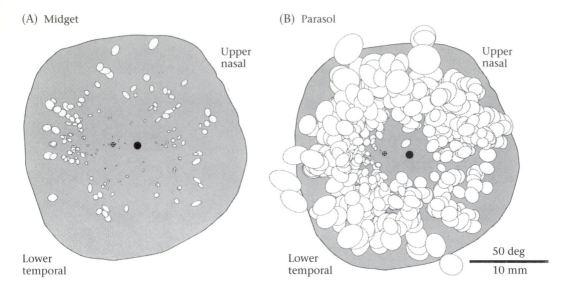

(A) Midget

(B) Parasol

Upper nasal

Upper nasal

Lower temporal

Lower temporal

50 deg

10 mm

5.8 MIDGET AND PARASOL DENDRITIC FIELDS, represented here by white ellipses, both sample the entire retinal image. The dendritic fields of the midget ganglion cells (A) are small compared to those of the parasol cells (B). Parasol cells have much larger dendritic fields at each retinal location, so that fewer are needed to cover the entire retina. The black spot symbolizes the optic disk; the cross represents the fovea. Source: Watanabe and Rodieck, 1989.

al., 1984; Sterling et al., 1994). The midget ganglion cells encode the spatial image up to the full sampling resolution of the photoreceptors, roughly 60 cpd. The less abundant parasol cells are capable of encoding the signal up to a spatial resolution of 20 cpd.

Central Projections

A second method of identifying visual streams originating in the ganglion cell layers is to consider how different types of retinal ganglion cells are connected to the brain. By injecting tracer substances that are carried from the brain back to the retina, we can identify where different types of retinal ganglion cell send their output.

Perry et al. (1984) studied where different cell types send their axons using a tracer substance called horseradish peroxidase. Horseradish peroxidase absorbed by a neuron is transported throughout the cell. Thus, if horseradish peroxidase is absorbed in the axon, it is transported back to the cell body. Conversely, if the horseradish peroxidase is absorbed in the cell body, it will be transported to the axon terminals. The presence of horseradish peroxidase within a cell can be established by appropriate histochemistry.

Perry et al. first injected horseradish peroxidase into the optic nerve, near the retina. From these injections, they could identify all of the different retinal ganglion cell types and how they appeared when stained with this tracer substance. Then they introduced horseradish peroxidase into the **lateral geniculate nucleus (LGN)**, a structure located in the thalamus which is a major recipient of axons from the retina. The majority of the retinal ganglion cells make a connection with this nucleus so that the horseradish peroxidase was transported to many retinal ganglion cells. Perry et al. estimated that 90 percent of monkey retinal ganglion cells send their axons to the LGN layers. While the preponderance of retinal ganglion cells containing horseradish peroxidase could be classified as either parasol or midget cells, there is also evidence that at least two other types of retinal ganglion cells also send their output to the LGN (Rodieck and Watanabe, 1993).

There is considerable regularity in the distribution of axons from the parasol and midget neurons within the primate LGN. The primate LGN contains six different layers (Figure 5.9). The four superficial layers

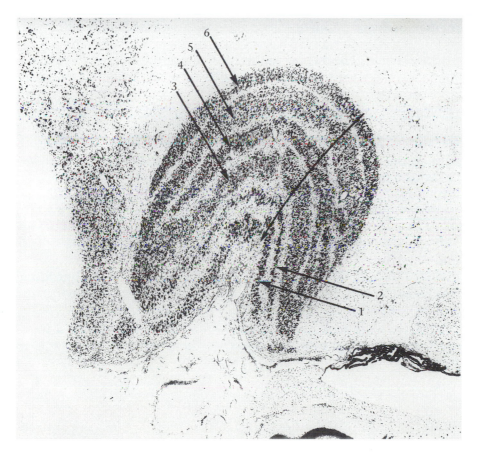

5.9   THE LATERAL GENICULATE NUCLEUS, or LGN, is located in a region of the brain called the thalamus. In primates, the majority of retinal ganglion cell axons terminate in this nucleus. When stained with Golgi material, the nucleus appears to have six separate layers. The four superficial layers have neurons with small cell bodies and are called the parvocellular layers. The two deep layers have neurons with large cell bodies and are called the magnocellular layers. There are also cell bodies that fall between these layers in regions called the intercalated zones. Each layer contains a map of the visual field, and these maps are in register. Hence, the LGN neurons located near the radial arrow respond to stimuli at a common location in the visual field. From Hubel and Wiesel, 1977.

contain neurons with small cell bodies and are called the **parvocellular layers**. The two deeper layers contain neurons with large cell bodies and are called the **magnocellular layers**. The axons of parasol and midget retinal ganglion cells make connections in different layers: the axons of the midget retinal ganglion cells terminate in the parvocellular layers, while the axons of the parasol cells terminate in the magnocellular layers. In addition to the cell bodies within parvocellular and magnocellular layers, there are also cell bodies that fall in between in regions called the **intercalated zones**. These zones may receive signals from yet another class of retinal ganglion cells.

The consistency in the shape of the retinal ganglion cells and their central projections suggests that the midget and parasol cells form separate visual streams. The pathway that begins with the midget ganglion cells and terminates within the parvocellular layers of the LGN is called the **parvocellular pathway**, while the pathway that begins within the parasol cells and terminates within the magnocellular layers of the LGN is called the **magnocellular pathway**. The significance of these pathways for visual perception is the source of much current experiment and speculation. How far within the visual pathways are these signals segregated? Do the signals on these pathways carry information with different and specialized perceptual significance? In the next sections I will review some of the differences in how these neurons respond to light. I will discuss experiments that address the broader topic of the perceptual significance of these pathways at several points throughout the book.

Although the majority of retinal ganglion cells send their outputs to the LGN, there are many other destinations for the optic tract fibers. For example, Perry and Cowey (1980) introduced horseradish peroxidase into the monkey **superior colliculus** (or SCN), a nucleus in the midbrain that is known to receive input from retinal ganglion cells. They found that about 10 percent of the retinal ganglion cells send axons that terminate in the superior colliculus. None of the labeled cells were midget or parasol ganglion cells. Rodieck and Watanabe (1993) review a broad range of measurements concerning visual streams of retinal origin. They conclude that each subcategory of ganglion cell sends its output to a single destination in the brain, making the morphology of retinal ganglion cells a very important clue in determining the organization of the visual streams that originate in the retina.

Again, most of the retinal output is sent to the LGN. But the retinal connections in the LGN account for only about 10 percent of the synapses there; nearly 60 percent of the synapses in the LGN are signals from the cortex, and the remaining synapses are connections with other parts of the brain (Sherman and Koch, 1990).

Conduction Time and Contrast Gain

There are several differences in the way neurons in the parvocellular and magnocellular pathways code information. These differences are clues about the kinds of visual information represented by these visual streams and the function these streams serve in vision.

First, the conduction time for electrical signals traveling from the retina to the parvocellular layers of the LGN is longer than the conduction time to the magnocellular layers. The **optic chiasm** is a location where the optic nerve axons from the two retinae join and are then reorganized into two separate groups that encode information about the right and left visual fields (these two groups make connections with the two different cerebral hemispheres, as is explained in Chapter 6). Schiller and Malpeli (1978) measured the conduction time for an electrical stimulus originating in the optic chiasm to travel to different layers in the LGN. They found that the signal arrives later in the parvocellular layers than it does in the magnocellular layers. Their conduction time measurements are shown in Figure 5.10.

Second, the response of neurons in these two pathways to contrast patterns differs reliably. Kaplan and Shapley (1982, 1986) observed that as the stimulus contrast of a sinusoidal grating pattern increases, the response of neurons in the magnocellular pathway changes more rapidly than does the response of neurons in the parvocellular pathway. Figure 5.11 compares the **contrast-response curves** of a neuron in the parvocellular pathway and a neuron in the magnocellular pathway. The horizontal axis measures the stimulus contrast, and the vertical axis measures the neuron's response as a percentage change from the spontaneous response level. The contrast-response curve of the neuron in the magnocellular pathway rises more rapidly with stimulus contrast and also saturates at a lower contrast. The slope of the contrast-response curve is called the neuron's **contrast-gain**. We can summarize the results in Figure 5.11 by saying that magnocellular neurons have higher contrast-gain than parvocellular neurons; the contrast–gain ratio is approximately eight.

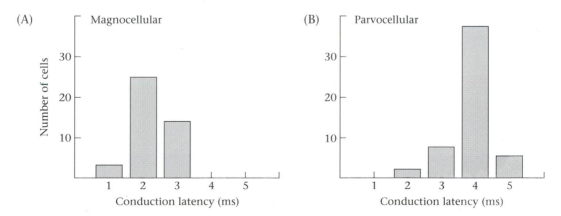

5.10   THE CONDUCTION TIME for an electrical stimulus to travel from the optic chiasm to the magnocellular and parvocellular layers of the LGN. The responses of neurons in the magnocellular layers (A) occur sooner than those of neurons in the parvocellular layers (B). Source: Schiller and Malpeli, 1978.

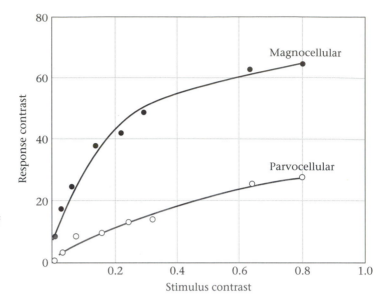

5.11   CONTRAST-RESPONSE FUNCTIONS of neurons in the LGN. The contrast responses of magnocellular neurons (filled circles) increase more rapidly than the contrast responses of parvocellular neurons (open circles). Source: Shapley, 1990.

While they originally observed the difference in contrast-gain in the LGN, Kaplan and Shapley went on to show that this difference can be traced to differences in the response gains of the midget and parasol neurons within the primate retina. Quite possibly, the differences in these signals may begin at the bipolar connection to the cones themselves.

Visual Information Encoded by the Parvocellular and Magnocellular Pathways

Anatomical and physiological measurements suggest that the parvocellular and magnocellular pathways carry different types of information to the brain. We can try to evaluate this hypothesis by using a lesion to disrupt one of the pathways and observing the lesioned animal's performance.

When we perform a lesion, we must be careful not to damage fibers that are merely passing by, or else we will have affected remote sites that are the source or destination of those fibers. The substance ibotenic acid is particularly useful for lesion studies because it destroys cell bodies of neurons but spares axons, and it has been used to lesion neurons in the magnocellular or parvocellular layers. By studying changes in performance after ibotenic lesions of the parvocellular and magnocellular pathways, we learn something about the information present in these two visual streams (Schiller and Logothetis, 1990; Merigan et al., 1991a, b; Lynch et al., 1992).

When cells in the parvocellular layers of a monkey's LGN are destroyed, performance deteriorates for a variety of tasks, such as color discrimination and pattern detection. Since the parvocellular pathway includes more than 70 percent of the retinal ganglion cells, perhaps this result is not terribly surprising. When cell bodies in the magnocellular layers are destroyed, many visual performances are unaffected. The results of several behavioral measurements before and after these lesions are summarized in Figure 5.12 (Merigan et al., 1991a).

The most informative result is that when neurons in the magnocellular layers are destroyed, the animal is less sensitive to rapidly flickering low-spatial-frequency targets. This loss of sensitivity shows that the magnocellular pathway contains the best information about this aspect of the image, and suggests that the magnocellular pathway is a specialization that improves the ability to perform tasks requiring high temporal frequency information.

What types of behaviors depend on the low-spatial-frequency and high-temporal-frequency information represented by the magnocellular pathway? Two examples of visual tasks that require precise and rapid information about rapidly varying image signals are motion detection and motion tracking. The central projections of the magnocellular pathway (which I will describe below), coupled with the significance of the perceptual signals, suggest that the magnocellular pathway plays an important role in providing high-quality information used in motion perception. However, the signals of the magnocellular pathway are not absolutely necessary to perform motion tasks. Merigan et al. (1991a),

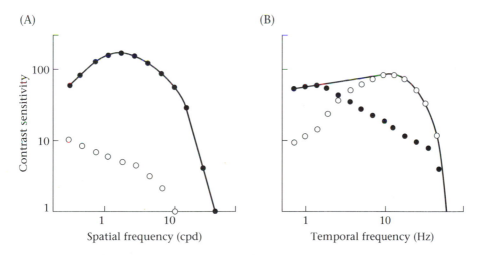

5.12 BEHAVIORAL EFFECTS OF LESIONS in the parvocellular and magnocellular layers of the monkey LGN. (A) The smooth curve defines the control monkey's performance when detecting a stationary grating. Filled circles show performance following lesioning of the magnocellular pathway. Open circles show performance following lesioning of the parvocellular pathway. (B) The smooth curve defines the control monkey's performance when detecting a low-spatial-frequency target at various flicker rates. Filled circles show performance following lesioning of the magnocellular pathway, and open circles show performance following lesioning of the parvocellular pathway. Source: Merigan and Maunsell, 1993.

who studied motion perception in monkeys with magnocellular pathway lesions, found that they could compensate for performance deficits on motion tasks simply by increasing the stimulus contrast; in other words, one can compensate for loss of information on the magnocellular pathway by improving the quality of the information on the parvocellular pathway. Discovering where the signals of the magnocellular and parvocellular pathways are sent in the central brain should provide us with some useful ideas about where we compute and perceive motion, as well as other visual tasks requiring this type of information.

Retinal Ganglion Cell Response to Light

Retinal ganglion cells form part of a pathway that transforms light into a temporal series of discrete electrical impulses called **action potentials** or **spikes**. We measure ganglion cell responses by recording the temporal pattern of action potentials caused by light stimulation. The properties of the neural transformation from a light signal to a pattern of action potentials is one of the main types of evidence we have about a neuron's functional significance and, hence, the pathway's role in vision.

Within the field of electrophysiology, the field that studies the electrical response of neurons, the transformation associated with a neuron is called the neuron's **receptive field**. The receptive-field concept, first used in vision by Hartline (1940), is a cornerstone of the electrophysiolgist's description of the action of visual neurons. The receptive-field concept, like the notion of a transformation, is quite general. Hence, the receptive-field notion is used also to describe neural properties in other sensory and motor areas (Mountcastle, 1957).

Classically, the visual receptive field of a neuron was defined as the retinal area in which light influences the neuron's response. This region can be defined by positioning small flashes of light and simple moving bars and determining when the neuron responds and fails to respond. The responses of many neurons in the visual pathway are influenced only by light falling within narrow regions of the retina, and hence small regions of the visual field. This description is relatively easy to obtain and provides a useful preliminary description of the neuron's transformation.

Although we refer to a *neuron's* receptive field, in fact the receptive field depends on the properties of the entire visual pathway, beginning with the optics and including the transformation by the neuron itself. In some cases, when there is feedback descending upon the neuron from central brain regions, the receptive field we measure at a neuron includes contributions from many places within the visual pathways (though there is no feedback to the retinal ganglion cells).

Center-Surround Organization

Several important properties of ganglion-cell receptive fields were discovered by measuring the classically defined receptive field. In this section we will consider how one important property, **center-surround organization**, was measured.

There are two locations in the visual pathways where one can conveniently record spiking activity of retinal ganglion cells (Figure 5.13). One can measure the electrical activity from the cell bodies of the retinal ganglion cells, which are on the surface of the retina closest to the cornea, or one can insert the microelectrode in the optic nerve which contains the axonal fibers that emerge from the cell bodies and carry the signal to the cortex. When the electrode is positioned properly with respect to the cell body of a neuron, or an axon in the optic nerve, one can record action potentials.

When the stimulus is a large uniform field, most retinal ganglion cells respond with a random stream of action potentials. A typical retinal ganglion cell's response to uniform illumination might consist of 50 spikes per second. For most retinal ganglion cells, the temporal sequence of the spiking activity has no systematic temporal structure, so the chance of a spike occurring in the next brief interval of time is approximately constant. We call the average number of action potentials per unit time in the presence of a constant field the **spontaneous firing rate** of the retinal ganglion cell.

Kuffler (1953) was the first to define the receptive field of mammalian retinal ganglion cells. He used small points of light flashed at different retinal positions and recorded the difference between the spontaneous firing rate and the response when the point of light was

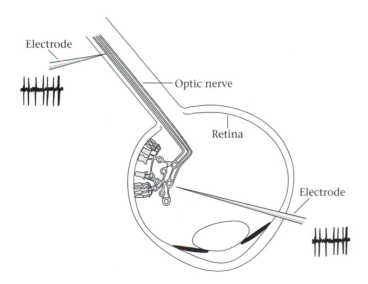

5.13 RETINAL GANGLION CELL ACTION POTENTIALS can be recorded with a microelectrode near the cell bodies in the ganglion cell layer of the retina, or near the optic nerve. Source: Enroth-Cugell and Robson, 1984.

presented. An example from Kuffler's measurements is shown in Figure 5.14. A small spot of light flashed within a central region of the receptive field causes an increase in firing relative to the spontaneous activity. When the spot is placed on a surrounding area, there is a measurable decrease in the cell's activity. The intermediate region shows some excitation at the beginning of the stimulus and some inhibition at stimulus extinction (Kuffler, 1953; Barlow et al., 1957).

The responses illustrated in Figure 5.14 define an **on-center, off-surround** receptive field. About half of the retinal ganglion cells respond this way. The remaining ganglion cells are inhibited by light falling on the center and excited by light falling on the surround. These are called **off-center, on-surround** cells. Most mammalian retinal ganglion cells exhibit one of these basic center-surround organizations.

The dendritic fields of retinal ganglion cells with on-center receptive fields are segregated in the inner plexiform layer of the retina from retinal ganglion cells with off-center receptive fields. Ganglion cells that make connections in the upper portion of the inner plexiform layer have off-center receptive fields, while neurons that synapse in the lower half of the inner plexiform layer have on-center receptive fields. Hence, the anatomy and electrophysiology suggest that there are at least two types of visual pathways, on-center and off-center, emerging from the retina.

Measurements of Receptive Fields

The classical receptive field is only a partial description of a neuron's response properties. To understand a neuron's transformation of the

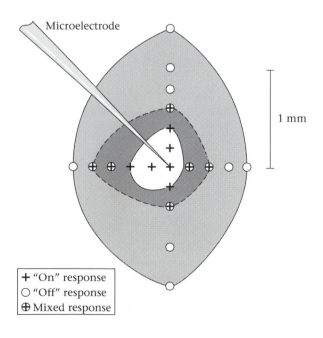

5.14 CENTER-SURROUND ORGANIZATION of the receptive field of mammalian retinal ganglion cells. In a small central region of the retina, light stimulation may excite or inhibit a neuron. In a surrounding annular region, light stimulation will have an opposing effect to that of the center. The cell shown here has an on-center and an off-surround receptive field. Source: Kuffler, 1953.

Microelectrode

1 mm

+ "On" response
○ "Off" response
⊕ Mixed response

light signal completely, we would like to predict the pattern of action potentials in response to any visual stimulus. To describe the transformation from light to neural activation completely, we need to develop a more systematic method of measuring the neuron's response. Since there are many possible visual stimuli, we need to develop a method so that we can make a small set of measurements and then use these measurements to predict the responses to all other stimuli.

Linear-systems theory provides some guidance on the question of how to measure the receptive field completely. If a neuron's responses to light satisfy the principle of superposition, then we can use a few measurements to predict how the neuron will respond to many other visual stimuli. As we shall see, in the primate retina and LGN, linearity provides a satisfactory account for a large part of the neural response.

How do we test whether the input–output relationship of a retinal ganglion cell satisfies the principle of superposition? A simple and direct test, for one pair of stimuli, is shown in Figure 5.15. In this study, Enroth-Cugell and Pinto (1970) examined the center-surround antagonism of cat retinal ganglion cells. They studied the superposition of two stimuli: a spot placed in the center of the ganglion-cell receptive field and an annulus placed in the antagonistic surround. If the ganglion-cell response obeys the principle of superposition, we should be able to predict the temporal response when we present the spot and the annulus together. For this pair of stimuli, and this retinal ganglion cell, the principle of superposition predicts the neuron's complete response very well.

Steady-State Measurements

To build a complete description of the neural response properties, we must include time in our characterization of the neuron's receptive field. We will consider the full space–time receptive field later in this chapter, but it is simpler to begin with an example in which we eliminate time as a variable; we will consider only the response after the stimulus has been presented for several seconds and the neuron's response has stabilized. This asymptotic response is called the **steady-state response** of the neuron. By measuring the steady-state response of the neuron, we remove time as a factor in our analysis.

As in all cases of linear-systems studies, we must specify both the input and output signals carefully. One of the important advances in recent years has been formulating insightful definitions for the input and output stimuli we use to measure neurons' receptive fields. Both of these definitions are based on the notion of contrast.

THE STIMULUS. We use a spatial image as the input stimulus. We will represent the spatial image as the sum of two components. One part is the average light level of the stimulus, and the second part is the variation of the intensity about the mean. The mean level of the

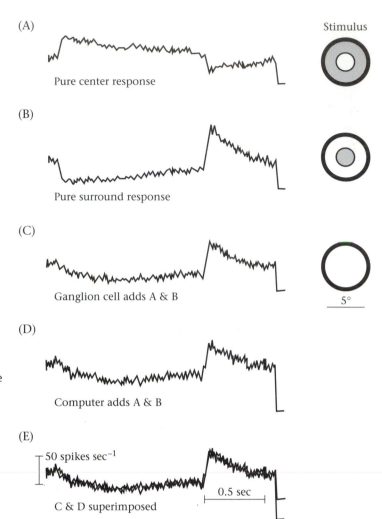

(A)

Pure center response

(B)

Pure surround response

(C)

Ganglion cell adds A & B

Stimulus

5°

(D)

Computer adds A & B

(E)

50 spikes sec^{-1}

0.5 sec

C & D superimposed

5.15 A TEST OF SUPERPOSITION of the response of a retinal ganglion cell. (A) The average response over time to a disk of light flashed in the center of the receptive field. (B) The response to an annulus flashed in the surround of the receptive field. (C) The response to simultaneous presentation of the disk and the annulus. (D) The computed sum of the responses in (A) and (B). (E) A comparison of the predicted and observed response to the sum of the stimuli. Source: Enroth-Cugell and Pinto, 1970.

stimulus is always a positive number. The variation around the average light level is the **stimulus contrast** pattern. The stimulus contrast contains both positive and negative values.

Consider the simple case of a one-dimensional stimulus that varies along one spatial dimension and is constant in the second dimension. We can specify the stimulus contrast with respect to a single spatial variable, say, x. The formula that relates the stimulus intensity to the mean background intensity and the stimulus contrast is

$$i_x = [1 + a_x]\, m \tag{5.1}$$

where i_x is the stimulus intensity, m is the mean background intensity, and a_x is the stimulus contrast.

THE RESPONSE. Suppose that a neuron's spontaneous firing rate is r_0. Now, suppose we introduce a contrast pattern, a, and the neuron's steady-state response becomes r spikes per second. We define the change in the retinal ganglion-cell rate of response, $\Delta r = r - r_0$, as the neuron's response. Thus, just as we consider the input to be the stimulus change from the mean background level, so too we consider the neuron's output to be the change from the average spontaneous response of the neuron.

TESTING CONTRAST LINEARITY. To test superposition, we must measure the response to two different contrast patterns and their sum. Suppose we use two contrast patterns, a_x and b_x, and corresponding changes in the steady-state response of Δr_a and Δr_b. To test superposition we combine the two contrast patterns to form a new stimulus,

$$[1 + a_x + b_x]\, m \qquad (5.2)$$

We expect that the steady-state response to the new test pattern will be $\Delta r_a + \Delta r_b$. Be sure to compare Equations 5.1 and 5.2; the new stimulus pattern is formed by adding together the **contrast terms**, a_x and b_x, not the two intensity patterns.

If the change in the neuron's response satisfies the principle of superposition, we can predict the response to any contrast pattern by measuring the system matrix. Suppose that we represent the one-dimensional stimulus contrast pattern as a column vector, **a**, and the system matrix is a $1 \times N$ matrix, **R**. We can predict the response by multiplying the input times the system matrix, $\Delta r = \mathbf{R}$. In matrix tableau, the equation is

$$\Delta r = (r_1 \ldots r_i \ldots r_N) \begin{pmatrix} a_1 \\ a_2 \\ \vdots \\ a_{N-1} \\ a_N \end{pmatrix}$$

We say that the entries of the matrix **R** define the **linear, steady-state receptive field** of the neuron.

We can estimate the entries of the system matrix by measuring the contrast response to a set of stimuli whose contrast vectors are zero at all but one entry, such as $(0, \ldots, 0, a_i, 0, \ldots 0)$. These stimuli are simply lines at different positions on the retina. The slope of the contrast response to the *ith* line is the *ith* entry in the system matrix. The curve in Figure 5.16 is a graphical representation of the entries of the system matrix of a typical center-surround neuron. The curve represents the neuron's one-dimensional receptive field.

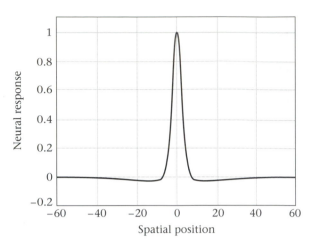

5.16 THE ONE-DIMENSIONAL STEADY-STATE CONTRAST RESPONSE of a primate retinal ganglion cell. When a neuron's response to contrast patterns is linear, we can measure a system matrix that maps the stimulus contrast of one-dimensional patterns onto the change in firing rate of the neuron. The curve, which is a graphical representation of the system matrix, represents the neuron's one-dimensional steady-state receptive field.

The Two-Dimensional Receptive Field

By measuring with points of light rather than lines, we can measure a two-dimensional steady-state receptive field. Figure 5.17 shows two ways to represent the two-dimensional receptive field of a retinal ganglion cell. The height of the curve in Figure 5.17A shows the change in a neuron's light response as we stimulate with a point of light at different locations in the visual field. The large positive values in the center of the diagram indicate that this neuron is excited by stimuli in a central region. The negative values in the surrounding region show the inhibition by point stimuli surrounding the central region. Notice that

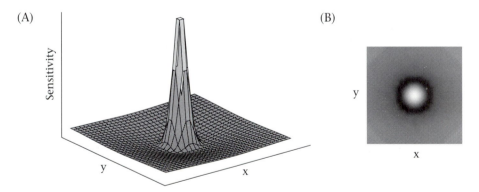

5.17 THE TWO-DIMENSIONAL STEADY-STATE RECEPTIVE FIELD of an on-center off-surround retinal ganglion cell is represented in two different ways. (A) A surface plot shows the spatial sensitivity by the height of the surface. The inhibitory surround covers a large area compared to the center, but its general effect on the neuron's response is small compared to the center. (B) An image shows the spatial sensitivity of the receptive field by the image intensity. A light color denotes a retinal location where light excites the neuron, a dark color is a location where light inhibits the neuron, and gray locations are places where light has no influence on the neuron's response.

the effect at each point in the inhibitory surround is very small, but the inhibitory surround covers a large area compared to the excitatory center. The picture captures quantitatively the center-surround antagonism that Kuffler (1953) measured in cat retinal ganglion cells. Figure 5.17B represents these measurements as an image. Light regions show where the neuron is excited by a spot, and dark regions show where the neuron is inhibited.

Contrast-Sensitivity Functions

Often, it is useful to characterize the response of a linear system in terms of the system's response to harmonic functions. Similarly, to understand the information encoded by neurons, it is helpful to measure their response to harmonic functions by determining the amount of stimulus contrast necessary to elicit a criterion level of response from the neuron. When a contrast pattern is ineffective at influencing the neuron, we need to present the pattern at high contrast to elicit the response. When a pattern is well-suited to the neuron's receptive field, a small amount of contrast will elicit the criterion response level. We call the amount of necessary to elicit the criterion response the **contrast threshold**. The inverse of contrast threshold is called **contrast sensitivity**.

From Figure 5.18, you can see how a center-surround ganglion cell will respond to cosinusoidal patterns whose peak is centered over the receptive field of the neuron. When the spatial frequency is very low, a bright bar in the stimulus covers both the excitatory center and the inhibitory surround, and the steady-state response is small. The most effective spatial frequency has bright bars imaged on the excitatory part of the linear receptive field, and dark bars on the opposing surround. This spatial frequency is well matched to the receptive field, and we will observe a strong neural response. If the frequency is higher still, parts of the cosinusoid greater and less than the mean both fall within the excitatory and inhibitory regions. The net effect of the stimulus averages out to a small response, so that high spatial frequencies are ineffective stimuli.

We summarize the neuron's response to harmonic functions at a range of spatial frequencies using the **contrast-sensitivity function**. Different aspects of the function provide us with information about the neuron's spatial receptive field. The most effective spatial frequency provides information about the overall size of the receptive field. The extent of the decline in sensitivity at low spatial frequencies provides information about the strength of the opposing surround. Finally, the decline in sensitivity at high spatial frequencies describes the size of the receptive-field center, since the highest spatial frequency to which the cell responds is limited by the size of the receptive-field center. Neurons with small receptive-field centers respond well to high-spatial-frequency targets, while neurons with large centers do not.

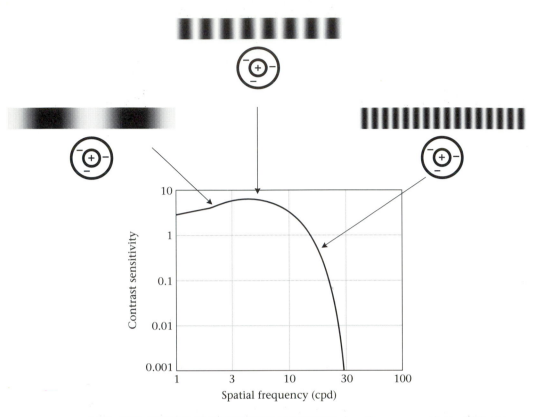

5.18 THE CONTRAST-SENSITIVITY FUNCTION describes a neuron's sensitivity to harmonic stimuli. In the example illustrated, a linear on-center neuron responds best to an intermediate spatial frequency whose bright bars fall on-center and whose dark bars fall over the opposing surround. When the spatial frequency is low, the signals from the center and surround oppose one another, thus diminishing sensitivity. When the spatial frequency is high, the stimulus is averaged by the center, again diminishing the response. From the response to harmonic stimuli, one can derive the spatial structure of the receptive field.

Figure 5.19 shows a contrast-sensitivity function from a linear cell in the parvocellular layers of a monkey LGN. The receptive fields of these neurons are indistinguishable from the receptive fields of midget ganglion cells.[3]

The contrast-sensitivity function of a retinal ganglion cell is an alternative way to represent the cell's receptive field. Retinal ganglion cell contrast-sensitivity functions are generally single-peaked. Single-

---

[3] To describe a general linear receptive field, we must measure the neuron's response using both sinusoidal and cosinusoidal contrast patterns. The receptive fields of retinal ganglion cells can be measured using only cosinusoids centered on the peak because the receptive fields are *even-symmetric*. A function is said to have even symmetry if $f(x) = f(-x)$. A function has *odd symmetry* if $f(x) = -f(-x)$. When a receptive field is even-symmetric, it will have zero response to any odd-symmetric inputs, so we need to measure only the response to even-symmetric inputs. For retinal ganglion cells, then, the contrast-sensitivity function is a complete description of the receptive field.

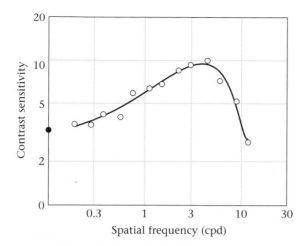

5.19 CONTRAST-SENSITIVITY MEASUREMENTS of a neuron in the parvocellular layers of the monkey LGN. This neuron responds best to a spatial frequency near 5 cpd. Notice that the opposing surround reduces the sensitivity to low-spatial-frequency patterns. Each grating pattern drifted across the retina at a velocity such that each point on the retina saw 5.2 cycles of the pattern each second. The symbol on the vertical axis is the contrast sensitivity to a uniform spatial pattern flickering at 5.2 Hz. Source: Derrington and Lennie, 1984.

peaked contrast-sensitivity functions are called **bandpass**, and the peak-frequency is called the **center frequency**.

Why Contrast Patterns Are Important

In early studies of the neural response to light, the stimulus intensity, i, was treated as the input variable. In this case, the linear-systems methods fail severely. If we wish to apply linear methods to characterize the responses of retinal ganglion cells, it is important to fix the mean level and to treat the stimulus contrast, a, as the input.

Formulating our experiments in terms of contrast does not make a nonlinear system linear. The nonlinear behavior of neurons becomes quite clear when we compare measurements at different mean levels. But by organizing our measurements around the contrast responses at a fixed mean level, we can use linear methods to characterize the receptive field for perturbations around the mean level. To describe the neuron fully, we must combine the neuron's response across many mean intensity levels. This forces us to acknowledge the nonlinear aspects of the neuron's response.

The change in the system performance as we vary the mean stimulus level is called **visual adaptation**. We can measure the effects of visual adaptation in individual neurons, beginning in the retina, as well as in the behavior of animals and people. Visual adaptation is one of the most important topics in vision. By formulating our stimulus in terms of a mean intensity level and a contrast pattern, we segregate the effects of visual adaptation from the local contrast effects. Formulating our experimental input this way is an important decision that has ramifications for how we study many important aspects of vision.

Most of modern vision science uses contrast as the key experimental parameter. The linearities that I will describe in this chapter and the following chapters are usually measured in the contrast domain, at a fixed mean level. As we change the mean level, the properties of the linear system we estimate change as well. This is a fundamental nonlinearity in the system's behavior. A complete theory must weave together how the locally linear responses, on a single mean background, vary with the mean. We will review adaptation at the end of this chapter and then again in later chapters.

Connections to Different Cone Types

In the primate fovea, the center response of the midget ganglion cells depends on the light captured by a single cone. Hence, the centers will inherit the wavelength sensitivity of the photopigment in that cone's outer segment. Parvocellular pathway neurons with receptive fields near the primate fovea often have a center response that is roughly equal to the optical blur imposed by diffraction (2.4–4.2 minutes of arc), which is consistent with the center response being due to a single cone.

There are two views concerning the connections of the different cone types to the surround region in ganglion cell receptive fields. Lennie (1980) suggested that the surround is driven by a random collection of cones, including both the L and M types. Reid and Shapley (1992) attempted to measure the surround and concluded that only a single class of cones contributes to the surround response. When the center response of a cell in the parvocellular pathway is from an L-cone, the surround response is due to M-cones. Conversely, when the center is from the M the surround is from the L. At the moment, the question of the segregation of cone signals in the surround of parvocellular-pathway neurons is unresolved (see Gouras and Evers, 1989).

There is some agreement that the centers and surrounds of neurons in the magnocellular pathway receive a signal from both cone types. An on-center parasol cell receives an excitatory signal from the L- and M-cones, while the the surround signal is inhibitory and originates in both of these cone classes. The relative strength of the signals from these cone classes to the surround may vary (Derrington et al., 1984).

Mariani (1984) and Dacey and Lee (1994) have shown that the signals from the S-cones are coded within a specialized visual stream. Neurons that receive a signal from the S-cones have large receptive fields (18 min). As noted in Chapter 2, the chromatic aberration of the optics is very strong in the short-wavelength region. Since the image from a short-wavelength light source will be blurred, the large size of these receptive fields is not necessarily a disadvantage.

Mariani's anatomical studies described the existence of bipolar neurons that make contact with a few widely spaced cones that appeared to be consistent with the S-cone mosaic. His observations suggest that the spatial connectivity of the S-cone signals also plays a role in creating large center receptive fields (also see Kouyama and Marschak, 1992).

Dacey and Lee have confirmed the existence of a visual stream specialized for carrying information about the S-cone signal and made several important and novel observations. First, Dacey showed that there is a morphologically distinct type of retinal ganglion responsible for carrying the S-cone signal. These **bistratified ganglion cells** have dendritic trees that are stratified into two tiers near the inner and outer borders of the inner plexiform layer where the on- and off-center receptive-field neurons stratify. Based on their anatomical connectivity, Dacey suggested that these neurons carry an S-cone excitatory signal. Using electrophysiological measurements, Dacey and Lee made two additional and surprising observations. First, their sample of midget and parasol ganglion cells contained no input from the S-cones. Second, they showed that all of the bistratified ganglion cells had an S excitatory input (Dacey, 1993; Dacey and Lee, 1994).

The bistratified neurons send their outputs to the parvocellular layers of the LGN (Rodieck and Watanabe, 1993). Using electrophysiological methods, one can measure receptive fields in that nucleus whose excitatory centers are driven by signals from the S-cones. It is also possible that these neurons project to the intercalated zones of the LGN. Because the sampling resolution of the S-cone mosaic is poor, we do not expect these neurons to make up a large fraction of the total population. Nonetheless, they are important, since at present they are the only cell class known to carry the S-cone signal (Wiesel and Hubel, 1966; Gouras, 1968; Derrington et al., 1984).

Spatio-temporal Analysis: Lines and Spots

Up to now, we have considered only the steady-state response, thus excluding time in order to simplify our analysis. Now we consider how to include the temporal response of the neuron in our measurement of the receptive field.

Figure 5.15 illustrates an average temporal response of a cat retinal ganglion cell to a flashed target. To obtain the curves shown in the figure, the experimenters presented the test light and recorded the resulting neural activity. If the test flash is presented repeatedly, the resulting pattern of spikes will differ slightly each time. The differences will be small, however, so that one can sum together all of the responses obtained from, say, 50 repetitions of the test flash. We can compute the average number of action potentials at each moment in time following the flash, and plot this as a curve. This curve is called the **peri-stimulus time histogram (PSTH)**.

The data in Figure 5.15 and other experimental measurements have shown that for certain cells in the cat retina, linearity holds rather well (Enroth-Cugell and Robson, 1984). Linearity has not been extensively tested in the primate retina. However, to a fair approximation, linearity has been confirmed in measurements in the parvocellular pathway within the primate LGN (Derrington and Lennie, 1984). Hence, based on linear methods we can measure the responses to a collection of basic stimuli and use these responses to predict the responses to many other stimuli.

Figure 5.20A shows two simulated PSTHs for an on-center cell response to a briefly flashed line. One PSTH shows the simulated response to a line flashed over the center of the receptive field, and the second PSTH is for a line flashed over the opposing surround. By measuring the responses to briefly flashed lines at many receptive-field positions, we can specify the **space–time receptive field** of the neuron (Stevens and Gerstein, 1976). I have collected a series of these simulated responses in the surface plot shown in Figure 5.20B. One axis of the figure measures time, and the second axis describes spatial position of the test line. Each curve along the time axis shows a simulated PSTH for a single spatial position of the line. When the position of the line is in the receptive field's center, the simulated response is large and begins soon after the stimulus. When the line is positioned over the receptive-field surround, the simulated response is weaker, delayed, and of opposite sign.

Since any one-dimensional time-varying stimulus is the sum of a set of briefly flashed lines, a collection of measurements like the simulations in Figure 5.20B permits us to predict the response to any such stimulus. Such measurements define the space–time receptive field of this simulated neuron for one spatial dimension. This method of defining space–time receptive fields has been applied mainly to study the cat visual pathway (Stevens and Gerstein, 1976; Palmer and Davis, 1981; Emerson et al., 1992).

Spatio-temporal Measurements: Harmonic Functions

It is also possible to measure receptive-field properties using harmonic functions, though in this case, we need to use harmonic functions in

(A)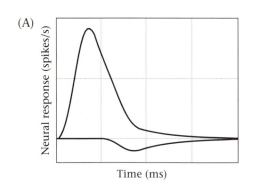

(B)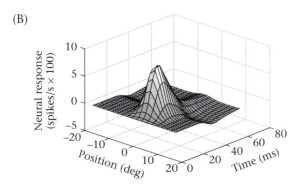

5.20 THE SPACE–TIME RECEPTIVE FIELD of a linear neuron can be estimated by measuring the temporal responses to briefly flashed lines. (A) A simulation of the temporal response to briefly flashed lines positioned either in the center or the surround portion of the receptive field. (B) A surface plot showing simulated temporal responses to individual lines at different positions within the receptive field. Such a collection of measurements can be used to predict a linear neuron's response to any one-dimensional time-varying stimulus. Hence, these measurements provide one way to define the space–time receptive field of the neuron.

space and time. We can create space–time harmonic functions by multi-plying cosinusoidal contrast patterns in space and time, creating a stim-ulus called a **contrast-reversing grating**. Such a pattern is the product of a spatial harmonic with frequency f_x cpd and a temporal harmonic with frequency f_t Hz. The formula for a contrast-reversing grating made from cosinusoids is

$$i_{x,t} = [1.0 + \cos(2\pi f_t t) \cos(2\pi f_x x)]m \tag{5.3}$$

where m is the mean background intensity.

Figure 5.21 shows the contrast-reversing in two different forms. At each moment in time, the grating is a one-dimensional spatial fre-quency grating, with spatial frequency f_x. At each point in space, the time-varying contrast is a cosinusoidal function of time, with tem-poral frequency f_t. In Figure 5.21A the function is shown as a sur-face plot. One axis of the plot represents time, and the other repre-sents space. Individual lines in both of these dimensions are sinusoidal. In Figure 5.21B the function is shown as an intensity image. Again, one dimension of the image represents time, and the other represents space. The image intensity is bright at those points where the function has positive contrast and dark where the function has negative con-trast.

Neurons in the LGN respond linearly for stimuli as high as 30-percent contrast. Hence, it is appropriate to use linear methods to mea-sure the spatial-receptive fields of these neurons. Moreover, since the re-ceptive fields of retinal and LGN neurons in the parvocellular pathway are even-symmetric, we can measure the space–time contrast-sensitivity function using only cosinusoidal functions centered on the receptive field. Because the neurons are linear and temporally shift-invariant, the

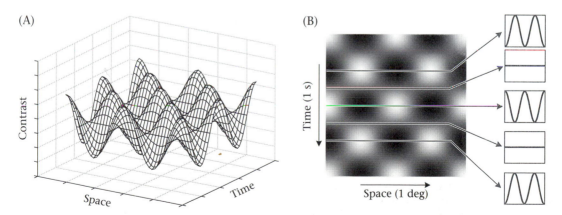

(A)   (B)

Contrast   Space   Time   Time (1 s)   Space (1 deg)

5.21 SPACE–TIME REPRESENTATIONS OF A CONTRAST-REVERSING GRATING. At each moment in time this image is a cosinusoidal spatial pattern; the amplitude of the spatial pattern varies cosinusoidally over time. The contrast-reversing space–time pattern is represented as a two-dimensional surface plot (A) and as an intensity image (B).

PSTH is a harmonic function at the same temporal frequency of the input stimulus, f_t. The amplitude and phase of the PSTH modulation depends on the temporal and spatial frequency of the contrast-reversing pattern used as an input.

The response to contrast-reversing patterns of a parvocellular neuron in the monkey LGN is shown in Figure 5.22. This cell responded to temporal and spatial modulations up to 15 Hz and 15 cpd. From the shape of the plot we can make several observations about the neuron's responsivity. First, the reduced sensitivity at low spatial frequencies shows that the neuron has a significant opponent surround. Second, the neuron responds well to all tested temporal frequencies when a low-spatial-frequency stimulus is used, but the neuron responds poorly at high temporal frequencies when a high-spatial-frequency stimulus is used. Since the response to the high-spatial-frequency stimulus is mediated through the on-center, the data show that the temporal sensitivity from the on-center and opposing surround may be different. It is time to consider the general question of the interdependence of spatial and temporal sensitivity.

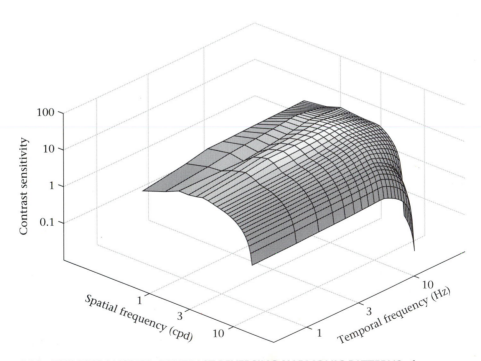

5.22 THE RESPONSE TO CONTRAST-REVERSING HARMONIC PATTERNS of a neuron in the parvocellular layers of the monkey LGN. The two horizontal axes measure the spatial and temporal frequency of the contrast-reversing pattern. The height of the surface measures the response amplitude of the neuron's PSTH. Notice that the loss of temporal frequency sensitivity depends on the spatial frequency: the temporal sensitivity falls off more rapidly at higher spatial frequencies. The surface plot was created by interpolating measurements reported by Derrington and Lennie (1984).

Space–Time Separability

We have defined the neuron's receptive field using two complementary representations. In one case, we have defined the receptive field using briefly flashed lines, and in the second case we have defined the receptive field using space–time harmonic functions. We can use either method to measure and describe a linear neuron's receptive field.

No matter which description we use, the neuron's sensitivity depends jointly on space and time. When our description of the receptive field includes both space and time, how can we define a neuron's spatial receptive field? Or, how can we define its temporal receptive field?

Suppose that we refer to the neuron's space–time receptive field, illustrated in Figure 5.20B, using the function $R(x, t)$. This function defines the response of the neuron to a line briefly flashed at position x at time t following the flash. We can ask whether a neuron has a unique *spatial* receptive field by examining this function at several different moments in time. That is, we might fix time at a value of t_1 and consider the function of position, $R(x, t_1)$, that defines the spatial receptive field at time t_1. We can compare this spatial receptive field with the measurements at a second time, say, $R(x, t_2)$. We would say that the neuron has a unique spatial receptive field when the two functions are essentially the same, say,

$$R(x, t_1) = a\, R(x, t_2) \tag{5.4}$$

where a is a scalar constant. If the spatial receptive field at each moment in time is the same except for a constant scale factor, then we say the neuron has a "well-defined" spatial receptive field.

A neuron will only have a well-defined spatial receptive field when the space–time receptive field is a *separable* function of space and time. Separability means that the receptive-field function can be written as the product of two functions, one that depends only on space and the other that depends only on time, namely,

$$R(x, t) = S(x)T(t) \tag{5.5}$$

If the space–time receptive field is separable, then it follows from the definition that the spatial receptive fields at two times will always be related by the scale factor $T(t_1)/T(t_2)$. In this case the function $S(x)$ is a meaningful definition of the neuron's spatial receptive field. The function $T(t)$ is a meaningful definition of the neuron's temporal impulse response function. If the space–time receptive field is separable, then it is possible to show that the space–time contrast-sensitivity function will also be separable.

As the plots in Figure 5.20B and Figure 5.22 show, the space–time receptive fields of neurons in the parvocellular pathway are not space–time separable. Hence, these neurons do not have unique spatial or temporal response properties.[4] In part because of this complexity, it is important to go beyond the descriptions of the neuron's response we obtain from linear measurements, and to build a model to predict the neuron's response to space–time patterns.

The Difference of Gaussian Model

In the mid-1960s, Rodieck and Enroth-Cugell, and Robson introduced a linear receptive-field model that has served as the basis for most subsequent models of linear retinal ganglion cells. The basic model is important in vision science broadly, since the ideas in the model have been used in many different areas, including work in the visual psychophysics of spatial perception and in computer vision work addressed to edge-detection and image segmentation. The receptive-field model is now called the **Difference of Gaussian model** (Rodieck, 1965; Enroth-Cugell and Robson, 1966; Enroth-Cugell et al., 1983).

The Difference of Gaussian model supposes that the neural response results from the combined signal of two separate mechanisms called the center and the surround. The center mechanism receives all of its input from a small central region, and the surround mechanism receives its input from a region that includes the center and the surrounding region. Both the center and surround are assumed to respond to contrast stimuli as space–time separable linear systems. Because each mechanism is separable, we can describe them as having meaningful spatial and temporal sensitivities. The curves describing the spatial sensitivities of the center and surround mechanisms are shown in Figure 5.23A. Both curves follow the shape of a **Gaussian distribution**, also known as the normal curve.

According to the Difference of Gaussian model, the output of the neuron can be predicted by summing together the temporal response from the center mechanism with a temporal signal from the surround mechanism. The model further assumes that the temporal response from the surround is different from the temporal response of the center, generally being slower to develop over time. Because of this delay between the center and surround responses, the behavior of the cell as a whole is not space–time separable, even though the responses of the component mechanisms are space–time separable. Hence, the model neuron does not have a unique spatial receptive field, nor does it have a unique temporal response function.

The Difference of Gaussian model has been useful to vision scientists in several different ways. First, the model simplifies our calculations and thinking about receptive fields. The Difference of Gaussian model predicts the response of neurons from a calculation that requires us to specify only a few unknown parameters, such as the widths of the

---

[4] Although I will not go into the details here, by considering the connections to specific cone types you can convince yourself that the receptive fields will not be separable with respect to space and wavelength.

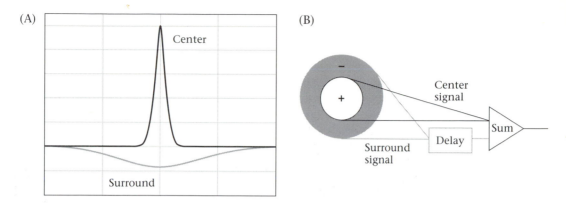

(A)

Center

Surround

(B)

Center
signal

Surround
signal

Delay

Sum

5.23   A LINEAR MODEL OF THE SPACE–TIME RECEPTIVE FIELD. The neural response
depends on the linear sum of two independent mechanisms: a center and an opposing
surround. (A) The spatial sensitivities of the center and surround mechanism both follow
a Gaussian curve. The linespreads of the two mechanisms are shown here. (B) The signals
are summed separately within the center mechanism and the surround mechanism. The
signal from the surround mechanism is temporally delayed and added to the signal from
the center mechanism. After Enroth-Cugell et al., 1983.

center and surround mechanisms' receptive fields. The model provides
a very efficient method of describing neural space–time receptive fields,
and thus a convenient way of comparing the receptive fields of neurons.

Just as important, the model provides a framework for posing new
and interesting questions. You should notice that the idea of opposing center and surround mechanisms is entirely theoretical. I have
not offered any direct proof of their existence. By building a model
to efficiently describe the results, we have generated a new hypothesis
about how the responses of neurons are created. In probing to identify
whether these are merely useful theoretical tools, or whether there are
true anatomical center and surround pathways, we will be led to explore
new and interesting aspects of the visual encoding of light in the retina.

Finally, the model is specified in enough detail that it can be used
in a variety of branches of vision science. As we shall see in later chapters, the Difference of Gaussian model has been used as a key element to
describe some of the limitations in human visual sensitivity to patterns.
The model has also been used to describe certain aspects of computational models of how images are represented in the visual pathways.

Retinal Light Adaptation

We have divided the study of receptive fields into two parts. We began
by studying the neuron's response to contrast patterns presented on a
fixed mean background. Contrast patterns are perturbations about the
mean background field; by studying the responses to these stimuli we
have been able to apply linear methods successfully to specify the transformation from light signal to neural impulses.

When we measure with respect to contrast instead of absolute intensity, tests of linearity have a better chance of succeeding. To a significant degree, this is because contrast stimuli limit the range of intensities in the image. For example, the peak intensity in a 100-percent contrast sinusoidal pattern is only a factor of 2 greater than the mean background intensity. The range of contrasts that we encode in a typical image, from the least contrast we can detect to 100-percent contrast, is no more than 2 orders of magnitude.

Through the course of a day, however, the range of image absolute intensities we experience typically exceeds six orders of magnitude. The visual pathways do not remain linear over this enormous range. When we study the response to contrast stimuli, we are attending to the local response of a globally nonlinear system. To fully understand the properties of neurons, we must also analyze how their responses change as we vary the mean background level. The changing of neural and behavioral responses as a function of mean background intensity is called visual adaptation. In this section we will consider how the locally linear measures we have developed using contrast must be extended when we consider the visual pathways over a wider range of mean signal levels.

Contrast Sensitivity: Dependence on Mean Intensity

Figure 5.24A shows several contrast-sensitivity functions from a cat retinal ganglion cell. These functions were measured on a wide range of mean intensities. When the mean intensity is relatively low, the neuron responds poorly to relatively high spatial frequencies.[5] At low background intensities the contrast sensitivity function shows little bandpass behavior, suggesting that there is little effect of the inhibitory surround. As the background intensity increases, the contrast sensitivity function changes shape. The reduced sensitivity to low-frequency sensitivity stimuli becomes apparent, indicating that the opponent surround is more significant.

The change in the contrast-sensitivity function with mean background intensity is a clue about how visual adaptation compensates for the change in mean background intensity. At low mean levels the neuron simply sums all of the quanta incident within the receptive field. At these low levels there is little surround inhibition, and thus there is little fall-off in the low-frequency portion of the contrast-sensitivity function. At higher mean levels, when quanta are more abundant, the spatial receptive field of the neuron becomes relatively more sensitive to stimuli whose intensity varies within the receptive field. The presence of the opposing surround means that the neuron no longer sums the response to every quantum. Instead, the neuron responds better when there is variation in the intensity level within the spatial receptive field.

---

[5] In general, cats have very poor spatial resolution compared to primates. This is reflected in their performance, as measured behaviorally. The spatial frequency range of the cat retinal ganglion cell is far below the normal range for primate visual acuity.

At the high mean background intensities, the contrast-sensitivity functions are rather similar. For example, the three highest mean intensities used in the measurements in Figure 5.24 differ by a factor of 100. Yet, in the low spatial frequency range the contrast-sensitivity curves measured at these levels differ only by about a factor of 3. Figure 5.24B shows the relatively small change in contrast sensitivity with mean background by comparing the cell's contrast sensitivity to a 0.2-cpd pattern measured on different background intensities. As mean intensity changes over five orders of magnitude, the contrast sensitivity to this pattern varies one order of magnitude.

The relative constancy in contrast sensitivity reinforces the view that the response of the neuron is more closely coupled to the stimulus contrast than the absolute intensity level. This suggests that the contrast variable may be the key stimulus variable represented by the neuron's activity.

Image contrast and image intensity are interrelated quantities. The relatively constant sensitivity to contrast implies that the neuron's sensitivity to absolute light level varies with changes in mean intensity level; Figure 5.25 shows this variation in sensitivity to light. The vertical axis of the graph measures the logarithm of the light intensity of an incremental flash needed to cause a fixed increase in firing rate from the spontaneous rate. This is a measurement of the threshold sensitivity to the incremental test flash. The horizontal axis of the graph is the logarithm of the mean background intensity. Since the slope of the increasing portion of the graph is close to 1, we can conclude that the threshold increases roughly in proportion to mean background intensity. This relationship between threshold and background level was

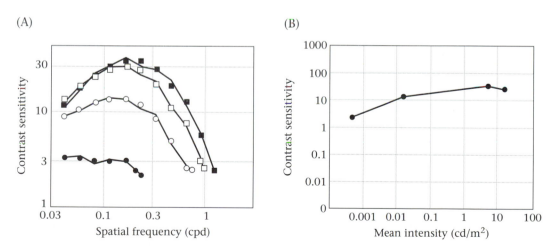

5.24 CONTRAST-SENSITIVITY FUNCTION OF A CAT RETINAL GANGLION CELL measured at different mean intensity levels. (A) The curves correspond to contrast-sensitivity measurements made on backgrounds with mean luminance levels of 16, 5.1, .016, and .0005 cd/m^2 running from top to bottom. (B) The contrast sensitivity to a 0.2 cpd spatial pattern varies by less than a factor of 10 as the mean level varies over almost five orders of magnitude. Source: Enroth-Cugell and Robson, 1966.

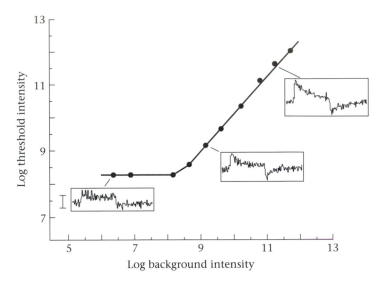

5.25 THRESHOLD SENSITIVITY AS A FUNCTION OF BACKGROUND INTENSITY measured in a cat retinal ganglion cell. The threshold intensity of an incremental test flash required to elicit a criterion peak firing rate in a retinal ganglion cell was measured; the test flash was presented on a large steady background. The logarithm of the threshold intensity of the test flash grows linearly with the logarithm of the mean background intensity, and the slope is close to 1. Hence, the threshold intensity is proportional to the background intensity. The insets within the figure show the PSTHs and demonstrate that the time course of the ganglion cell changes with intensity level. On higher-intensity backgrounds, transient overshoots and undershoots are evident. Source: Enroth-Cugell et al., 1977.

first discovered from measurements of human behavior, and is called **Weber's law** to honor the scientist who first discovered the principle.

As the mean intensity of the background varies, we can find other aspects to the change in the neural response as well. Plotted as insets to the figure are the PSTHs of the measurements to these incremental threshold flashes. The time course of the response to the incremental flash varies with mean intensity level, becoming somewhat brisker with sharper signals at the onset and offset of the test flash. Thus, we see that the temporal response of the neuron, like the spatial contrast sensitivity, varies with mean intensity level. These adaptations probably occur to take advantage of the improved quality of the signal available at higher light levels.

Comparison with Behavioral Contrast Sensitivity

Sensitivity to contrast and sensitivity to absolute light level are complementary measures. When the threshold to the absolute light level is proportional to the background, as Weber's law predicts, sensitivity to contrast will be precisely constant. In most cases, however, Weber's law is only a rough approximation. For example, consider the contrast-sensitivity functions plotted in Figure 5.24. Were Weber's law exact, all of the contrast-sensitivity functions would overlap. Plainly, this is not so. Moreover, the quality of the Weber's law approximation depends on the spatial pattern of the stimulus. The approximation is better for low-spatial-frequency patterns than for high-spatial-frequency patterns.

Reasoning based on this type of approximation is part of the challenge confronting the student of biological systems. The laws we discover do not have the same precision as physical laws. It is often a question of judgment as to whether the approximation to a law we see in a biological measurement is adequate to support a principled view about the function of a neuron or a visual pathway. In this case, there is some consensus that contrast is a key variable encoded by the retinal ganglion cells. In part, the consensus has developed from the neural-response data we have reviewed in this chapter. And, secondly, the consensus depends on the analysis that we will undertake later in this volume, in which we consider the important signals for visual function.

There is a third type of evidence that we should consider as well: this is the extent to which the properties of the contrast-sensitivity function we measure at the level of individual neurons can be detected in the properties of an animal's behavior. In Chapters 2, 3, and 4 we have seen several successful comparisons between human behavior and physiological measurements.

The retinal ganglion cell contrast-sensitivity functions have counterparts in behavioral contrast-sensitivity functions. Pasternak and Merigan (1981) measured behavioral contrast-sensitivity functions of the cat on a variety of mean background intensities (Figure 5.26). The behavioral contrast-sensitivity functions parallel neural contrast-sensitivity

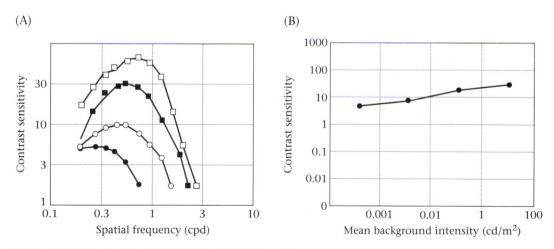

5.26 BEHAVIORAL CONTRAST-SENSITIVITY FUNCTIONS OF THE CAT. (A) Measurements on mean background intensities of 16 (open squares), 16×10^{-2} (filled squares), 16×10^{-4} (open circles), and 16×10^{-6} (filled circles) candelas per meter squared (cd/m²). Individual behavioral contrast-sensitivity functions show the same qualitative properties as the contrast-sensitivity functions of individual retinal ganglion cells. As the mean background intensity increases, the contrast-sensitivity function becomes increasingly bandpass. (B) As the mean background intensity varies over six orders of magnitude, the contrast sensitivity of a 0.3 cpd target changes by only one order of magnitude. Source: Pasternak and Merigan, 1981.

functions. For example, as the mean background intensity increases, the behaviorally measured contrast-sensitivity functions become more bandpass. Also, as the mean background intensity varies over six orders of magnitude, the contrast sensitivity changes by only one order of magnitude. Hence, there is good qualitative agreement between the response sensitivities of individual retinal ganglion cells and the animal's behavior.

The agreement between neural measurements and behavioral measurements demonstrates that the information present in the responses of individual neurons is similar to the information available to the cat when it makes behavioral judgments concerning the presence of the contrast pattern. This does not mean, however, that the responses of individual retinal ganglion cells govern the animal's behavior. We have already seen, for example, that the information encoded about wavelength by the cone photoreceptors is equivalent to the information available to a human making a color-match. Yet it is certain that when we formulate our conscious decisions about a color-match we do not have access to the information encoded by the cones themselves. The agreement between neural and behavioral responses is an abstract one, an agreement at a theoretical level. We shall see this type of comparison again as we move on to study the visual cortex and human behavior. As we do, remember that a good method of comparing neural and behavioral responses is to analyze the information available at a point in the visual pathway with the information available to the human making a behavioral decision.

Exercises

1. Suppose that a monkey retinal ganglion cell has a center that is fed by L-cones and an inhibitory surround that is fed by M-cones.

   (a) Suppose we measure the retinal ganglion cell's receptive field using a 670-nm light. Draw the one-dimensional receptive field you will measure.

   (b) Draw the one-dimensional receptive field you will measure using a 560-nm light.

   (c) Draw the contrast-sensitivity function you will measure using contrast patterns at each of these two different wavelengths presented on a neutral background.

2. Robson (1980) writes about physiological measurements of neural response,

   > if a cell's responses to a stimulus are so unreliable that we have to average responses to dozens or even hundreds of stimulus presentations in order to see that the cell *is* responding to the stimulus, then what do our measurements have to do with vision?

   Write an answer to his question.

3. In studies of the central fovea, determining the ratio of photoreceptors to ganglion cells and the ratio of ganglion cells to cortical cells has preoccupied anatomists. What are the current best estimates? What features of the fovea make these numbers hard to estimate?

4. Answer these questions about the parvocellular and magnocellular pathways.

   (a) Based on the properties of the neurons described in this chapter, what hypothesis do you have about the functions of the parvocellular and magnocellular pathways?

   (b) Design an experimental test of your hypothesis.

   (c) Do you think that the signals from the parvocellular and magnocellular pathways will remain segregated further along in the visual pathways? If so, to what end?

   (d) Livingstone et al. (1991) have argued that developmental dyslexia is due to a dysfunction in the magnocellular pathway. Read their paper and read about dyslexia. What more do you need to learn to decide whether they are right? If they are, what types of cures do you think might be possible?

5. Answer the following questions about receptive fields.

   (a) The outputs of individual retinal ganglion cells synapse on neurons in the LGN pathway. The receptive fields of neurons in the LGN, however, are quite similar to the receptive fields of retinal ganglion cells. What implication does this have for the connectivity pattern between retinal ganglion cells and LGN neurons?

   (b) The receptive fields of neurons in the superficial layers of the visual cortex do not have the same center-surround organization as LGN neurons. Suppose that the response of a cortical neuron is the weighted sum of the responses of two nearby retinal ganglion cells. What will be the shape of the cortical receptive field?

   (c) What advantage is there to having a center-surround organization?

   (d) In a classic study of the frog retina, Lettvin et al. (1959, p. 1942) describe how they analyzed the receptive fields of retinal ganglion cells in the frog:

   > We decided then how we ought to work. First, we should find a way of recording from single myelinated and unmyelinated fibers in the intact optic nerve. Second, we should present the frog with as wide a range of visible stimuli as we could, not only spots of light but things he would be disposed to eat, other things from which he would flee, sundry geometrical figures, stationary and moving about, etc. From the variety of stimuli we should then try to discover what common features were abstracted by whatever groups of fibers we could find in the optic nerve. Third, we should seek an anatomical basis for the grouping.

   > In the primate retina, their approach is not particularly useful since linearity holds so well. Beyond the retina, however, there are many neurons whose responses are nonlinear and which we do not undersand. Explain whether you think Lettvin et al.'s approach is attractive for the study of those areas.

(e) Later in their discussion section Lettvin et al. write:

> One might attempt to measure numerically how the response of each kind of fiber varies with various properties of the successions of patterns of light which evoke them. But to characterize a succession of patterns in space requires knowledge of so many independent variables that this is hardly possible by experimental enumeration of cases. . . . We would prefer to state the operations of ganglion cells as simply as possible in terms of whatever *quality* they seem to detect. . . .

Comment on how they might have obtained added efficiencies in their measurement procedures.

6. Answer these questions about visual adaptation.

   (a) Weber's law does not hold equally well when we measure using contrast patterns with different spatial frequencies. What type of neural adaptation mechanism could achieve this effect?

   (b) Explain whether the spatial and wavelength sensitivities of visual adaptation have to be the same as the spatial and wavelength properties of a system that communicates information about the pattern on the retina.

6

The Cortical Representation

In this chapter we will review the representation of information in the visual cortex. There have been many advances in our understanding of the visual cortex over the last 25 years. Even today, our view of the visual cortex is changing rapidly; new results that change our overall view sometimes seem to appear weekly. In the beginning of this chapter, I will review what is commonly accepted concerning the visual cortex. Toward the end, I will introduce some of the broader claims that have been made about the relationship between the visual cortex and perception. We will take up the issue of connecting the cortex, computation, and seeing again in the later chapters.

Overview of the Visual Cortex

The most prominent feature in the lateral view of the brain shown in Figure 6.1 is the cortex. The human cortex is a 2-mm-thick sheet of neurons with a surface area of 1,400 cm^2. Rather than lining the skull, as the retina lines the eye, the cortex is like a crumpled sheet stuffed into the skull. Each location where the folded cortex forms a ridge visible from the exterior is called a **gyrus**, while each shallow furrow that separates a pair of gyri is called a **sulcus**. The pattern of sulci and gyri differ considerably across species: the human brain contains more sulci than other primate brains. There are also significant differences between human brains, although the broad outlines of the sulcal and gyral patterns are usually present and recognizable across different people. The gyri

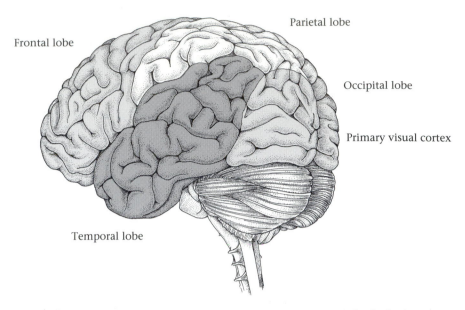

Frontal lobe

Parietal lobe

Occipital lobe

Primary visual cortex

Temporal lobe

6.1 CORTICAL REGIONS. Based on its overall shape, anatomists divide the human brain into four regions called the occipital, temporal, parietal, and frontal lobes. Based on its internal connections, the cortex can be further divided into many anatomically distinct areas. Visual input to the brain arrives in primary visual cortex, or area V1, which is located in the occipital lobe.

and sulci are convenient landmarks, but they probably have no functional significance.

The most visible sulci are used as markers to partition the human brain into four **lobes**. The lobes are called **frontal**, **parietal**, **temporal**, and **occipital** to describe their relative positions (see Fig. 6.1). Each lobe contains many distinct brain areas, that is, contiguous groups of cortical neurons that appear to function in an interrelated manner. A cortical area is identified in several ways, though perhaps the most significant is by its anatomical connections with other parts of the brain. Each brain area makes a distinctive pattern of anatomical connections with other brain areas. The inputs arriving to one area come from only a few other places in the brain, and the outputs emerging from that area are sent to a specific set of destination areas.

In primates, the great part of the visual signal from the retina and the LGN arrives at a single area within the occipital lobe of the cortex called **area V1**, or the **primary visual cortex**. This is a large cortical area, comprising roughly 1.5×10^8 neurons, many more than the 10^6 neurons in the LGN. Area V1 can be identified by a prominent striation made up of a dense collection of myelinated axons within one of the layers of visual cortex. The striation is coextensive with area V1 and appears as a white band to the naked eye.[1] Because of its promi-

---

[1] Because area V1 was defined by the presence of this striation, it is sometimes called *striate cortex*.

nence, important anatomical location, and large size (24 cm^2), area V1 has been the subject of intense study, and we will begin this chapter with a review of the anatomical and electrophysiological features of area V1.

In addition to area V1, more than 20 other cortical areas that receive a strong visual input have been discovered. The anatomy, electrophysiology, and computational purpose of these areas are now under active study and will be an important topic for study for many years to come. We will review some of the preliminary experiments that have been performed in these visual areas at the end of this chapter. In later chapters concerning motion and color, we will return to consider the functional roles of these visual areas (Zeki, 1978, 1990; Felleman and Van Essen, 1991).

Most of what we know about cortical visual areas comes from experimental studies of cats and monkeys. There are significant differences in the anatomy and functional properties of the cortices of different species. These differences can be demonstrated in simple experimental manipulations. For example, Sprague et al. (1977) have shown that removal of the cat primary visual cortex does not blind the cat: the animal jumps, runs, and appears normal to the casual observer. Humphrey (1974) has studied the behavior of a monkey whose area V1 was removed. Initially the lesion appeared to blind the monkey completely. Over time, however, the monkey recovered some visual function and was able to walk around objects, climb a tree, and even find and pick up small candy pellets in her play area. In humans, however, the loss of area V1 is devastating to all visual function. Because of these differences, I have focused this review on experimental studies of primates, and describe measurements of the human brain whenever possible.

The Architecture of the Primary Visual Cortex

There is a great deal of precision in the interconnections of cortical visual areas. The specific pattern of connections received by area V1 from the two retinas via the LGN results in certain regularities of the architecture of the primary visual cortex. We review the anatomical structure of area V1 first. Then, we review how the pattern of connections from the two retinas imposes an overall organization on the visual information represented in cortical area V1.

The Layers of Area V1

Like the cortex in general, area V1 is a layered structure. Figure 6.2A shows a cross section of the visual cortex. Several major layers can be identified easily. Area V1 is segregated into six layers based on differences in the relative density of neurons, axons, and synapses, and differences in the interconnections to the rest of the brain. The superficial layer 1 has very few neurons but many axons, dendrites, and synapses,

(A)

(B)

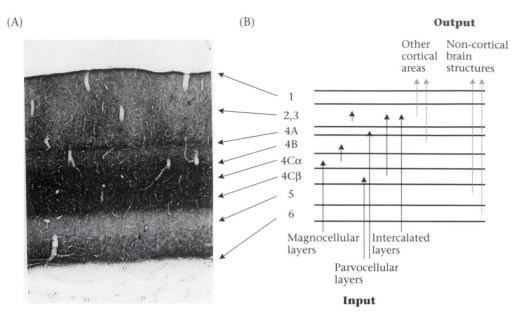

6.2   AREA V1 IS A LAYERED STRUCTURE. (A) A stained cross section of the visual cortex of a macaque shows the individual layers. Each layer has different proportions of cell bodies, dendrites, and axons and may be distinguished by the density of the staining and other properties. The light areas are blood vessels. (B) The organization of the neural inputs and outputs to area V1 are shown. The parvocellular and magnocellular inputs make connections in layer 4C. The intercalated neurons make connections in the superficial layers. The outputs are sent to other cortical areas, back to the LGN, and to other subcortical nuclei. Photomicrograph courtesy of Jennifer Lund.

which collectively are called **neuropil**. Layers 2 and 3 consist of a dense array of cell bodies and many local dendritic interconnections. These layers appear to receive a direct input from the intercalated layers of the LGN as well (Fitzpatrick et al., 1983; Hendry and Yoshioka, 1994), and the outputs from layers 2 and 3 are sent to other cortical areas. Layers 2 and 3 are hard to distinguish based on simple histological stains of the cortex. Frequently, layers 1–3 are grouped together and simply called the **superficial layers** of the cortex.

Layer 4 has been subdivided into several parts as the interconnections with other brain areas and layers have become clarified. Layer 4C receives the primary input from the parvocellular and magnocellular layers of the LGN. The magnocellular neurons send their output to the upper half of this layer, which is called 4Cα while the parvocellular neurons make connections in the lower half, called 4Cβ. Layer 4B receives a large input from 4Cα and sends its output to other cortical areas. Layer 4B can be defined anatomically by the presence of a large striation, called the **stria of Gennari**, which is composed mainly of cortical axons.

Layer 5 contains relatively few cell bodies compared to the surrounding layers. It sends a major output to the superior colliculus, a structure in the midbrain. Layer 6 is dense with cells and sends a large output back to the LGN (Lund et al., 1975). As a general though not absolute rule, forward outputs to new cortical areas tend to come from the superficial layers and terminate in layer 4. The feedback projections tend to come from the deep layers and terminate in layers 1 and 6 (Rockland and Pandya, 1979; Felleman and Van Essen, 1991).

The wiring diagram in Figure 6.2B shows that the signals to and from area V1 are complex and highly specific. One must suppose that the interconnections within area V1 are specific, too. Roughly 25 percent of the neurons in all layers are inhibitory interneurons, and their interconnections must be governed by the presence of biochemical markers that identify which neurons should connect and how. Anatomical classification of the cell types within the visual cortex, and identification of the local circuitry, will provide us with many more clues about the functional significance of this area.

The Pathway to Area V1

The structure of the anatomical pathways leading from the two retinas to the cortex defines many of the fundamental properties of area V1. Among the most significant properties is that area V1 in each hemisphere has only a restricted field of view: area V1 in the left hemisphere only receives visual input from the right half of the visual field; area V1 in the right hemisphere only receives input from the left visual field.

We can see how this arises by considering how retinal signals make their way to area V1. The optic tract fibers from the two retinas come together at the optic chiasm, as shown in Figure 6.3. There the fibers are sorted into two new groups that each connect to only one side of the brain. Axons from ganglion cells whose receptive fields are located in the left visual field send their outputs towards the LGN on the right side of the brain, while axons of ganglion cells with receptive fields in the right visual field communicate their output to the left side of the brain. Consequently, each LGN receives a retinal signal derived from both eyes, but from only one half of the visual field.

The signals reaching the cortex from the retina respect three other basic organizational principles. The interconnections are organized with respect to (a) the eye of origin, (b) the class of ganglion cell, and (c) the spatial position of the ganglion cell within the retina. Figure 6.3 illustrates the pattern of connections schematically, starting at the retinas and continuing to area V1.

EYE OF ORIGIN. Within the LGN, information about the eye of origin is preserved, since fibers from each eye make connections in different layers of the LGN. The parvocellular and magnocellular layers are numbered as 1–6: layers 1, 4, and 6 receive input from the retina on the same side of head, while layers 2, 3, and 5 receive input from the retina on the opposite side. The connections of these layers for the left LGN

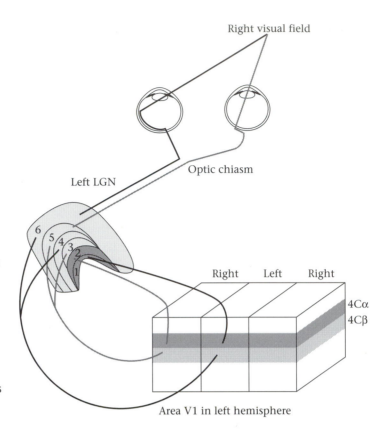

6.3 THE SIGNALS FROM THE TWO RETINAS ARE COMMUNICATED TO AREA V1 via the LGN. Points in the right visual field are imaged on the temporal side of the left eye and the nasal side of the right eye. Axons from ganglion cells in these retinal regions make connections with separate layers in the left LGN. Neurons in the magnocellular and parvocellular layers of the LGN send their outputs to cortical layers 4Cα and 4Cβ, respectively. The signals from each eye are segregated into different bands within area V1. Signals from these bands converge on individual neurons in the superficial layers of the cortex.

are illustrated in Figure 6.3. Why this particular pattern of ocular connections exists is a mystery. The eye of origin for the intercalated layers, which fall between the parvocellular and magnocellular layers, has not yet been ascertained.

The signals from the two eyes remain segregated as they arrive at the input layers of area V1. One can observe this segregation by measuring the electrophysiological responses of the units in layer 4C. As the recording electrode is moved within layer 4C, there is an abrupt shift as to which eye drives the unit. In layer 4C, the shift from one eye to the other takes place over a distance of less than 50 μm. Above and below layer 4C the signals from the two eyes converge onto single neurons, although there is still a tendency for individual neurons to receive inputs predominantly from one eye or the other, and this pattern is aligned with the input pattern. The transition between eyes of origin is less abrupt in the superficial layers, perhaps extending over 100 μm. The relative segregation of information across the visual cortex with respect to the eye of origin has led researchers to describe its organization in terms of **ocular dominance columns** (Hubel and Wiesel, 1977; Bishop, 1984).

In addition to evidence from electrophysiological measurements, one also can use anatomical methods to visualize the ocular dominance columns. After injection into one eye, the tritiated amino acid proline will be transported from the retina to the cortex across synaptic connections. By sectioning the visual cortex tangentially at layer 4C and exposing the sections to a photographic emulsion, one can develop a pattern of light and dark stripes that corresponds to the presence and absence of the tritiated proline. Figure 6.4 shows a pattern of light bands that mark regions receiving input from the injected eye; the intervening dark areas receive input from the opposite eye. In the monkey, these bands each span approximately 400 μm; in the human they span approximately 800 μm (Hubel et al., 1978; Horton and Hoyt, 1991).

In the superficial layers of area V1 many neurons respond to stimuli from both eyes; in a normal monkey, 80 percent of the neurons in the superificial layers of area V1 are binocularly driven. The development of the interconnections necessary to drive the binocular neurons depends upon experience during maturation. Hubel and Wiesel (1965) showed that artifically closing one eye or cutting an ocular muscle strongly affects the development of neurons in area V1. Specifically, the binocular neurons fail to develop. Behaviorally, if one eye is kept closed for a critical period during development, the animal will remain blind in this eye for the rest of its life. This is quite different from the result of closing an adult eye for a few months, which has no significant effect (Hubel et al., 1977a; Shatz and Stryker, 1978; Movshon and Van Sluyters, 1981; Mitchell, 1988). In the cat, normal development of ocular dominance columns and presumably the binocular interconnections as well depend upon neural activity originating in the two retinas (Stryker and Harris, 1986).

GANGLION CELL CLASSIFICATION. Information from different classes of retinal ganglion cells remains segregated along the path to the cortex. Neurons in the magnocellular layers receive fibers from the parasol cells; neurons in the parvocellular layers receive fibers from the midget

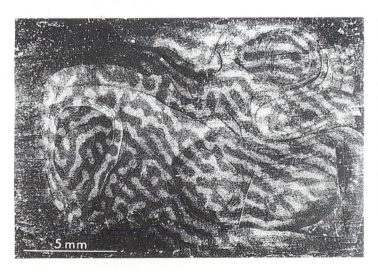

5 mm

6.4 THE OCULAR DOMINANCE COLUMNS IN AREA V1 can be visualized by using a radioactive marker, tritiated proline. When the marker is injected into one eye it is transported via the LGN nucleus to the cortex. The radioactive uptake is revealed in this dark-field photograph. The light bands in this tangential section show the places where the radioactive marker was located and thus reveal the ocular dominance columns. Source: Hubel et al., 1978.

ganglion cells. It is uncertain precisely which retinal ganglion cells project to the intercalated layers. The segregation of signals continues to the input of area V1. Within layer 4C, the upper half ($4C\alpha$) receives the axons from the magnocellular layers, while the lower half ($4C\beta$) receives the parvocellular input. The neurons in the intercalated layers send their output to the superficial layers 2 and 3.

RETINOTOPIC ORGANIZATION. The spatial position of the ganglion cell within the retina is preserved by the spatial organization of the neurons within the LGN layers. The back of the nucleus contains neurons whose receptive fields are near the fovea. Toward the front of the nucleus, the receptive field locations become increasingly peripheral. This spatial layout is called **retinotopic organization** because the topological organization of the receptive fields in the LGN parallels the organization in the retina.

The signals in area V1 are also retinotopically arranged. From electrophysiology in monkeys, one can measure the location of receptive fields with an electrode that penetrates tangentially through layer 4C, traversing through the ocular dominance columns. The receptive-field centers of neurons along this path correspond systematically to locations from the fovea to the periphery. This trend is interrupted locally by small, abrupt jumps at the ocular dominance borders. Within the first ocular dominance column the receptive-field center positions change smoothly; as one passes into the next ocular dominance region there is an abrupt shift of the receptive field positions equal to about half of the space spanned by receptive fields in the first column. Hubel and Wiesel (1977) refer to this organization as "two steps forward and one step back."

In the last 15 years, it has become possible to estimate spatially localized activity in the human brain. Beginning with **positron emission tomography (PET)** studies, and more recently by using **functional magnetic resonance imaging (fMRI)**, researchers have been able to measure activity in volumes of the cortex as small as 10 mm^3 containing a few hundred thousand neurons.[2]

Human area V1 is located within the **calcarine sulcus** in the occipital lobe. The calcarine sulcus in my brain, and its retinotopic organization, is shown in Figure 6.5. Neurons with receptive fields in the central visual field are located in the posterior calcarine sulcus, while neurons with receptive fields in the periphery are located in the anterior portions of the sulcus. At a given distance along the sulcus, the receptive fields are located along a semicircle in the visual field. Neurons with receptive fields on the upper, middle, and lower sections of

---

[2] Both of these methods are based on indirect measures of neural activation. With the PET method, an observer receives a low dose of radiation in his bloodstream, and neural activity is indicated by brain regions showing increased radioactivity. The fMRI signal detects differences in the local concentration of blood oxygen. Both the increased radioactivity and the change in local blood oxygenation are due to vascular responses to the neural activity (Kwong et al., 1992; Ogawa et al., 1992; Posner and Raichle, 1994).

(A)

(B)

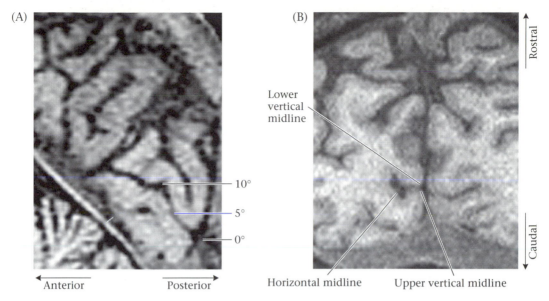

Lower
vertical
midline

Rostral

10°

5°

0°

Caudal

Anterior   Posterior

Horizontal midline   Upper vertical midline

6.5 HUMAN AREA V1 is located mainly in the calcarine sulcus, and in some individuals it may extend onto the occipital pole. (A) Seen in sagittal view, the calcarine is a long sulcus that extends roughly 4 cm. The visual eccentricities of the receptive fields of neurons at different locations are shown. (B) In the coronal plane the calcarine sulcus appears as an indentation of the medial wall of the brain. At a given distance along the sulcus, the receptive fields of neurons fall along a semicircle within the visual field. Each hemisphere represents one half of the visual field. Neurons with receptive fields on the upper, middle, and lower sections of a semicircle of constant eccentricity are found on the lower, middle, and upper portions of the calcarine sulcus respectively.

the semicircle are found on the lower, middle, and upper portions of the calcarine sulcus, respectively (Inouye, 1909; Holmes, 1918, 1945; Horton and Hoyt, 1991).

Engel et al. (1994) measured the human retinotopic organization from fovea to periphery by using the stimulus shown in Figure 6.6A. The stimulus consisted of a series of slowly expanding rings; each ring was a collection of flickering squares. The ring began as a small spot located at the fixation mark, and then it grew until it traveled beyond the edge of the visual field. As a ring faded from view, it was replaced by a new ring starting at the center. Because of the retinotopic organization of the calcarine sulcus, each ring causes a traveling wave of neural activity beginning in the posterior calcarine sulcus and traveling in the anterior direction.

We can detect the traveling wave of activation by measuring the fMRI signal at different points along the calcarine sulcus. Figure 6.6B is an image of the brain within the plane of the calcarine sulcus. Positions within the calcarine sulcus are indicated in black. The fMRI signal at each point within the sulcus, plotted as a function of time, is shown in the mesh plot in Figure 6.6C. Notice that the amplitude of the fMRI signal covaries with the stimulus; the fMRI signal waxes and wanes four times through the four periods of the expanding annulus.

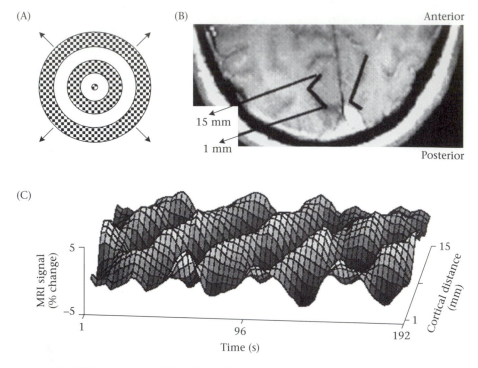

(A)

(B)

Anterior

15 mm

1 mm

Posterior

(C)

MRI signal (% change)

5

−5

1

96

192

Time (s)

Cortical distance (mm)

15

1

6.6 RECEPTIVE-FIELD LOCATIONS OF NEURONS IN THE HUMAN CALCARINE SULCUS measured by functional magnetic resonance imaging (fMRI). (A) The observer viewed a series of concentric expanding annuli presented on a gray background. Each annulus contained a high-contrast flickering radial checkerboard pattern. As an annulus expanded beyond the edge of the display, a new annulus emerged in the center creating a periodic image sequence. The sequence was repeated four times in a single experiment. (B) An image within the plane of the calcarine sulcus. The dark lines indicate points identified as within the calcarine sulcus. (C) The fMRI temporal signal at different points within the left calcarine sulcus. The fMRI signal follows the time course of the stimulus; the phase of the signal is delayed as one measures from the posterior to the anterior calcarine sulcus. After Engel et al., 1994.

The temporal phase of the fMRI signal varies systematically from the posterior to anterior portions of the sulcus. Activity in the posterior portion of the sulcus is advanced in time compared to activity in the anterior portion. This traveling wave occurs because the stimulus creates activity in the posterior part of the sulcus first, and then later in the anterior part of the sulcus.

In addition to fMRI, there are several other estimates of the mapping from visual-field eccentricity to locations in the calcarine sulcus. These estimates are compared in Figure 6.7. The fMRI measurements from two observers are shown as the black symbols. Estimates from direct electrical stimulation of the cortex are shown as gray squares (Dobelle et al., 1979). In these experiments the volunteer observer's brain was stimulated, and he indicated the location of the perceived visual stimulation within the visual field (see also Brindley and Lewin, 1968). The three gray diamonds are show measurements using PET. These data

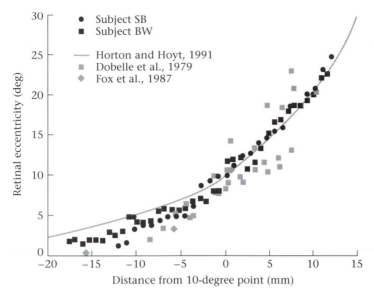

6.7 METHODS TO ESTIMATE THE RECEPTIVE-FIELD LOCATION OF NEURONS in the calcarine sulcus. The black symbols show measurements from two observers using the fMRI method (Engel et al., 1994). The shaded squares are from a microstimulation study on a blind volunteer (Dobelle et al., 1979). The shaded diamonds are measurements averaged from five observers using PET (Fox et al., 1987). The shaded curve is an estimate based on studying the locations of scotoma in stroke patients and single-cell data from nonhuman primates (Horton and Hoyt, 1991). Source: Engel et al., 1994.

represent the average of five different observers, normalized for differences in brain size. The shaded line shows an estimate Horton and Hoyt (1991) made by studying the positions of scotoma in observers with localized brain lesions and by extrapolating from data on monkeys. These estimates are in good agreement, and they all show that considerably more cortical area is allocated to the foveal representation than to the peripheral representation.

The allocation of more cortical area to the foveal representation than to the peripheral representation seems a natural consequence of the fact that more photoreceptors and retinal ganglion cells represent the fovea than the periphery. Wässle et al. (1990; see also Schein, 1988) suggested that the expanded foveal representation can be explained by assuming that every ganglion cell is allocated an equal amount of cortical area. More recently, Azzopardi and Cowey (1993) have suggested that there is a further expansion of the foveal representation, and that foveal ganglion cells are allocated 3–6 times more cortical area than peripheral ganglion cells.

Electrical Stimulation of Human Area V1

Direct electrical stimulation of the visual cortex causes the sensation of vision. When a visual impression is generated by nonphotic stimulation, say by pressing on the eyeball or by electrical stimulation, the resulting perception is called a **visual phosphene**. In order to develop visual prostheses for individuals with incurable retinal diseases, several research groups have studied the visual properties of phosphenes created by electrical stimulation of the visual cortex (Brindley and Lewin, 1968; Dobelle et al., 1979; Bak et al., 1990).

Brindley and Lewin (1968) describe experiments with a human volunteer who was diabetic and suffered from bilateral glaucoma and a right retinal detachment, and who was effectively blind. When she suffered a stroke, she required an operation that would expose her visual cortex. With the patient's consent, Brindley and Lewin built and implanted a stimulator that could deliver current to the surface of her brain, near the patient's primary visual cortex. They asked her to describe the appearance of the electrical stimulation following stimulation by the different electrodes, at various positions within her primary visual cortex. She reported that electrical stimulation caused her to perceive a phosphene that appeared to be a point of light or a blob in space. Her description of the visual impression caused by most of the electrodes was "like a grain of rice at arm's length." Occasionally one electrode might cause a slightly larger impression, "like half a matchstick at arm's length."

As might be expected from the retinotopic organization of the visual cortex, the position of the phosphenes varied with the position of the stimulating electrodes. The observer told the experimenters where she perceived the phosphenes to be using a simple procedure. She grasped a knob with her right hand and imagined she was fixating on that hand. She then pointed to the location of the phosphenes relative to the fixation point using her left hand.

Figure 6.8 shows the positions of the electrodes and the corresponding phosphenes. The pattern of results follows the expectations from the retinotopic organization of the calcarine sulcus. Stimulation by electrodes near the back of the brain created phosphenes in the central 5 degrees; stimulation by forward electrodes created phosphenes in more eccentric portions. More cortical area is devoted to the central regions of vision than to peripheral regions.

Brindley and Lewin tested the effects of superposition by stimulating with separate electrodes and then stimulating with both electrodes at once. When electrodes were far apart, the visual phosphene generated by stimulating both electrodes at once could be predicted from the phosphenes generated by stimulating individually. Superposition also held for some closely spaced electrodes, but not all. The test of superposition is particularly important for practical development of a prosthetic device. To build up complex visual patterns from stimulation of area V1, it is necessary to use multiple electrodes. If linearity holds, then we can measure the appearance from single electrode stimulations and predict the appearance corresponding to multiple stimulations. That superposition held approximately suggests that it may be possible to predict the appearance of the multiple electrode stimulation from measurements using individual electrodes. Without superposition, we have no logical basis for creating an image from the intensities perceived at single points.

There have been a few recent reports of stimulation of the human visual cortex. For example, Bak et al. (1990) used very fine (37.5-μm)

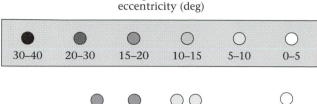

Phosphene
eccentricity (deg)

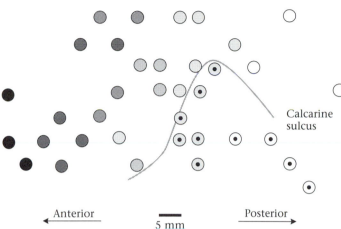

Calcarine
sulcus

Anterior · 5 mm · Posterior

6.8 ELECTRICAL STIMULATION OF HUMAN AREA V1 using implanted microelectrodes reveals the retinotopic organization of human cortex. The symbols are plotted at the electrode positions on the medial wall of the brain. The shading of the symbol indicates the visual eccentricity of the phosphene created by electrode stimulation. A dot within the symbol means that the phosphene was perceived in the upper visual field. The shaded curve shows the inferred position of the calcarine sulcus. Source: Brindley and Lewin, 1968.

microelectrodes inserted within the cortex. They experimented on patients who were having epileptic foci removed. These patients were under local anaesthesia and could report on their visual sensations. Bak et al. observed that, when the electrodes were embedded within the visual cortex, visual sensations could be obtained with quite low current levels. Brindley and Lewin (1968) had used about 2 mA of current, but Bak et al. found thresholds about 100 times lower, near 20 μA. The appearance of the visual phosphene was steady in these patients, and some of the phosphenes appeared to be colored. Time was quite limited in these studies, and only a few experimental manipulations were possible. But, Bak et al. report that when the microelectrodes were separated by more than 0.7 mm, the two phosphenes could be seen as distinct, while separations of 0.3 mm were seen as a single spot. For one subject, nearly all of the phosphenes were reported to be strongly colored, unlike the phosphenes reported by Brindley and Lewin's patient. While the subjects were stimulated, they could also perceive light stimuli. The phosphenes were visible against the backdrop of the normal visual field.

Receptive Fields in the Primary Visual Cortex

The receptive fields of neurons in area V1 are qualitatively different from those in the LGN. For example, LGN neurons have circularly symmetric receptive fields, but most V1 neurons do not. Unlike LGN neurons, some neurons in area V1 respond well to stimuli moving in one direction but fail to respond to stimuli moving in the opposite direction. Some area V1 neurons are binocular, responding to stimuli from both eyes. These new receptive-field properties must be related to the visual computations performed within the cortex such as the analysis of form and texture, the perception of motion, and the estimation of depth. We might expect that these new receptive-field properties have a functional role in these visual computations.

Much of what we know about cortical receptive fields comes from Hubel and Wiesel's measurements during their 25 years of collaboration. Others had accomplished the difficult feat of recording from cortical neurons first, but the initial experiments used diffuse illumination, say, turning on the room lights, as a source of stimulation. As we have seen, pattern contrast is an important variable in the retinal neural representation; consequently, cortical cells respond poorly to diffuse illumination (von Baumgarten and Jung, 1952). Hubel and Wiesel made rapid progress in elucidating the responses of cortical neurons by using stimuli of great relevance to vision and by being extremely insightful. Hubel and Wiesel's papers chart a remarkable series of advances in our understanding of the visual cortex. Their studies have defined the major ways in which area V1 receptive fields differ from LGN receptive fields. Their qualitative methods for studying the cortex continue to dominate experimental physiology (Hubel and Wiesel, 1959, 1962, 1968, 1977; Hubel, 1982).

Hubel and Wiesel recorded the activity of cortical neurons while displaying patterned stimuli, mainly line segments and spots, on a screen that was imaged through the animal's cornea and lens onto the retina. As the microelectrode penetrated the visual cortex, they presented line segments whose width and length could be adjusted. First, they varied the position of the stimulus on the screen, searching for the neuron's receptive field. Once the receptive-field position was established, they measured the response of the neuron to lines, bars and spots presented individually.

One important goal of their work was to classify the cortical neurons based on their responses to the small collection of stimuli. They sought classifications that represented the neurons' receptive field properties and that also helped to clarify the neurons' function in seeing. Recall that classification of the receptive-field types was also an important theme when we considered the responses of retinal ganglion cells. It is of great current interest to try to understand whether the classifications of cortical neurons and retinal neurons can be brought together to form a clear picture of this entire section of the visual pathways.

A second important aspect of characterizing cortical neurons is to measure the transformation from pattern contrast stimulus to firing activity. We used linear-systems methods to design experiments and create quantitative models of this transformation for retinal ganglion cells. Linearity is an important idea when applied to cortical receptive fields too. The most important application of linearity is Hubel and Wiesel's classification of cortical neurons into two categories, called **simple cells** and **complex cells**. This classification is based, in large part, on an informal test of linearity (Skottun et al., 1991). As Hubel writes, "For the most part, we can predict the responses of simple cells to complicated shapes from their responses to small-spot stimuli" (Hubel, 1988, p. 72). Complex cells, on the other hand, do not satisfy superposition. The response obtained by sweeping a line across the cell's receptive field cannot be predicted accurately from the responses to individual flashes of a line.

Orientation Selectivity

Because simple cell responses to light approximately satisfy homogeneity and superposition, their receptive fields can be measured using the linear methods described in Chapter 5. Simple-cell receptive fields differ from those of retinal ganglion cells or cells in the LGN. The receptive fields of simple cells consist of adjacent excitatory and inhibitory regions, as illustrated in Figure 6.9. Simple cells have oriented receptive fields, and hence they respond to stimuli in some orientations better than others. This receptive field property is called **orientation selectivity**. The orientation of the stimulus the evokes the most powerful response is called the cell's preferred orientation.

Orientation selectivity of cortical neurons is a new receptive-field property. LGN and retinal neurons have circularly symmetric receptive fields, and they respond almost equally well to all stimulus orientations. Orientation-selective neurons are found throughout layers 2 and 3, though they are relatively rare in the primary inputs within layer 4C.

Figure 6.9 shows several orientation-selective linear receptive fields and how these might be constructed from the outputs of LGN neurons. The simple-cell receptive fields consist of adjacent excitatory and in-

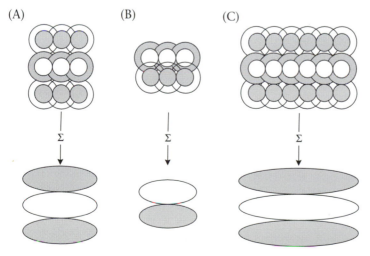

(A) (B) (C)

6.9 ORIENTATION-SELECTIVE RECEPTIVE FIELDS can be created by summing the responses of neurons with nonoriented, circularly symmetric receptive fields. The receptive fields of three hypothetical neurons are shown. Each hypothetical receptive field has adjacent excitatory and inhibitory regions. A comparison of (A) and (C) illustrates that the degree of orientation selectivity can vary depending on the number of neurons combined along the main axis.

hibitory regions that are longer in one direction than the other. The main axis of the receptive fields defines the preferred orientation; stimuli oriented along the main axis of these receptive fields are more effective at exciting or inhibiting the cell than stimuli in other orientations. The figure shows the excitatory regions as resulting from the combined output of neurons with excitatory centers and the inhibitory regions resulting from the combined output of neurons with inhibitory centers.[3]

By comparing the three panels in Figure 6.9 you will see that receptive fields sharing a common preferred orientation can differ in a number of other ways. Panels (A) and (B) show two receptive fields with the same preferred orientation but different spatial arrangements of the excitatory and inhibitory regions. Panels (A) and (C) show two receptive fields with the same preferred orientation and arrangement of excitatory and inhibitory regions, but differing in the overall length of the receptive field. The neuron with the longer receptive field will respond well to a narrower range of stimulus orientations than the neuron with the shorter receptive field.

Complex cells also show orientation selectivity. Complex cells are nonlinear, so to explain the behavior of complex cells, including orientation selectivity, will require more complex models than the simple sums of neural outputs used in Figure 6.9.

The preferred orientation of neurons varies in an orderly way that depends on the neuron's position within the cortical sheet. Figure 6.10 shows the preferred orientation of a collection of neurons measured during a single, long, tangential penetration through the cortex. In any small region of layers 2 and 3, the preferred orientation is similar. As the electrode passes tangentially through the cortical sheet, the preferred orientation changes systematically, varying through all angles. Figure 6.10A shows an extensive set of measurements of preferred orientation made during a single tangential penetration (Hubel and Wiesel, 1977). Upon later review, Hubel and Livingstone (1987) noted that during these measurements there were certain intervals during which the receptive-field orientation was ambiguous. Figure 6.10B shows a second penetration in which regions with no preferred receptive-field orientation are identified. As we shall see, Hubel and Livingstone also report that the regions lacking orientation selectivity coincide with locations in layers 2 and 3 of the cortex where an enzyme called **cytochrome oxidase** is present in high density. However, there is some debate whether these measurements represent true differences in the receptive fields of individual neurons, or whether they represent differences in the distribution of activity in local collections of neurons (Leventhal et al., 1993; O'Keefe et al., 1993).

---

[3] In principle, one might construct an oriented receptive field from the outputs of a single line of LGN neurons. But recall that the receptive fields of LGN neurons have a weak opposing surround. The inhibitory and excitatory regions of the cortical neurons often are more nearly balanced in their effect. Hence, I have constructed these regions by combining the outputs from separate groups of neurons.

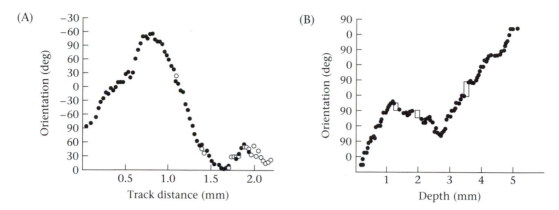

6.10 THE PREFERRED ORIENTATION OF NEURONS IN AREA V1 measured during single tangential penetrations. The horizontal axes show the distance along the tangential penetration, and the vertical axes show the orientation of the receptive field. (A) Data reported by Hubel and Wiesel (1977); (B) Data from a similar experiment by Hubel and Livingstone (1987). In this graph, open rectangles denote locations where responses to all orientations are equal.

The alternative interpretation is based on measurements of the spatial organization of cortical regions with common orientation preference. Obermayer and Blasdel (1993) measured regions with a common orientation preference using a high-resolution optical imaging method. In this method, a voltage-sensitive dye is applied to the cortex. Local neural activity causes reflectance changes in the dye, and these can be visualized by reflecting light from the exposed cortex. By stimulating with visual signals in different orientations and measuring the changes in reflectance, Obermayer and Blasdel (1993) visualized regions with common orientation preference; by stimulating with images originating in different eyes, they could identify ocular dominance columns (see also Hubel and Wiesel, 1977).

Figure 6.11 represents Obermayer and Blasdel's (1993) measurements as a contour plot. Regions with common orientation preference are shown as gray iso-orientation lines, and the boundaries of the ocular dominance columns are shown as dark lines. The figure shows that the variation in preferred orientation corresponds with the variation in ocular dominance. A full range of preferred orientations takes place within about 0.5 mm of the cortex, about equal to one ocular dominance column. Near the edges of the ocular dominance columns, the iso-orientation lines are arranged in linear, parallel strips extending roughly 0.5–1 mm. These linear strips are oriented nearly perpendicular to the edge of the ocular dominance edge. In the middle of the ocular dominance columns, the iso-orientation lines converge toward single points called **singularities**. In these regions, neurons with receptive fields with different preferred orientations are brought close to one another, and they may also be the position of the high density of cytochrome oxidase (Blasdel, 1992). These regions will have high

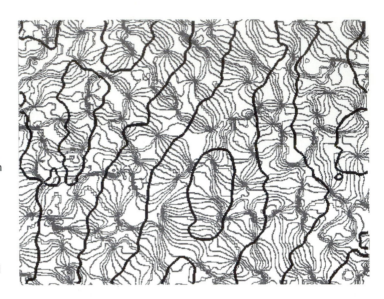

6.11 REGIONS WITH COMMON ORIENTATION PREFERENCE are shown as gray lines in this contour plot. The dark lines show the boundaries of ocular dominance columns. At the edges of the ocular dominance columns, regions with common orientation are arranged in parallel lines that are nearly perpendicular to the ocular dominance columns. These lines converge to singular points located near the center of the ocular dominance columns. From Obermayer and Blasdel, 1993.

metabolic activity since, for any stimulus orientation some of the neurons in the region will be active. This is an alternative explanation for why regions with high densities of cytochrome oxidase tend to exhibit reduced orientation selectivity of the neural response.

There are a number of broad questions that remain unanswered about the orientation selectivity in the visual cortex. First, we might ask how the receptive field properties of cortical neurons are constructed from the cortical inputs. Figure 6.9 shows that we can explain orientation selectivity theoretically, since combining signals from center-surround neurons with adjacent receptive-field locations results in an oriented receptive field. But there is no empirical counterpart to this theoretical explanation. Second, the regularity of the iso-orientation contours shows that the orientation preferences of neurons are created in a highly regular and organized pattern. What are the rules for making the interconnections that lead to this spatial organization of orientation selectivity? What functional role do they have in perceptual processing? Is this spatial organization essential for neural computations, or is it merely a convenient wiring pattern for an area whose output is communicated to other processing modules?

Direction Selectivity

Hubel and Wiesel (1968) found a second specialization that emerges in the receptive fields of area V1 neurons. Certain cortical neurons in the monkey respond well when a stimulus moves in one direction, and poorly or not at all when the same stimulus moves in the opposite direction. This feature is called **direction selectivity**. Figure 6.12 shows the response of a neuron in monkey area V1 to a line first moving in one direction and then in the opposite direction. Notice that the cell shows

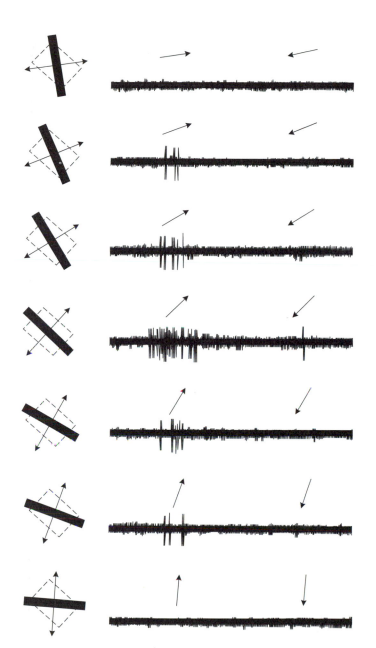

6.12 DIRECTION SELECTIVITY of a cortical neuron's response. The left-hand portion of each panel shows the receptive-field location, the orientation of the line stimulus, and the two motion directions. The action potentials shown on the right are the neuron's response to motion in each of the two opposite directions. The neuron's response depends upon the direction of motion and the orientation of the line. After Hubel and Wiesel, 1968.

orientation selectivity; it only responds well to the line in one orientation. In addition, the cell shows direction selectivity. When the line moves up and to the right the cell responds well, but when the same line moves down and to the left the cell responds poorly. Because of the low spontaneous response rate of this neuron, which is characteristic of many cortical neurons, we cannot tell from these measurements whether the neuron simply fails to respond or is actively inhibited by the stimulus moving in the wrong direction.

The direction-selective neurons are found mainly in certain layers of the cortex and are quite rare or absent from others. The main layers containing direction-selective neurons are 4A, 4B, 4Cα, and 6 (Hawken et al., 1988). These layers receive the main input from the magnocellular pathway and send their outputs to selected brain areas. Hence, these neurons may be part of a visual stream that is specialized to carry information about motion.

Direction selectivity of the receptive-field response may arise from neural connections that are analogous to the connections underlying orientation selectivity. A cell with a direction-selective receptive field can be built by sending the outputs of neurons with spatially displaced receptive fields onto a single cortical neuron and introducing temporal delays into the path of some of the input neurons. The temporal delays of the signal are displacements of the signal in time. As we will review in more detail in Chapter 10, the result of a combined spatial and temporal displacement is to create a cortical neuron that responds better to stimuli moving in one direction, when the delay reinforces the signal, than to stimuli moving in the opposite direction, when the delay works against the two signals. This scheme for connecting neurons is plausible, but like the mechanisms of orientation selectivity, the precise neural wiring used to achieve direction selectivity in primate cortical neurons is unknown.

Contrast Sensitivity of Cortical Cells

Perhaps the most straightforward way to classify simple and complex cells is based on their responses to contrast-reversing sinusoidal patterns. Examples of the response of a simple and a complex cell to a contrast-reversing pattern are shown in Figure 6.13.

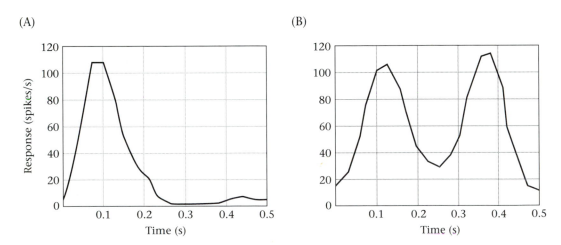

(A)   (B)

6.13 THE TIME COURSE OF RESPONSE OF CORTICAL CELLS to a contrast-reversing spatial frequency pattern at a period of 0.5 seconds. (A) The response of a simple cell is a half-wave rectified sinusoid. (B) The response of the complex cell is full-wave rectified. Consequently, the temporal response is at twice the frequency of the stimulus. Source: DeValois et al., 1982.

Recall from Chapter 5 that contrast-reversing patterns are periodic in both space and time. The stimulus used to create the neural responses shown in Figure 6.13 had a temporal period of 0.5 seconds. Figure 6.13A shows the firing rate of a simple cell averaged over many repetitions of the contrast-reversing stimulus. Were the simple cell perfectly linear, the variation in firing rate would be sinusoidal, and one period of the response would equal one period of the stimulus. This sinusoidal variation is impossible, however, because the spontaneous discharge rate of the neuron is close to zero; hence, the firing rate cannot fall below the spontaneous rate. The response shown in the figure is typical of cortical simple cells because many have a low spontaneous discharge rate. When a signal follows only the positive part of the sinusoid and has a zero response to the negative part, it is called **half-wave rectified**. The response of many simple cells shows this half-wave rectification.

Figure 6.13B shows the average response of a complex cell during one period of the stimulus. Unlike the simple cell, the complex cell's response does not vary at the same frequency as the input stimulus; the cell's response is elevated during both phases of the flickering contrast. This response pattern is called **full-wave rectification**, and the temporal response varies at twice the temporal frequency of the stimulus. This nonlinear **frequency doubling** is typical of complex cells. These cells make up a large proportion of the neurons in area V1.

DeValois et al. (1982) measured the spatial contrast-sensitivity functions of cortical neurons. Figure 6.14 shows a sample of these measure-

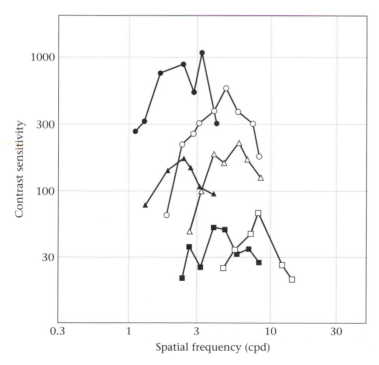

6.14 SPATIAL FREQUENCY SELECTIVITY of six neurons cells in area V1 of the monkey. These responses were recorded at nearby locations within the cortex, yet the neurons have different spatial frequency selectivity. Source: DeValois et al., 1982.

ments, for both simple and complex cortical neurons. The contrast-sensitivity functions of these neurons are narrower than those of retinal ganglion cells. Moreover, even though these measurements were made from neurons close to one another in the cortex, there is considerable heterogeneity in the most effective spatial frequency of the stimulus. This variation in spatial tuning is not found in retinal neurons from a single class. This may be due to a new specialization in the cortex, or it may be that we have not yet identified the classes of cortical neurons properly. In either case, the different peak spatial frequencies of the contrast-sensitivity functions raise the question of how the signals from retinal neurons within a small patch are recombined to form cortical neurons with such varied spatial receptive-field properties.

Movshon et al. (1978a, b) and Tolhurst and Dean (1987) tested the linearity of cat simple cells. Taking into account the low spontaneous rate and the resulting half-wave rectification, they found that they could predict quantitatively a range of simple-cell responses from measurements of the contrast-sensitivity function. The predictions work well for stimuli with moderate or weak contrast, that is, stimuli that evoke a response that is less than half of the maximum response rate of the neuron. There have not been extensive tests of linear receptive fields in the monkey cortex, but contrast-sensitivity curves are probably adequate to predict simple cell responses in the monkey, too.

Figure 6.14 also includes contrast-sensitivity functions of nonlinear complex neurons. Recall from our discussion in earlier chapters that when a system is nonlinear, its response to sinusoidal patterns is not a fundamental measurement of the neuron's performance: we cannot use it to predict the response to other stimuli. For these nonlinear neurons, the contrast-sensitivity function defines the response of the cell to an interesting collection of stimuli. These measurements may also help us understand the nature of the nonlinearity. However, the contrast-response function of a nonlinear system is not a complete quantitative measurement of the cell's receptive field.

Contrast Normalization

If one takes into account the low spontaneous firing rate, simple cells are approximately linear for moderate contrast stimuli. As one expands the stimulus range, however, several important response properties of cortical simple cells are nonlinear. One deviation from linearity, called **contrast normalization**, can be demonstrated by measuring the contrast-response function (cf. Figure 5.11).

Figure 6.15 shows the contrast-response function of a neuron in area V1 to four different sinusoidal grating patterns. The stimulus contrast and neuronal responses are plotted on logarithmic axes. The rightward displacements of the curves indicate that the neuron is differentially sensitive to the spatial patterns used as test stimuli. This shift is what we expect from a simple linear system followed by a static nonlinearity (see Chapter 4).

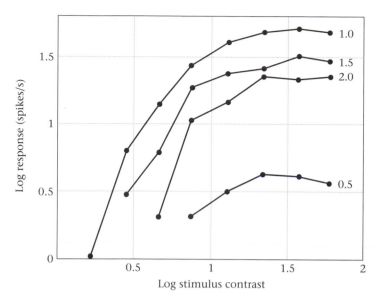

6.15 CONTRAST-RESPONSE FUNCTIONS of a neuron in area V1. Each curve shows the responses measured using a different spatial frequency grating. The spatial frequencies of the stimuli are shown at the right. The neuron's sensitivity and maximum response depend on the stimulus spatial frequency. Source: Albrecht and Hamilton, 1982.

The entire set of data is not consistent with such a model, however, because the response saturation level depends on the spatial frequency of the stimulus. Were the nonlinearity static, then the response saturation level would be the same no matter which stimulus we used. Since the saturation level is stimulus-dependent, it cannot be based on the neuron's intrinsic properties. Rather, it must be mediated through an active process (Albrecht and Geisler, 1991; Heeger, 1992).

Heeger (1992) has described a model of this process (Figure 6.16). The model assumes that the neuron's response is initiated by a linear process. This linear signal is divided by a second signal whose value de-

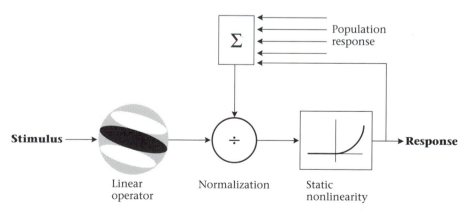

6.16 A MODEL OF CONTRAST NORMALIZATION is shown. According to this model, each neuron's response is derived from an initial linear encoding of the stimulus. The linear response is divided by a factor that depends on the activity of the neural population. Finally, the entire signal is modified by a static nonlinearity. Source: Heeger, 1992.

pends on the pooled activity of the population of cortical neurons. This is a nonlinear term. It is not a static nonlinearity because the divisive term depends on the contrast of the stimulus.

This model explains the data in Figure 6.15 as follows. First, the sensitivity of the neuron varies with the spatial frequency of the stimulus because the initial linear receptive field will respond better to some stimuli than others. This causes the response to be displaced along the horizontal axis in the log-log plot. Second, the response saturation level depends on the ratio of the neuron's intrinsic sensitivity to the stimulus and the neural population's sensitivity to the stimulus. This saturation level is set by the normalization process. If the neuron is relatively insensitive to the stimulus compared to the population as a whole, then the peak response of the neuron will be suppressed by the divisive signal. Finally, the overall shape of the response function is determined by the nature of the static nonlinearity that follows.

What purpose does the contrast-response nonlinearity serve? From the data in Figure 6.15, notice that the response ratio to different patterns remains approximately constant at all contrast levels. Without the contrast-normalization process, the neuron's response would saturate at the same level, independent of the stimulus. In this case, the response ratios at different contrast levels would vary. For example, at high contrast levels all area V1 neurons would be saturated, and their signals would be nondiscriminative with respect to the input signal. The normalization process adjusts the saturation level so that it depends on the neuron's sensitivity; in this way the ratio of the neuronal responses remains constant across a wide range of contrast levels.

Binocular Receptive Fields

At the input layers of the visual cortex, signals from the two eyes are spatially segregated. Within the superficial layers, however, many neurons respond to light presented to either eye. These neurons have **binocular receptive fields**. Cortical area V1 is the first point in the visual pathways where individual neurons receive binocular input. One might guess that these binocular neurons may play a role in our perception of stereo depth. What binocular information is present that neurons might use to deduce depth?

First, consider the two retinas as illustrated in Figure 6.17A. We can label points on the two retinas with respect to their distance from the fovea. We say that a pair of points on the two retinas fall at corresponding locations if they are displaced from the fovea by the same amount. Otherwise, the two points fall at noncorresponding positions.

Now, suppose that the two eyes are positioned so that a point F casts an image on the two foveas. By definition, then, the images of the point F fall on corresponding retinal locations. By tracing a ray from the corresponding retinal positions back into space, we can find the points in space whose images are cast on corresponding retinal positions (Fig-

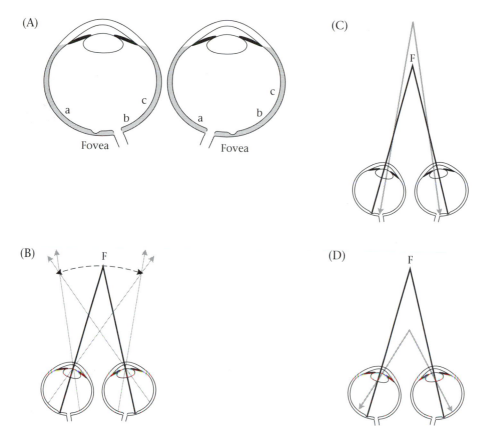

6.17 RETINAL DISPARITY AND THE HOROPTER. (A) The fovea and three pairs of points at corresponding retinal locations are shown. (B) When the eyes are fixated on a point F, rays originating at corresponding points on the two retinas and passing through the lens center intersect on the horopter (dashed curve). The images of points located farther away (C) or closer (D) than the horopter do not fall at corresponding retinal locations.

ure 6.17B). These points sweep out an arc about the viewer that is called the **horopter**.

The image of a point closer or farther away than the horopter will fall on noncorresponding retinal positions. The difference between the image locations and the corresponding locations is called the **retinal disparity**. Because the main separation between the two eyes is horizontal, the retinal disparities are mainly in the horizontal direction as well. The horopter is the set of points whose images have zero retinal disparity.

Panels C and D of Figure 6.17 show two examples in which image points fall on noncorresponding retinal points. Figure 6.17C shows an example when both images fall on the nasal side of the fovea, and Figure 6.17D shows an example when both images fall on the temporal side of the fovea. These panels show that the size and nature of the horizontal retinal disparity vary with the distance from the visual horopter.

Hence, the horizontal retinal disparity is a binocular clue for estimating the distance to an image point.[4]

Do binocular neurons represent stereo depth information by measuring horizontal disparity? There are two types of experimental measurements we can make to answer this question. First, we can measure the receptive fields of individual binocular neurons. If retinal disparity is used to estimate depth, then the receptive fields of the binocular neurons should show some selectivity for horizontal disparity. Second, we can look at the properties of the population of binocular neurons. While no single neuron alone can encode depth information, the population of binocular neurons should include enough information to permit the population to estimate image depth.

A complete characterization of binocular receptive fields requires many measurements. First, one would like to measure the spatial receptive fields of individual neurons when stimulated by each eye alone. These are called the **monocular receptive fields** of the binocular neurons. Then, we should characterize how binocular neurons respond to simultaneous stimulation of the two eyes. In practice there have been very few complete measurements of binocular neurons' receptive fields. The vast majority of investigations have been limited to localization of the monocular receptive-field centers which are then used to derive the retinal disparities between the monocular field centers.

Given the variability inherent in biological systems, the two monocular receptive fields will not be in perfect register. We would like to decide whether the observed horizontal disparities serve a purpose, or whether they are due to unavoidable random variation. To answer this question several groups have measured both the horizontal and the vertical disparities of binocular neurons in the cat cortex (Barlow et al., 1967; Joshua and Bishop, 1970; von der Heydt et al., 1978). The histograms in Figure 6.18A show the initial measurements from Barlow et al. (1967). They observed more variability in the horizontal disparity than in vertical disparity, and they concluded that the horizontal variation was purposeful and used for processing depth. Joshua and Bishop (1970) and von der Heydt et al. (1978) saw no difference in the range of disparities in the horizontal and vertical directions. A scatterplot of the retinal disparities observed by Joshua and Bishop (1970) is shown in Figure 6.18B. While these data do not show any systematic difference between the horizontal and vertical disparity distributions, the authors do not dispute Barlow et al.'s hypothesis that variations in the horizontal disparity are used for stereo depth detection.[5]

---

[4] You can demonstrate the relative shift in retinal positions to yourself as follows. Focus on a nearby object, say your finger placed in front of your nose. Then, alternately look through one eye and then the other. Although your finger remains focused in the fovea, the relative positions of points nearer or farther away than your finger will change as you look through each eye in turn.

[5] A frequently suggested alternative is that these disparity cues serve to converge the two eyes. Since the same cues are used to converge the eyes and estimate depth, this alternative hypothesis is virtually impossible to rule out.

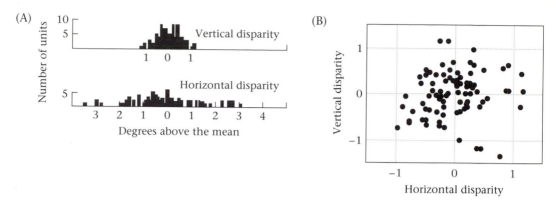

6.18   THE HORIZONTAL AND VERTICAL DISPARITIES OF BINOCULAR NEURONS in the cat visual cortex are shown. (A) Histograms of the horizontal and vertical disparities of binocular neurons in cat cortex. (B) A scatter diagram of the vertical and horizontal disparities of cells in cat cortex with receptive fields located within 4 degrees of the cat's best region of visual acuity. Sources: A from Barlow et al., 1967; B from Bishop, 1973.

For the moment, accept the premise that the variation in horizontal disparity of these binocular neurons is a neural basis for stereo depth. How might we design the binocular response properties of these neurons to estimate depth?

One possibility is to create a collection of neurons that each respond to only a single disparity. One might estimate the local disparity by identifying the neuron with the largest response. An alternative possibility, suggested by Richards (1971), is that one might measure disparity by creating a few **pools** of neurons with coarse disparity tuning. One pool might consist of neurons that respond when an object feature is beyond the horopter, and a second pool might consist of neurons that respond when the feature is in front of it. The third pool might respond only when the feature is close to the horopter. To estimate depth, one would compare the relative responses in the three neural pools.

Some support for Richards's hypothesis comes from measurements of individual neurons in area V1 and an adjacent area of a monkey brain. Poggio and Talbot (1981; see also Ferster, 1981) measured how well individual neurons respond to stimuli with different amounts of disparity. They used experimental stimuli consisting of bar patterns whose width and velocity were set to generate a strong response from the individual neuron. The experimenters varied the retinal disparity between the two bars presented to the two eyes. They plotted the binocular neuron's response to the moving bars as a function of their retinal disparity. The curves in Figure 6.19, plotting response as a function of retinal disparity, are called **disparity-tuning curves**.

Poggio and Talbot (1981) found that the disparity-tuning curves could be grouped into a small number of categories. Typical tuning curves from each of these categories are are illustrated in the separate panels of Figure 6.19. The two neurons illustrated in the left panels re-

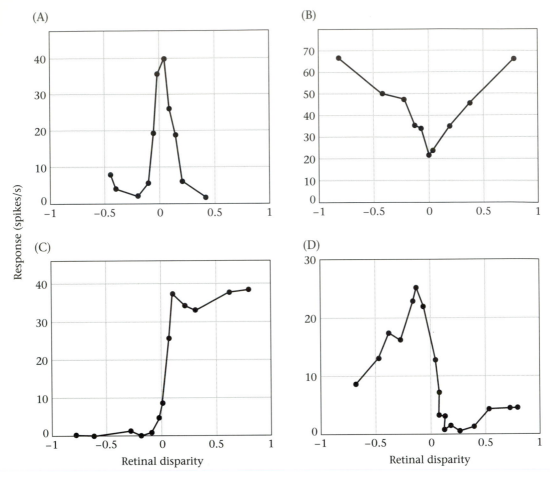

6.19 DISPARITY-TUNING CURVES of binocular neurons in areas V1 and V2 in a monkey. Each panel plots the response of a different neuron to moving bar patterns. The independent variable is the retinal disparity of the stimulus. Panels (A) and (B) show the responses of neurons that respond best to stimuli with near zero disparity, that is, near the horopter. Responses of a neuron that responds best to stimuli with positive disparity (C) and a neuron with negative disparity (D) are also shown. The curves represent data measured using binocular stimulation. Source: Poggio and Talbot, 1981.

spond to disparities near the fixation plane; for these neurons, stimuli near the horopter stimulate or inhibit the cell. The two panels on the right illustrate neurons with opponent tuning. One neuron is excited by a bar whose disparity places the object beyond the horopter and is inhibited by bars in front of the horopter. The second neuron shows approximately the complementary excitation pattern: it is excited by objects nearer than the horopter and inhibited by objects farther away. Poggio and his colleagues view their measurements in monkeys as support for Richards's hypothesis that the encoding of binocular depth is based on the response of neurons organized in disparity pools (also see Ferster, 1981).

We have been paying attention mainly to the retinal disparity of the binocular neurons. But disparity tuning is only one measure of the receptive-field properties of these neurons. In addition, the receptive fields must have spatial, temporal, and chromatic selectivities. To fully understand the responses of these neurons we must make some progress in measuring all of these properties.

To obtain a more complete description of binocular neurons, Freeman and Ohzawa (1990; also see DeAngelis et al., 1991) studied the monocular spatial receptive fields of cat binocular neurons. They found that the spatial receptive fields measured in the two eyes can be quite different. Figure 6.20 shows an example of the differences they observed between the monocular spatial receptive fields. The left-eye spatial receptive field and the right-eye field are displaced relative to one another. If we only concern ourselves with disparity, we will report that this cell's receptive field has significant horizontal disparity. Notice, however, that the spatial receptive fields are different from one another. The spatial receptive field in the left eye is a mirror-reversal of the field in the right eye.

Freeman and Ohzawa suggest that these different monocular spatial receptive fields are important to the way stereo depth is estimated by the nervous system. They hypothesize that stereo depth depends on having neurons with different monocular spatial receptive fields. Perhaps most important, however, their measurements remind us that, in order to understand the biological computation of stereopsis, we must

(A)   (B)

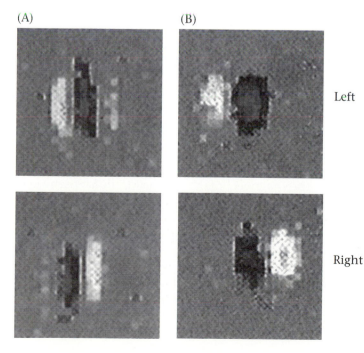

Left

Right

6.20 MONOCULAR SPATIAL RECEPTIVE FIELDS of two binocular neurons in cat cortex. Panels (A) and (B) show examples of left and right monocular receptive fields whose centers are displaced horizontally and thus have nonzero retinal disparity. In addition to the disparity, the left and right monocular spatial receptive fields differ. Source: Freeman and Ohzawa, 1990.

study more than just the center position of the monocular receptive fields.

Visual Streams in the Cortex

We have reviewed two major principles that characterize the flow of information from retina to cortex. First, visual information is organized into separate visual streams. These streams begin in the retina and continue along separate neural pathways into the brain. Second, the receptive-field properties of neurons become progressively more sophisticated. Receptive fields of cortical neurons show selective responses to stimulus properties that are more complex than retinal neurons. The new receptive-field properties are clues about the specialization of the computations performed within the visual cortex.

As we study visual processing within the cortex we should expect to see both of these principles extended. First, we should expect to find new visual streams that play a role in the cortical computations. Some new visual streams will arise in the visual cortex, and some, like the rod pathway in the retina, will have served their purpose and will merge with other streams. Second, as we explore the cortex we should expect to find neurons with new receptive-field properties. We will need to characterize these receptive fields adequately in order to understand their computational role in vision.

Our understanding of cortical visual areas is in an early and exciting phase of scientific study. In this section, we will review some of the basic organizational principles of the cortical areas. In particular, we will review how information from area V1 is distributed to other cortical areas, and we will review the experimental and logical methods that relate activity within these cortical areas to what we see. We will review some of the more recent data and speculative theories in Chapters 9 and 10.

The Fate of the Parvocellular and Magnocellular Pathways

The segregation of visual information into separate streams is an important organizing principle of neural representation. Two of the best-understood streams are the magnocellular and parvocellular pathways, whose axons terminate in layers $4C\alpha$ and $4C\beta$ within area V1. What happens to the signals from these pathways within the visual cortex?

Along one branch, signals from the magnocellular pathway continue from area V1 directly to a distinct cortical area. The magnocellular pathway in layer $4C\alpha$ makes a connection to neurons in layer 4B where there are many direction-selective neurons. These neurons then send a strong projection to cortical **area MT** (medial temporal). It seems reasonable to suppose, then, that the information contained within the magnocellular stream is of particular relevance for the visual processing in area MT. As we saw in Chapter 5, the magnocellular pathway has particularly good information about the high-temporal-frequency components of the image. Earlier in this chapter we saw that neurons in layer 4B show strong direction selectivity, as do the neurons in area MT (Zeki, 1974, 1990a,b). Taken together, these observations have led to the hypothesis that area MT plays a role in motion perception. We will discuss this point more fully in Chapter 10.

While one branch of the magnocellular stream continues on an independent path, another branch of this stream converges with the parvocellular pathway in the superficial layers of area V1. Malpeli et al. (1981) and Nealey and Maunsell (1994) made physiological measurements demonstrating that signals from the parvocellular and magnocellular streams converge on individual neurons. In these experiments parvocellular or magnocellular signals were blocked by application of either a local anaesthetic, lidocaine hydrochloride (Malpeli et al., 1981), or the neurotransmitter γ-aminobutyric acid (GABA) (Nealey and Maunsell, 1994) to small regions of the LGN. Both studies report instances of neurons whose responses are influenced by both parvocellular and magnocellular blocking. Anatomical paths for this signal have also been identified. Lachica et al. (1992) injected retrograde anatomical tracers (i.e., tracers that are carried from the injection site toward the inputs to the injection site) into the superficial layers of the visual cortex. They concluded that the magnocellular and parvocellular neurons contribute inputs into overlapping regions within the superficial layers of the visual cortex. Hence, these anatomical pathways could be the route for the physiological signals.

Just as the rod pathways are segregated for a time, and then merge with the cone pathways, so too signals from the magnocellular stream merge with parvocellular signals. The purpose of the peripheral segregation of the parvocellular and magnocellular signals, then, may be to communicate rapidly certain types of image information to area MT. After the signal has been efficiently communicated, the same information may be used by other cortical areas, in combination with information from the parvocellular pathways.

Cytochrome Oxidase Staining

Livingstone and Hubel (1984a, b, 1987a, b, 1988) have argued that several new visual streams begin in area V1. Their argument begins with a discovery made by Wong-Riley (1979), who used a histochemical marker to detect the presence of an enzyme called cytochrome oxidase, and found that the enzyme is present mainly in a continuous and heavy pattern in layer 4, but is present mainly as a set of patches in the superficial and deeper layers. These patches can be seen by staining for cytochrome oxidase and viewing the superficial layers in tangential section. In that case, the regions of high cytochrome oxidase density appears as a set of darkened spots (Figure 6.21). These darkened regions

(A)

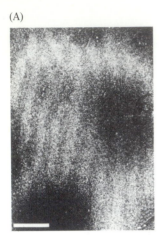

(B)

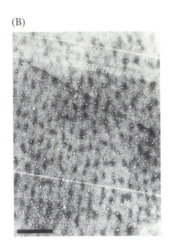

(C)

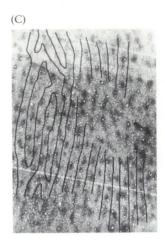

6.21 CYTOCHROME OXIDASE PUFFS ARE LOCATED IN THE MIDDLE OF OCULAR DOMINANCE COLUMNS. The three panels show tangential sections of area V1. (A) The locations of the ocular dominance columns in layer 4C correspond to the light and dark patterns. The columns were identified by a monocular injection of the radioactive tracer tritiated proline. (B) The puffs are the darkened spots identified by a high concentration of cytochrome oxidase. The image is a tangential section in the superficial layers. (C) An overlay of (A) and (B), placed in register by comparing the positions of larger blood vessels, shows that the puffs are located in the center of the ocular dominance columns. Scale bar = 1 mm. Source: Horton and Hubel, 1981.

are called variously "puffs," "blobs," or "CO-rich" areas. These puffs are visible in several, but not all, primate species, including humans. Cytochrome oxidase density is correlated with regions of high neuronal activity, though the enzyme itself is not known to have any specific significance for visual function (Wong-Riley, 1979; Humphrey and Hendrickson, 1980; Livingstone and Hubel, 1982; Hendrickson, 1985).

Several lines of evidence suggest that cytochrome oxidase labeling is correlated with the presence of new visual streams in the cortex. First, Horton and Hubel (1981) discovered that the cytochrome oxidase staining pattern is related to at least one aspect of visual function: the ocular dominance columns. Figure 6.21A shows the ocular dominance columns measured by injecting one eye of a monkey with a radioactive tracer, tritiated proline. The section is through layer 4C (and a little bit of layer 5) where the ocular dominance columns are best segregated. The data in this figure replicate the demonstration of ocular dominance columns depicted in Figure 6.4. Figure 6.21B shows the puffs in a tangential section from layers 2 and 3, just above the region shown in Figure 6.21A. Figure 6.21C shows an overlay of the ocular dominance columns and the puffs. The images were placed into spatial register by finding blood vessels common to the two images and aligning their positions. Figure 6.21C demonstrates that the puffs trace a path down the center of the ocular dominance columns.

The second suggestion that the presence of cytochrome oxidase identifies new visual streams comes from studying the connectivity between neurons within area V1. Burkhalter et al. (1989) report that the neurons within the V1 puffs in humans are connected to other neurons in the puffs, while neurons between the puffs are connected to other neurons between the puffs (Rockland and Lund, 1983).

A third piece of evidence is the relationship between cytochrome oxidase puffs and connections to other cortical areas. Like area V1, cytochrome oxidase is distributed unevenly in a second cortical area, **V2**, which is adjacent to area V1. In area V2, staining for cytochrome oxidase yields a regular three-striped pattern defining regions that stain to different degrees. The three types of stripes are labeled **thick stripes**, **thin stripes**, and **interstripes**. The thick and thin stripes contain more cytochrome oxidase than the interstripe regions. This pattern of stripes is visible in human area V2 as well as in some species of monkey.

Livingstone and Hubel (1982, 1987a) demonstrated the specificity of these interconnections. Regions with a high density of cytochrome oxidase in area V1, that is, regions with high metabolic activity, are connected to high-density regions in area V2. Neurons in layer 4B of area V1 send outputs to the thick stripes of area V2. Neurons in the puffs send outputs to the thin strips. Neurons in between the puffs send outputs to the interstripes.

Finally, the pattern of cytochrome oxidase staining of area V2 correlates with the connections from area V2 to other visual areas. In monkeys, visual area MT receives a strong projection from the thick stripes in area V2. **Area V4** receives signals mainly from the thin stripes and the interstripes (Deyoe and Van Essen, 1988; Merigan and Maunsell, 1993). These measurements suggest that there is considerable organization of the signals communicated within individual cortical areas.

Areas Central to Primary Cortex

Figure 6.22 shows a few of the many cortical visual areas. Often, the connections between areas are reciprocal; ascending axons make connections with the primary input layer, 4C, and descending axons make connections in layers 1 and 6. A single visual area can have connections with several other cortical areas (Rockland and Pandya, 1979; Felleman and Van Essen, 1991).

Figure 6.22 is arranged to emphasize one aspect of the segregation of visual information within the cortex, namely, that information from the visual areas in the occipital lobe separates into two visual streams. One stream sends its outputs mainly to the posterior portion of parietal lobe, while the second stream makes its connection mainly in the inferior portion of the temporal lobe.

There are several known connections between these two streams, but a study by Baizer et al. (1991) shows that the segregation is impressive. These authors injected large amounts of two retrograde tracers into individual monkey brains: one tracer was injected into the posterior parietal lobe and the other into the inferior temporal cortex. They

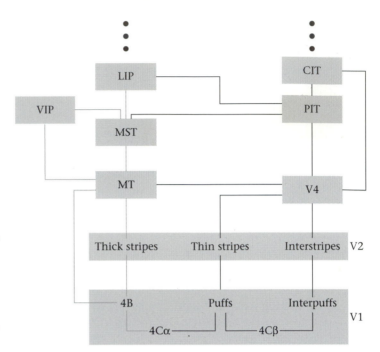

6.22 AN OVERVIEW OF THE ORGANIZATION OF VISUAL AREAS is shown. The signals from the occipital lobe areas are sent along two major streams. One stream passes into the posterior parietal lobe and a second to the inferior temporal lobe. The visual signals in the temporal and parietal lobe areas appear to arise from different neurons within the occipital lobe. MST = medial superior temporal area, MT = medial temporal area, VIP = ventral intraparietal area, PIT = posterior inferotemporal area, LIP = lateral intraparietal area, CIT = central infero-temporal area. Source: Merigan and Maunsell, 1993.

examined where the two types of tracers could be found in visual areas within the occipital lobe, including areas V1, V2, V4, and MT. They report finding almost no neurons that contained both tracers, suggesting that the signals from individual neurons are communicated mainly to either the parietal or temporal lobes. Baizer et al. also report that neurons in the parietal lobe received information mainly from neurons with receptive fields located in the periphery, while neurons in the temporal lobe received information mainly from neurons with receptive fields located near the fovea.

Baizer et al.'s observations support Ungerleider and Mishkin's (1982) proposal that the parietal and temporal streams serve different visual functions. Ungerleider and Mishkin observed that clinical damage to the parietal stream of one hemisphere causes difficulties in visual and motor orientation. It also causes **hemineglect**, a condition in which the observer appears to be unaware of stimulation arising in the hemifield that projects to that parietal lobe. Such patients also have trouble orienting toward or reaching for objects in the visual periphery. The clinical symptoms associated with damage to the temporal stream are quite different. In this case, patients have impaired form discrimination or recognition. They also have problems with visual memory. These behavioral deficits are very different, so that neurologists have supposed that the visual function of the parietal and temporal lobes are quite different. One brief characterization of the distinction is this: the parietal system defines *where*, while the temporal system defines *what* (Ungerleider and Mishkin, 1982; Merigan and Maunsell, 1993).

The anatomical segregation of the neural signals coming from the occipital lobe into these two streams shows that the temporal and parietal areas receive different information about the visual image. Hence, it seems likely that the computations in these two portions of the brain must serve different goals, though a more refined analysis of these differences will be helpful.

Cortical Representations and Perception

The brilliant visual scientist William Rushton enjoyed needling his colleagues. On one occasion, he challenged neuroscientists with the assertion that only the hope of understanding perception and consciousness makes neuroscience worth doing. Much of the work I have reviewed was inspired by the desire to understand conscious perception. In this sense, some neuroscientists think of themselves as philosophers studying the mind–body problem. They form a field one might call experimental philosophy; it is the expensive branch of philosophy.

More recently Crick (1993) has taken up Rushton's call and pressed us to consider the question: what aspect of the cortical response corresponds to conscious experience? Since neuroscientists nearly all make the assumption that consciousness is a correlate of cortical activity, Crick points out that identifying the relationship between consciousness and neural activity is properly an experimental question.

What experimental tests might we perform to answer questions about the relationship between our conscious awareness and the activity of our brains? One way to study this question is to compare the information available within a cortical area with the visual experience we have. An interesting example of an experiment concerning consciousness is the comparison of conscious awareness with the information available in area V1. From the anatomy and physiology of area V1, we have learned that there is plenty of information there that we can use to deduce which eye is the source of a visual signal. Within layer 4C, entirely different sets of neurons, confined to different ocular dominance columns, respond depending on which eye sends the signal. Is this information available to us?

We can answer this question experimentally by asking subjects to discriminate between visual signals originating in the right and left eyes. If we can accurately decide on the eye of origin, then we might conclude that the information in area V1 is part of our conscious experience. If we cannot, then we should conclude that information within layer 4C can be lost prior to reaching our conscious experience.

Notice that eye-of-origin information is certainly available to us unconsciously. For example, Helmholtz (1896) pointed out that eye-of-origin information is necessary and used for the computation of stereopsis. The question, therefore, is not whether the information is present, but whether it is accessible to conscious experience. Based on

his own introspections, Helmholtz answered the question in the negative. And, while there have been occasional reports that some discriminations are possible, Ono and Barbeito's (1985) careful experiments suggest that no reliable eye-of-origin discriminations are possible. Hence,
the massive information available in the input layers of area V1 (and
earlier) about the eye-of-origin is not part of our conscious experience.
Through this negative result, we have made a small amount of progress
in localizing consciousness.

The Function of the Visual Areas

Even when the computation performed in a visual area is not part of
our conscious experience, we would still like to know what the area
does. Over the last 15 years, there have been a broad variety of hypotheses concerning the perceptual significance of the cortical areas. Mainly,
we have seen a flurry of proposals suggesting that individual visual areas are responsible for the computation of specific perceptual features,
such as color, stereo, form, and so forth.

What is the logical and experimental basis for reasoning about the
perceptual significance of visual areas? Horace Barlow (1972) has set
forth one specific doctrine to relate neurons to perception, the **neuron
doctrine**. This doctrine asserts that a neuron's receptive field describes
the percept caused by excitation of the neuron. You will see the idea
expressed many times as you read through the primary literature and
study how investigators interpret the perceptual significance of neural
responses.

Our understanding of the peripheral representation lends little support to the neuron doctrine. For example, the principle does not serve
us well when analyzing color appearance. In that case, we know with
some certainty that a large response from an L photoreceptor does not
imply that the observer will perceive red at the corresponding location
in the visual field. Rather, the color appearance depends upon stimulation at many adjacent points of the retina. The conditions for a red
percept include a pattern of peripheral neural responses, including more
L- than M-cone excitation. Data from the periphery are generally more
consistent with the notion of a representation in which an experience
depends on the response of a collection of neurons.

Oddly, the failure of the neuron doctrine in the periphery is often
used to support the neuron doctrine. After all, the argument goes, the
periphery is not the site of our conscious awareness, so failures of the
doctrine in the periphery are to be expected. The neuron doctrine's significance depends on the idea that there will be a special place, probably located in the cortex, where the receptive field of a neuron predicts conscious experience when that neuron is active. This location in
the brain should only exist at a point after the perceptual computations
needed to see features we perceive (e.g., color, form, depth) have taken
place.

In the past, secondary texts sometimes cited Hubel and Wiesel's work in area V1 as providing an example of a location where the neuron doctrine might hold. The receptive fields in area V1 seem like basic perceptual features; orientation, motion selectivity, binocularity, and complex cells all emerge for the first time in area V1. Consequently, these texts often described our knowledge of receptive fields in area V1 as if it were a theory of vision, with the receptive fields defining salient perceptual features.

However, by 1979 the significance of the other cortical areas had become undeniable (Zeki, 1974, 1978; Felleman and Van Essen, 1991; Van Essen et al., 1992). In reviewing the visual pathways, Hubel and Wiesel (1979) wrote:

> The lateral geniculate cells in turn send their axons directly to the primary visual cortex. From there, after several synapses, the messages are sent to a number of further destinations: neighboring cortical areas and also several targets deep in the brain. One contingent even projects back to the lateral geniculate bodies; the function of this feedback path is not known. The main point for the moment is that the primary visual cortex is in no sense the end of the visual path. It is just one stage, probably an early one in terms of the degree of abstraction of the information it handles.

Acknowledging this point leads one to ask, What is the function of these other cortical areas? The answer to this question has relied mainly on the neuron doctrine. For example, when Zeki (1980, 1983, 1993) found that color contrast was a particularly effective stimulus in area V4, he argued that this area is responsible for color perception. Since movement was particularly effective in stimulating neurons in area MT, that became the motion area (Dubner and Zeki, 1971). The logic of the neuron doctrine permits one to interpret receptive-field properties in terms of perceptual function.

A particularly vigorous application of the neuron doctrine is contained in articles by Livingstone and Hubel (1984a,b, 1987a,b, 1988). They supported Zeki's basic views and added new hypotheses of their own. Their hypothesis, which continues to evolve, is summarized in the elaborate anatomical/perceptual diagram shown in Figure 6.23. In this diagram, anatomical connections in visual cortex are labeled with perceptual tags, including color, motion, and form. The logical basis for associating perceptual tags with these anatomical streams is the neuron doctrine. Receptive fields of neurons in one stream were orientation-selective; hence the stream was tagged with form perception. Neurons in a different stream were motion-selective, and hence the stream was tagged with motion perception.

The perceptual-anatomical hypotheses proposed by Zeki and by Livingstone and Hubel define a new view of cortex. On this view, the relationship between cortical neurons and perception should be made at the level of perceptual features. These investigators did not study the computation within the neural streams, but rather they summa-

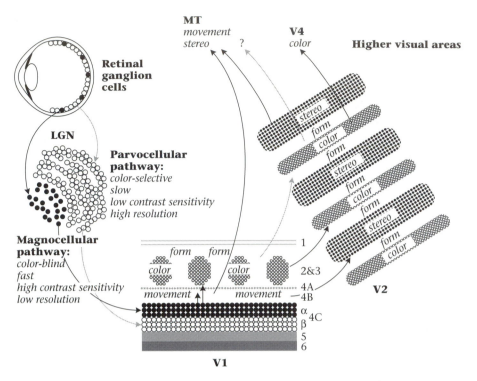

6.23 AN ANATOMICAL/PERCEPTUAL MODEL OF THE VISUAL CORTEX. In this speculative model, visual streams within the cortex are identified with specific perceptual features. The anatomical streams are identified using anatomical markers; the perceptual properties are associated with the streams by applying the neuron doctrine. Source: Livingstone and Hubel (1988).

rized the receptive field properties and based their interpretations on the neuron doctrine (see Hubel and Wiesel [1977] for a description of this approach).

The use of the neuron doctrine to interpret brain function is very widespread, but there is very little evidence in direct support of the doctrine (Martin, 1992). The main virtue of the hypothesis is the absence of an articulated alternative. The most frequently cited alternative is the proposal that perceptual experience is represented by the activity of many neurons, so that no individual neuron's response corresponds to a conscious perceptual event. Such models are often called **distributed processing models**; they are not widely used by neurophysiologists since they do not provide the specific guidance for interpreting experimental measurements from single neurons, the neurophysiologist's stock-in-trade. The neuron doctrine, on the other hand, provides an immediate answer.

In my own thinking about brain function, I am more inclined to wonder about the brain's computational methods than the mapping between perceptual features and tentatively identified visual streams. I find it satisfying to learn that the magnocellular pathway contains the best representation of high temporal frequencies, but less satisfying to summarize the pathway as the motion pathway, since high temporal frequency information may also be used in many other types of performance tasks. The questions I find fundamental concerning computation are "how?" not "where?" How are essential signal-processing tasks, such as multiplication, addition, and signal synchronization, carried out by the cortical circuitry? What means are used to store temporary results, and what means are used to represent the final results of computations? What decision mechanisms are used to route information from one place to another?

Although the neuron doctrine is widely used because it is an easy tool to relate perception and brain function, my own view is that the doctrine distracts us from the most important question about visual function: how do we *compute* perceptual features like color, stereo, and form? Even if it turns out that a neuron's receptive field is predictive of experience, the question we should be asking is how the neuron's receptive-field properties arise. Answering these computational questions will help us most in designing practical applications that range from sensory prostheses to robotics applications. We should view the specific structures within the visual pathways as a means of implementing these principles, rather than as having an intrinsic importance.

Hubel and Wiesel (1979) once expressed something like this view. While reviewing their accomplishments in the study of area V1, they wrote (p. 23):

> What happens beyond the primary visual area, and how is the information on orientation exploited at later stages? Is one to imagine ultimately finding a cell that responds specifically to some very particular item? (Usually one's grandmother is selected as the particular item, for reasons that escape us.) Our answer is that we doubt there is such a cell, but we have no good alternative to offer. To speculate broadly on how the brain may work is fortunately not the only course open to investigators. To explore the brain is more fun and seems to be more profitable.
>
> There was a time, not so long ago, when one looked at the millions of neurons in the various layers of the cortex and wondered if anyone would ever have any idea of their function. Did they all work in parallel, like the cells of the liver or the kidney, achieving their objectives by pure bulk, or were they each doing something special? For the visual cortex the answer seems now to be known in broad outline: Particular stimuli turn neurons on or off; groups of neurons do indeed perform particular transformations. It seems reasonable to think that if the secrets of a few regions such as this one can be unlocked, other regions will also in time give up their secrets.

In the remaining chapters, we will see how other areas of vision science, based on behavioral and computational studies, might help us to unlock the secrets of vision.

Exercises

1. Answer these questions about forming cortical receptive fields from the inputs of LGN neurons.

   (a) What is an orientation column?

   (b) Suppose the cortical cell response is the sum of two LGN neurons' outputs. Describe the LGN neurons' receptive fields needed for the cortical cell receptive field to be circularly symmetric?

   (c) Use a matrix representation to describe how the receptive field of a linear cortical neuron depends on the linear receptive fields of a collection of LGN neurons.

   (d) Use the matrix representation to design a weighted combination of LGN responses that indicates how much each LGN neuron's response should contribute to the cortical cell's response in order to achieve different receptive-field functions.

2. Answer these questions about retinotopic organization.

   (a) What is a retinotopic map?

   (b) Certain neurons in the central nervous system have very large receptive fields, spanning 20 degrees of visual angle. Can visual areas containing such neurons have retinotopic maps? Experimentally, how would you convince yourself that such an area had a retinotopic organization?

   (c) Draw a picture describing the logical organization of an area of visual cortex that is retinotopic and also has orientation columns. Are the two types of organization necessarily linked to one another, or can you imagine that each would follow its own independent layout?

   (d) How many different kinds of organization can be simultaneously superimposed within a single cortical region?

3. Lesion studies have been an important source of information about neural function. The logical foundation of lesion studies, however, is quite involved. Often, it is difficult to be precise about the conclusions one may draw from a lesion study. The problems of interpreting lesion studies can be illustrated by this old joke:

   > A scientist once decided to study binocular vision. He removed the right eye of a cat and observed that the cat lost its stereo vision. He then wrote an article describing how stereovision was localized to the right eye.
   >
   > To follow on his groundbreaking work, this scientist studied the animal's behavior again and noted that the animal could perform monocular tasks. He enucleated the left eye and observed that the animal could no longer perform such tasks. The scientist wrote a second paper describing how monocular vision is localized to the left eye.

   Write a paragraph that describes what conclusions the scientist should have drawn. Choose your words carefully.

4. Answer these questions about color coding.

   (a) How would you measure the wavelength responsivity of a cortical neuron?

(b) Recall the definition of separability for space and time in the receptive fields of neurons from Chapter 5. Make an analogous definition for wavelength–space separability.

(c) Suppose you measure the wavelength encoding of four neurons in the cortex. Recall that the initial encoding of wavelength is based on three types of cones. Do the wavelength encoding properties of any two of the neurons have to be precisely the same?

(d) If the four neurons have different wavelength encoding properties, will this have any implications for trichromacy?

(e) Suppose the neurons respond linearly to wavelength mixtures. Describe how you might be able to infer the connections between the neurons and the three different cone classes.

5. "Functional specialization" refers to the notion that different brain areas are specialized for certain visual functions, such as the perception of motion or color.

(a) What interconnections would you anticipate finding between different brain areas if each one is specialized to represent a different perceptual function?

(b) What properties do you think a neuron should exhibit before we believe that it is specialized for a visual function?

(c) What special role might the LGN play? Could it be connected with eye movements? Saccadic suppression? Attentional gating? Synchronization of the images from the two eyes? How would you study this question?

7

Pattern Sensitivity

In this chapter we will consider measurements and models of human visual sensitivity to spatial and temporal patterns. We have covered topics relevant to pattern sensitivity in earlier chapters as we reviewed image formation and the receptor mosaic. Here, we will extend our analysis by reviewing a collection of behavioral studies designed to reveal how the visual system as a whole detects and discriminates spatiotemporal patterns.

The spatial-pattern vision literature is dominated by detection and discrimination experiments, not by experiments on what things look like. There are probably two reasons why these measurements make up such a large part of the literature. First, many visual technologies (e.g., televisions, printers, etc.) are capable of reproducing images that appear similar to the original, but not exactly the same. The question of which approximation to the original is visually best is important and often guides the engineering development of the device. As a result, there is considerable interest in developing a complete theory to predict when two different images will appear very similar. When we cannot reproduce the image exactly, a theory of discrimination helps the device designer; the theory identifies which of the images that the device can reproduce will appear most similar to the original. Threshold and discrimination experiments are indispensable to the design of discrimination theories.

Second, many authors believe that threshold and discrimination tasks can play a special role in analyzing the neurophysiological mechanisms of vision. The rationale for using threshold and discrimination to analyze the physiological mechanisms of vision is rarely stated and thus rarely debated, but the argument can be put something like this. Suppose the nervous system is built from a set of components, or mechanisms, that analyze the spatial pattern of light on the retina. Then we should identify and analyze these putative mechanisms to understand how they contribute to perception of spatial patterns. Threshold performance offers us the best chance of isolating the mechanisms because, at threshold, only the most sensitive mechanisms contribute to visibility. If threshold performance depends upon the stimulation of a single mechanism or small number of mechanisms, then threshold studies can serve as a psychologist's dissecting instrument: at threshold we can isolate different parts of the visual pathways. After understanding the component mechanisms, we can seek a unified theory of the visual system's operation.

I am not sure whether this rationale in terms of visual mechanisms adequately justifies the startling emphasis on threshold measurements. But it is plain that by now we have learned a lot from detection and discrimination experiments (DeValois and DeValois, 1988; Graham, 1989). Many of the basic ideas used in image representation and computer vision were derived from the work on detection and discrimination of spatial patterns. This chapter is devoted to an exposition of some of those experiments and ideas. In Chapters 9, 10, and 11 we will take up the question of what things look like.

A Single-Resolution Theory

The problem of predicting human sensitivity to spatial contrast patterns has much in common with other problems we have studied: image formation, color-matching, or single-unit neurophysiological responses. We want to make a small number of measurements, say, sensitivity to a small number of spatial contrast patterns, and then use these measurements to predict sensitivity to all other spatial contrast patterns.

In 1956, Otto Schade had some ideas about how to make these predictions, and he set out to build a photoelectric analog of the visual system in order to predict visual sensitivity. His idea was to use the device to predict whether small changes in the design parameters of a display would be noticeable to a human observer. For example, in designing a new display monitor an engineer might want to alter the spatial resolution of the device. To answer whether this difference is noticeable to a human observer, Schade needed a way to predict the sensitivity of human observers to the effect of the engineering change.

Figure 7.1 shows a schematic diagram of Schade's computational eye. I include the diagram to show that Schade created a very extensive

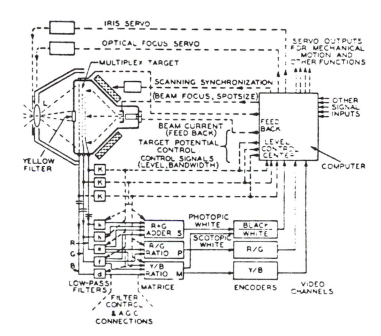

7.1 A COMPUTATIONAL MODEL OF THE HUMAN VISUAL SYSTEM. Otto Schade designed a visual simulator to predict human visual sensitivity to patterns. His model incorporated many features of the visual pathway, and it may be the earliest computational model of human vision. From Schade, 1956.

model that incorporated many visual functions, such as optical image formation, transduction, integration of signals from the different cone types, adaptation, spatial integration, negative feedback, and even some thoughts about correction, interpretation, and correlation of the signals with stored information (i.e., memory). In this sense, his work was a precursor to the computational vision models set forth by Marr (1982) and his colleagues.

The Neural Image

A fundamental part of Schade's computation—and one that has been retained by the field of spatial-pattern vision—is his suggestion that we can summarize the effects of the many visual components using a single representation now called the **neural image**.[1] A real image and a couple of neural images are drawn suggestively in Figure 7.2. The idea is that there is a collection of neurons whose responses, taken as a population, capture the image information available to the observer. The responses of a collection of neurons with similar receptive fields, differing only in that the receptive fields are centered at various positions, make up a neural image.

Figure 7.2 shows how the neural-image concept permits us to visualize the neural response to an input image. At several places within

---

[1] To the best of my knowledge, John Robson first suggested this term.

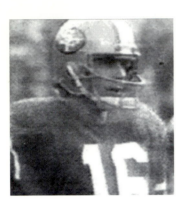

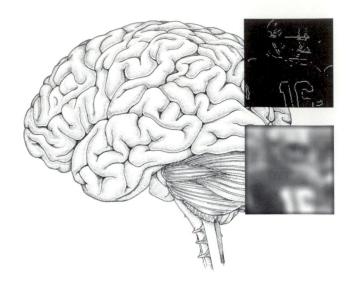

7.2 A NEURAL IMAGE represents the activity of a group of neurons. A real image, shown on the left, will be encoded by many distinct populations of neurons within the brain. The intensity at each point in a neural image, illustrated by the images on the right, represents the activity of a single neuron in the population. Each population of neurons may encode a different property of the original image. One of the neural images represents the edge locations. The other image represents an encoding of the local mean intensity, such as might be used to regulate adaptation. Other neural images, not shown, might represent aspects of color, motion, and depth.

the figure, I have represented the neural responses as an image. The intensity at each point in these neural images represents the response of a neuron single whose receptive field is centered at the corresponding image point. A bright value represents a neuron whose response is increased by the stimulus, and a dark value represents a neuron whose response is decreased.

The assumptions we make concerning the receptive-field properties of neurons comprising the neural image permit us to calculate the neural image using linear methods. For example, suppose the receptive fields of a collection of neurons are identical except for the position of the receptive-field centers; further, suppose these are uniformly spaced. In that case, we can calculate the mapping from the real image to the responses of these neurons using a shift-invariant linear mapping (i.e., convolution).

The neural images shown in Figure 7.2 illustrate the idea that different populations of neurons may represent different types of information. One neural image is shown representing the coarse aspects of the original. The values in this image were obtained by forming a local average of the original image intensities. The average local intensity represented in this image might be used for various purposes, such as regulating visual adaptation to illumination variation in the image. The second neural image in the figure represents positions where there are likely to be edges in the original image. This image may be used as part of an object recognition system. There may be many other neural images in the cortex as well that represent different aspects of the image including color, motion, and depth. Of course, the information represented in a cortical neural image depends on transformations of the signal that take place all along the visual pathway, including lens defocus, sampling by the photoreceptor mosaic, wavelength encoding by the cones, and so forth.

Schade's Single-Resolution Theory

Schade's theory of pattern sensitivity is formulated mainly for foveal vision. Schade assumed that foveal pattern sensitivity could be predicted by the information available in a single neural image. He assumed that, for this portion of the visual field, the relevant neural image could be represented by a shift-invariant transformation of the retinal image, much like the neural image shown near the bottom of the visual cortex in Figure 7.2. In this section we review the significance of this hypothesis and also some empirical tests of it.

We know that a neural image spanning the entire visual field cannot really be shift-invariant. In earlier chapters, we reviewed measurements showing that the fovea contains many more photoreceptors and retinal ganglion cells than the periphery, and also that there is much more cortical area devoted to the fovea than to the periphery. Consequently, a neural image can have a shift-invariant representation only over a relatively small portion of the visual field, say, within the fovea or a small patch of the peripheral visual field.

Still, a model of pattern discrimination in the fovea is a good place to begin. First, the theory will be much simpler because we can avoid the complexities of visual-field inhomogeneities. Second, because of our continual use of eye movements in normal viewing, the fovea is our main source of pattern information. So, we begin by reviewing theory and measurements of pattern sensitivity in the fovea. We will consider how acuity varies across the visual field later in this chapter.

There are several ways the shift-invariant neural-image hypothesis helps us predict contrast sensitivity. Perhaps the most important is an idea we have seen several times before: if the mapping from image to neural image is shift-invariant, then the mapping from image to neural image is defined by knowing the shape of a single receptive field. In a shift-invariant neural image there is only one basic receptive-field shape. Neurons that make up the neural image differ only with respect to their receptive-field positions.

The analogy between shift-invariant calculations and neural receptive fields is useful. But we should remember that we are reasoning about behavioral measurements, not real neural receptive fields. Hence, it is useful to phrase our measurements using the slightly more abstract language of linear computation. In these calculations, the linear receptive field is equivalent to the **convolution kernel** of the shift-invariant mapping. The shift-invariance hypothesis tells us that to understand the neural image, we must estimate the convolution kernel. Its properties determine which information is represented by the neural image and which information is not.

As we have done several times earlier in this book, we will begin our analysis using one-dimensional stimuli: vertical sinusoids varying only in the x-direction. If we use only one-dimensional stimuli as inputs, then we can estimate only the one-dimensional receptive field of the transformation. We can write the shift-invariant transformation that maps the one-dimensional contrast stimulus, a_x, to the one-dimensional neural image, n_x, using the summation formula,

$$n_x = \sum_{\langle y \rangle} l_{x-y} a_y \tag{7.1}$$

where l_x is the one-dimensional receptive field.[2] We can also express the transformation in matrix tableau:

$$
\begin{pmatrix} n_0 \\ n_1 \\ \vdots \\ n_{N-1} \\ n_N \end{pmatrix}
=
\begin{pmatrix}
l_0 & \ldots & l_{-N/2} & \ldots & l_{-N} \\
\ldots & \ldots & \ldots & \ldots & \ldots \\
l_{N-2} & \ldots & l_0 & \ldots & l_{-N/2} \\
\ldots & \ldots & \ldots & \ldots & \ldots \\
l_N & \ldots & l_{N/2} & \ldots & l_0
\end{pmatrix}
\begin{pmatrix} a_0 \\ a_1 \\ \vdots \\ a_{N-1} \\ a_N \end{pmatrix}
$$

In matrix tableau it becomes clear that the system matrix is very simple; the rows and columns are all equal to the receptive field (i.e., convolution kernel) except for a shift or a reversal. Hence, by estimating the convolution kernel, we will be able to predict the transformation from contrast image to neural image.

The overall plan for predicting an observer's pattern sensitivity is as follows. First, we will measure sensitivity to a collection of harmonic contrast patterns. These measurements will define the observer's contrast sensitivity function (see Chapters 5 and 6). Because of the special relationship between harmonic functions and shift-invariant linear systems described in the earlier chapters and Appendix A, we can use the contrast-sensitivity function to estimate the convolution kernel of the shift-invariant linear transformation from image to neural image, l_x. Finally, we will use the estimated kernel to calculate the neural image and predict the observer's sensitivity to other one-dimensional contrast patterns. This final step will provide a test of the theory.

---

[2] See Appendix A for a discussion of the circular convolution formula and the meaning of the bracket notation, $\langle y \rangle$.

Shortly, it will become clear that we must make a few additional assumptions before we can use the observer's contrast-sensitivity measurements to estimate the convolution kernel. But first I will review some measurements of the human spatial contrast-sensitivity function.

Spatial Contrast-Sensitivity Functions

Schade measured the contrast-sensitivity function by asking observers to judge the visibility of sinusoidal patterns of varying contrast. The observer's task was to decide what contrast was necessary to render the pattern just barely visible. Because of optical and neural factors, observers are not equally sensitive to all spatial-frequency patterns; the threshold contrast depends upon the pattern's spatial frequency.

To get a sense of the informal nature of Schade's (1956) experiments, it is interesting to read his description of the methods (p. 739):

> The test pattern is faded in by increasing the electrical modulation at a fixed rate and observed on the modulation meter; the observer under test gives a signal at the instant he recognizes the line test pattern, and the person conducting the test reads and remembers the corresponding modulation reading. The modulation is returned to zero, and within seconds it is increased again at the same fixed rate to make a new observation. By averaging 10 to 15 readings mentally and recording the average reading directly on graph paper, the [contrast sensitivity] function . . . can be observed in a short time and inconsistencies are discovered immediately and checked by additional observations.

The contrast-sensitivity function he measured is shown in Figure 7.3. The horizontal axis is spatial frequency as measured in terms of the display device. The vertical axis is contrast sensitivity, namely

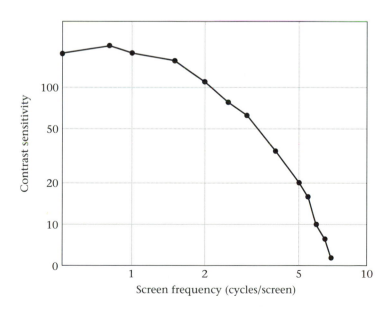

7.3 CONTRAST-SENSITIVITY measurements of a human observer. The contrast thresholds are plotted with respect to spatial frequency on the display rather than cycles per degree of visual angle. Source: Schade, 1956.

$\log(1/c) = -\log c$, where c is the contrast of the pattern at the detection threshold. The contrast-sensitivity function has two striking features. First, there is a fall-off in sensitivity as the spatial frequency of the test pattern increases. This effect is large, but it should not surprise you since we already know many different components in the visual pathways are insensitive to high-spatial-frequency targets: the optical blurring of the lens reduces the contrast of high-spatial-frequency targets; also, retinal ganglion cells with center-surround receptive fields are less sensitive to high-spatial-frequency targets.

Second, and somewhat more surprisingly, there is no improvement of sensitivity at low spatial frequencies; there is even a small loss of contrast sensitivity at the lowest spatial frequency. The eye's optical image-formation does not reduce sensitivity at low frequencies, so the fall in contrast sensitivity at low spatial frequencies is due to neural factors. Center-surround receptive fields are one possible reason for this low-frequency fall-off.

Schade's measurements were made using a steadily presented test pattern or a drifting pattern. Robson (1966; see also Kelly, 1961) made additional measurements using flickering **contrast-reversing gratings**. Contrast-reversing patterns are harmonic spatial patterns with harmonic amplitude variation (see Chapter 5). For example, suppose the mean illumination is m. Then the *intensity* of the contrast-reversing stimulus at spatial frequency f_x, temporal frequency f_t, and contrast a is

$$[\, 1.0 + a\cos(2\pi f_t t)\cos(2\pi f_x x)\,]m \qquad (7.2)$$

The intensity is always positive (cf. Equation 5.3). The spatiotemporal *contrast* of the pattern is

$$a\cos(2\pi f_t t)\cos(2\pi f_x x) \qquad (7.3)$$

The contrast can be both positive and negative.

As the data in Figure 7.4 show, the spatial sensitivity falls at low frequencies when we measure at a low temporal frequency (1 Hz). At high temporal frequencies, such as one might encounter during a series of rapid eye movements, there is no low-frequency sensitivity loss. As we shall see later, the contrast-sensitivity function also varies with other stimulus parameters such as the mean illumination level and the wavelength composition of the stimulus.

The Psychophysical Linespread Function

We will now return to the problem of using the contrast-sensitivity data to calculate the convolution kernel, l_x. Because this kernel defines both the rows and the columns of the shift-invariant linear transformation, it is also called the **psychophysical linespread function**, in analogy with

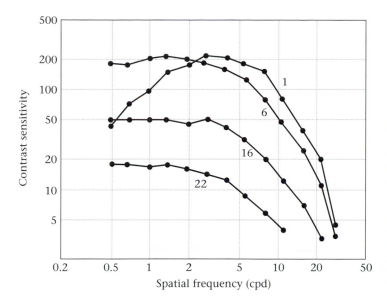

7.4 TEMPORAL VARIATIONS CHANGE THE SHAPE OF THE HUMAN SPATIAL CONTRAST-SENSITIVITY FUNCTION. The contrast-sensitivity functions shown here were measured with contrast-reversing targets at several different temporal frequencies. At low temporal frequencies (1 Hz) the contrast-sensitivity function is bandpass. At high temporal frequencies (22 Hz) the function is lowpass. Source: Robson, 1966.

the optical linespread function (see Chapter 2). By now you have probably noticed that each time we apply linear-systems theory, some special feature of the measurement situation requires us to devise some slightly different approach to calculating the system properties. The calculations involved in using contrast-sensitivity measurements to predict sensitivity to all contrast patterns are no exception.

We should now determine what we need to do to estimate the psychophysical linespread function. The general linear problem was illustrated in the matrix tableau representation near Equation 7.1, where the input stimulus is shown as a column vector, specifying the one-dimensional spatial contrast pattern. The matrix describes how the stimulus is transformed into the neural image. We want to make a small number of measurements in order to estimate the entries of the system matrix.

We have solved this problem before, but in this case we have a special challenge. In our previous attempts to estimate linear transformations we have been able to specify both the stimulus and the response. When we obtain the contrast-sensitivity measurements, however, we never measure the output neural image. We only measure the input threshold stimulus. Hence, we have fairly limited information available.

Because we assumed that the neural image is a shift-invariant mapping, we do know something about the neural image: when the input stimulus is a harmonic function, the output must be a harmonic function at the same frequency. But we do not know the amplitude or phase of the harmonic function in the hypothetical neural image. To estimate the psychophysical linespread function, we must make additional assumptions about the properties of a neural image that render it at detection threshold. From these assumptions, we will then specify the phase and amplitude of the neural image at detection threshold.

Two additional assumptions are commonly made. First, we assume that the spatial phase of the neural image is the same as the spatial phase of the input spatial contrast pattern.[3] Specifically, when the input pattern is a one-dimensional cosinusoid, $\cos(2\pi f i/N)$, we assume that the neural image output pattern is a scaled copy of the input pattern, $n_i = a_f \cos(2\pi f i/N)$. The scale factor, a_f, depends on the frequency of the input signal.

Second, we must specify the amplitude of the neural image at detection threshold. The amplitude of the neural image should be related to the visibility of the pattern, and we can list a few properties that should be associated with pattern visibility. For example, whether the change introduced by the signal increases or decreases the firing rate should be irrelevant; any change from the spontaneous rate ought to be detectable. Also, detectability should depend on responses pooled across the neural image, rather than the response of a single neuron. The squared **vector-length** of the responses of the neural image is a measure that has both of these properties. The squared vector-length of the neural image, d^2, is defined by the formula

$$d^2 = \sum_{i=1}^{N} n_i^2 \tag{7.4}$$

This formula satisfies both of our requirements since (a) the signs of the individual neural responses, n_i, are not important (because the neural image entry is squared), and (b) the formula incorporates the responses from different neurons. Other measures are possible. For example, one might assume that at detection threshold the sum of the absolute values of the neural image is equal to a constant, or one might make up a completely different rule. But, one must make some assumption, and the vector-length rule is a useful place to begin.

If we assume that at contrast detection threshold all neural images have the same vector-length, then we can specify the amplitude of the harmonic functions in the neural image. Hence, at this point we have made enough assumptions so that we can specify the complete neural image and solve for the psychophysical linespread function. Figure 7.5 shows three linespread functions estimated using these assumptions. Figure 7.5A shows a psychophysical linespread computed from Schade's measurements (note that the spatial dimension is uncalibrated). Figure 7.5B and Figure 7.5C show psychophysical linespreads, plotted in terms of degrees of visual angle, derived from Robson's measurements using 1-Hz and 6-Hz contrast-reversing functions. No single linespread

[3] We used the same assumption to infer the properties of the lens in Chapter 2.

(A)

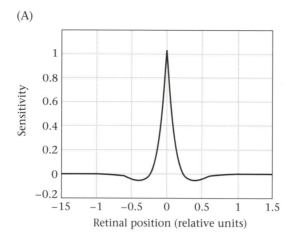

(B)   (C)

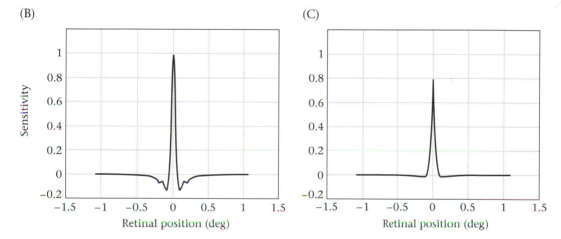

7.5 THE PSYCHOPHYSICAL LINESPREAD FUNCTION can be estimated from the contrast-sensitivity function. (A) A linespread estimated from Schade's measurements. The horizontal axis is in arbitrary units because the spatial frequency of the contrast-sensitivity function was reported in arbitrary units. Parts (B) and (C) show, respectively, linespread functions for contrast-reversing targets at 1 Hz and 6 Hz derived from Robson's measurements; the horizontal axis is in degrees of visual angle.

function applies to all stimulus conditions. We will consider how the linespread function changes with the stimulus conditions later in this chapter.

Schade (1956) suggested that the general shape of the psychophysical linespread function can be described using the difference of two Gaussian functions. This description is the same one used by Rodieck (1965) and Enroth-Cugell and Robson (1966) to model receptive fields of retinal ganglion cells. The correspondence between the psychophysical linespread function, derived from the behavioral measurement of contrast sensitivity, and the receptive-field functions of retinal ganglion cells, derived from retinal physiology, is encouraging.

Discussion of the Theory: Static Nonlinearities

To estimate the convolution kernel of Schade's hypothetical neural image, without being able to measure the neural image directly, we have been forced make several assumptions. It is wise to remember the three strong assumptions we have made:

1. The neural image is a shift-invariant linear encoding.

2. There is zero phase shift of the linear encoding.

3. The vector-length rule determines visibility.

Taken as a whole, this is a nonlinear theory of pattern sensitivity. Although the neural image is a linear representation of the input (indeed, it is even a shift-invariant representation), the vector-length rule linking the neural image to performance is nonlinear. You can verify this by noting that when a stimulus vector s_1 has length d_1 and vector s_2 has length d_2, the vector $s_1 + s_2$ need not have length $d_1 + d_2$. Thus, even when s_1 and s_2 are at one-half threshold, $s_1 + s_2$ may not be at threshold.[4]

The vector-length calculation is a static nonlinearity applied after a linear calculation (see Chapter 4). This is a relatively simple nonlinearity, so that it is straightforward to make certain general predictions about performance even though the theory is nonlinear. In the next section, we consider some of these predictions as well as experimental tests of them.

Experimental Tests

The contrast-sensitivity function by itself offers no test of Schade's theory other than reasonableness: do the inferred linespread functions seem plausible? We have seen that the linespread functions are plausible since they are quite similar to the receptive fields of visual neurons. But, because we have made so many assumptions, it is important to find general properties of the theory that we can test experimentally and in that way gain confidence in the theory's usefulness.

Harmonic functions will play a special role in testing the theory. There are two separate reasons why harmonics are important for our new test: (a) Given the assumed shift-invariance, the neural image of a harmonic is also a harmonic. We have seen this property many times before and it will be important again; (b) Harmonic functions at different frequencies are orthogonal to one another. Geometrically, orthogonality means that the vectors are oriented perpendicular to one another. Algebraically, we say two vectors **a** and **b** are orthogonal when

---

[4] The only case in which the lengths will sum to $d_1 + d_2$ is when the vectors representing the neural images point in the same direction.

$0 = \sum a_x b_x$. Sinusoids and cosinusoids are orthogonal to one another, and any pair of harmonic functions at different frequencies are orthogonal to one another. We will use these two properties, combined with the vector-length rule, to test Schade's basic theory.

Suppose we create a stimulus equal to the sum of two sinusoids at frequencies, f_i, and contrasts, c_i, for $i = 1, 2$ (Figure 7.6). According to the shift-invariant theory, the neural image of these two sinusoids is the weighted sum of two sinusoids. Each sinusoid is scaled by a factor, s_i,

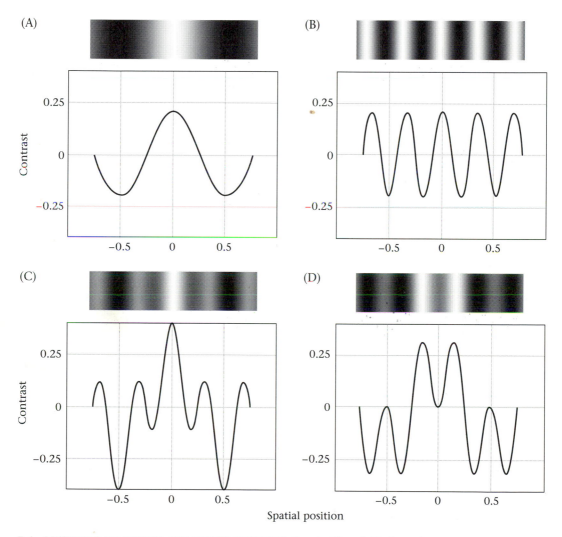

7.6 MIXTURES OF SPATIAL CONTRAST PATTERNS. Panels (A) and (B) show the contrast of cosinusoidal stimuli at 1 and 3 cpd. Mixtures of these two stimuli are shown in a spatial phase in which the peaks add (C) and a spatial phase in which the peaks subtract (D). The general appearance of the stimuli is indicated by the images shown above each panel.

that defines how well the stimulus is passed by the shift-invariant system. The squared vector-length of the neural image created by the sum of the two sinusoids is

$$d^2 = \sum_{i=1}^{N} [c_1 s_1 \sin(2\pi f_1 i/N) + c_2 s_2 \sin(2\pi f_2 i/N)]^2 \qquad (7.5)$$

The squared term in the summation can be expanded into three terms

$$d^2 = [c_1 s_1 \sum_{i=1}^{N} \sin(2\pi f_1 i/N)]^2 + [c_2 s_2 \sum_{i=1}^{N} \sin(2\pi f_2 i/N]^2$$

$$+ 2c_1 c_2 s_1 s_2 \sum_{i=1}^{N} \sin(2\pi f_1 i/N) \sin(2\pi f_2 i/N) \qquad (7.6)$$

Because sinusoids at different frequencies are orthogonal functions, the third term is zero, leaving only

$$d^2 = [c_1 s_1 \sum_{i=1}^{N} \sin(2\pi f_1 i/N)]^2 + [c_2 s_2 \sum_{i=1}^{N} \sin(2\pi f_2 i/N)]^2 \quad (7.7)$$

We can group some terms to define a new equation,

$$d^2 = (c_1 a_1)^2 + (c_2 a_2)^2 \qquad (7.8)$$

where a_i is a constant, namely, $s_i \sum_{i=j}^{N} \sin(2\pi f_i j/N)^2$.

Equation 7.8 tells us when a pair of contrasts of the two sinusoids, (c_1, c_2), should be at detection threshold. Figure 7.7 is a graphical representation of these predictions. The axes of the graph represent the contrast levels of the two sinusoidal components used in the mixture. The solutions to Equation 7.8 sweep out a curve called a **detection contour**.

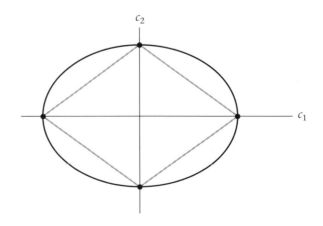

7.7 THE SPATIAL TEST-MIXTURE EXPERIMENT provides a test of contrast-sensitivity models. We measure the visibility of a test-mixture whose sinusoidal components have contrasts c_1 and c_2. The set of contrast pairs such that the mixture stimulus is at detection threshold defines the detection contour. Schade's hypothesis predicts that the detection contour is an ellipse aligned with the axes of the graph, as shown by the solid curve. If the peak stimulus contrast determines contrast sensitivity to the pair, then the detection contour should fall along the contour indicated by the shaded lines.

As shown in Figure 7.7, Equation 7.8 is the equation of an ellipse whose principal axes are aligned with the axes of the graph. The two unknown quantities, the scale factors a_i, are related to the lengths of the principal axes. Hence, if we scale the contrast of the sinusoidal components so that threshold contrast for each sinusoidal component is arbitrarily set to 1, the predicted detection contour will fall on a circle (Graham and Nachmias, 1971; Nielsen and Wandell, 1988).

Many alternative theories are possible. For example, had we supposed that threshold is determined by the peak contrast of the pattern, then the detection contour would fall on the diamond shape shown in Figure 7.7. The important point is that the shape of the detection contour depends on the basic theory. The prediction using Schade's theory is clear, so that we can use the prediction to test the theory.

Graham et al. (1978; see also Graham and Nachmias, 1971) measured sensitivity to mixtures of sinusoidal gratings at 1 cpd and 3 cpd. They measured thresholds using a careful psychophysical threshold estimation procedure called a **two-interval, forced-choice design**. In this procedure each trial is divided into two temporal periods, usually indicated by a tone that defines the onset of the first temporal period, a second tone that defines the onset of the second temporal period, and a final tone that indicates the end of the trial. A test stimulus is presented during one of the two temporal intervals, and the observer must watch the display and decide which interval contained the test stimulus. When the contrast of the test pattern is very low, the observer is forced to guess, and so performance is at chance. When the contrast is very high, the observer will nearly always identify the correct temporal interval. Hence, as the test-pattern contrast increases, performance varies from 0.5 to 1.0. The threshold performance level is arbitrary, but for technical reasons described in their paper, Graham et al. (1978) defined threshold to be the contrast level at which the observer was correct with probability 0.81.

The test-mixture data in Figure 7.8 do not fall precisely along the circular detection contour predicted by Schade's single-resolution theory. Specifically, thresholds measured in the 45° direction tend to fall just outside the predicted detection contour; thresholds are a little too high compared to the prediction. The theory predicts that the threshold contrasts of the individual components should be reduced by a factor of 1.414, but thresholds are reduced by only a factor of 1.2. These data are typical for these types of experimental measurements.

Is this an important difference? The point of this theory is to measure sensitivity to a small number of spatial patterns and to use these measurements to predict sensitivity to all other spatial patterns. If we see failures when we measure sensitivity to a mixture of only two test patterns, we should be concerned: The theory must be precise enough to tolerate decomposition of an arbitrary pattern into a sum of many sinusoidal patterns and then predict sensitivity to the mixtures of the multiple components. If we already see failures with two components,

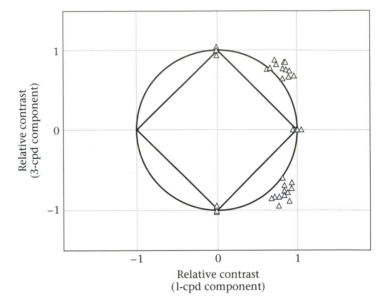

7.8   SPATIAL TEST-MIXTURE THRESHOLDS measured using a 1- and 3-cpd grating. The thresholds fall outside of the detection contour predicted by the shift-invariant hypothesis and vector-length rule. Source: Graham et al., 1978.

we should worry about how well the theory will do when we measure with three components.

The data in Figure 7.9 illustrate sensitivity measurements to the combination of three sinusoidal gratings. In this case, the data are plotted as three **psychometric functions**. Shown in this format, the dependence of performance on contrast is explicit. The data points connected by the dashed curves show the observer's probability of correctly detecting the individual sinusoidal grating patterns at 1.33, 4.0, or 12 cpd.

7.9   A THREE-COMPONENT SPATIAL TEST-MIXTURE EXPERIMENT. The probability of correct detection in a two-interval forced choice is shown as a function of normalized contrast. The shaded lines on the right show detection for three simple sinusoidal gratings at frequencies of 1.33, 4, and 12 cpd. The two solid lines show the probability of detecting mixtures of these three components in cosine phase and sine phase. The shaded curve on the left shows the predicted sensitivity using the shift-invariant model and the vector-length rule. Source: Graham, 1989.

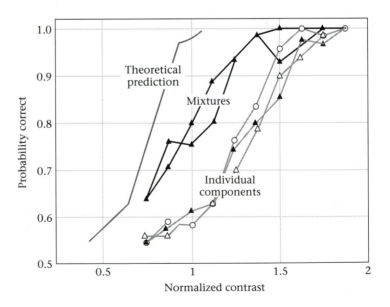

The horizontal axis measures the scaled contrast of the sinusoids in which the scale factor has been chosen to make the three curves align.

The visibility of two patterns formed by the mixtures of all three sinusoidal patterns, whose contrast ratios have been adjusted to make the three sinusoidal patterns equally visible, are shown as solid lines. One sum was formed with the peak contrasts all aligned (cosine phase) and the other with their zero-crossings aligned (sine phase).

Again, because the input signals are sinusoids or sums of sinusoids, we can predict performance based on the shift-invariant neural image and the vector-length rule. The neural image of the sum of three sinusoidal gratings will be the weighted sum of three sinusoidal neural images. The predicted threshold to the mixture of the three patterns is shown by the dot-dashed curve at the left of Figure 7.9. The vector-length rule also predicts that the probability correct will be the same in both sine and cosine phase.

The model prediction is not completely wrong; the phase relationship of the gratings does not have a significant influence on detection threshold for the mixture of three targets. But the mixture patterns are less visible than predicted by the theory: The contrasts of the three component mixtures are reduced by a factor of about 1.4 compared to their individual thresholds, while the theory predicts a contrast reduction of 1.73. The basic theory has some good features, but the quantitative predictions fail more and more as we apply the theory to increasingly complex patterns.

Intermediate Summary

We have begun formulating psychophysical theory using the simple computational ideas of shift-invariance followed by a static nonlinearity. These ideas are reminiscent of the properties of certain neurons in the visual pathway. While this theoretical formulation is a vast simplification of what we know about the nervous system, it is a reasonable place to begin. The nervous system is complex and contains many different types of computational elements. While Schade's effort to capture all of the nuances of the neural representation is inspiring, it was perhaps a bit premature. Much of the neural representation must be irrelevant to the tasks we are studying. Nonetheless, by beginning with simpler formulations, we can use psychophysical models to discover those aspects of the neural representation that are essential for predicting behavior. By comparing and contrasting the behavioral data and the neural data, we can discern the important functional elements of the neural representation for different types of visual tasks.

While the shift-invariant theory did not succeed, it has served the useful purpose of organizing some of our thinking and suggesting some experiments we should try. For the purpose of making some approximate predictions quickly, there are some good aspects of the calculation. For example, the inferred psychophysical linespread is similar to the receptive fields of some peripheral neurons. Also, for simple mixtures, the theoretical predictions are only off by by a modest factor. Still, the shift-invariant theory plainly does not fit the data very well, and its performance will only deteriorate when we apply it to complex stimuli, such as natural images. We need to find new insights and experiments that might suggest how to elaborate the theory.

Multiresolution Theory

Schade's single-resolution theory of pattern sensitivity does not predict the pattern-sensitivity data accurately. But the theory is not so far wrong that we should abandon it entirely. The question we consider now is how to generalize the single-resolution theory, keeping the good parts.

Modern theories generally use an initial linear encoding consisting of a collection of shift-invariant linear transformations, not just a single one. Each shift-invariant linear transformation has its own convolution kernel and hence forms its own neural image. We will refer to the data represented by the individual shift-invariant representations as a **component-image** of the full theory.

To specify the properties of the more general theory, we need to select convolution kernels associated with each of the shift-invariant linear transformations and the static nonlinearities that follow. Also, we need to specify how the outputs of the different component images are combined to form a single detection decision.[5]

Pattern Adaptation

The motivation for building a multiresolution theory comes from a collection of empirical observations, such as the one illustrated in Figure 7.10. That figure demonstrates a phenomenon called **pattern adaptation**. To see the illusion, first notice that the bars in the patterns on top and bottom of Figure 7.10B are the same width. Next, stare at the fixation target between the patterns in Figure 7.10A for a minute or so. These patterns are called the **adapting patterns**. When you stare, allow your eye to wander across the dot between patterns, but do not let your gaze wander too far. After you have spent a minute or so examining the adapting patterns, look at the patterns in Figure 7.10B again. Particularly at first, you will notice that the bars at the top and bottom of the middle pattern will appear to have different sizes. You can try the same experiment by fixating between the adapting patterns in Figure 7.10C for a minute or so. When you examine the bars in the middle, the top

---

[5] For reasons I will explain in the next section, the properties of the convolution kernels of the component images are usually selected so that the expanded theory is a multiresolution representation of the image, a term I will define shortly.

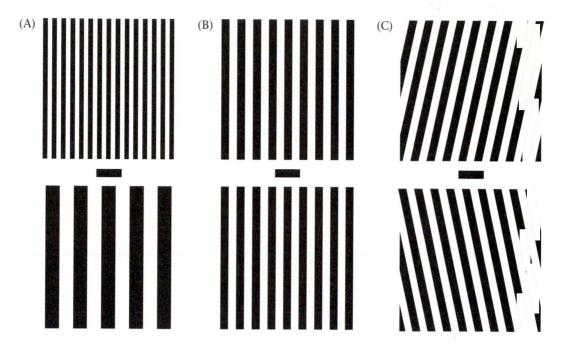

7.10   A SIZE ILLUSION AND AN ORIENTATION ILLUSION SHOWING VISUAL PATTERN ADAPTATION. The bar widths and orientations of the two square-wave patterns in the middle are the same. Stare at the fixation point between the two patterns in (A) for a minute, adapting to the two patterns in your upper and lower visual fields. When you shift your gaze to the patterns in (B) the patterns will appear to have different bar widths. Then, stare at the fixation point between the two patterns in (C) and then examine the middle pattern. When you shift your gaze to (B) the patterns will appear to have different orientations. After Blakemore and Sutton, 1969; see also DeValois, 1977a, b.

and bottom will appear to have different orientation (Gilinsky, 1968; Pantle and Sekuler, 1968; Blakemore and Campbell, 1969; Blakemore and Sutton, 1969; Blakemore, Nachmias and Sutton, 1970).

The effect of pattern adaptation can be measured by comparing the contrast-sensitivity function before and after adaptation. The curve through the filled circles in Figure 7.11A shows the contrast-sensitivity function prior to pattern adaptation. After adapting for several minutes to a sinusoidal contrast pattern, much as you adapted to the patterns in Figure 7.10A, the observer's contrast sensitivity to stimuli near the frequency of the adapting pattern is reduced, while contrast sensitivity to other spatial frequency patterns remains unchanged. The ratio of contrast sensitivity before and after adaptation is shown in Figure 7.11B. When this experiment is repeated, using adapting patterns at other spatial frequencies, contrast sensitivity falls for test patterns whose spatial frequency is similar to that of the adapting pattern (Blakemore and Campbell, 1969).

The results of the pattern-adaptation measurements suggest one way to generalize the neural image from a single-resolution theory to

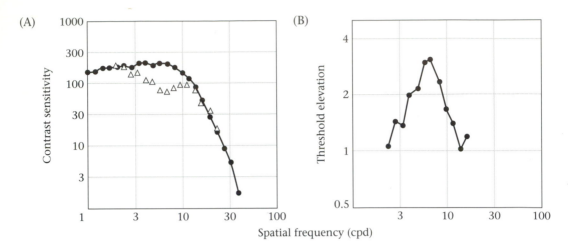

7.11 THE EFFECT OF PATTERN ADAPTATION ON THE CONTRAST-SENSITIVITY FUNCTION. (A) The curve through the filled circles shows the observer's contrast-sensitivity function before pattern adaptation. The open triangles show contrast sensitivity following adaptation to a sinusoidal pattern of 7.1 cpd. (B) Threshold elevation, that is, the ratio of contrast sensitivity before and after adaptation, is plotted as a function of spatial frequency. The threshold elevation occurs at test frequencies near the frequency of the adapting stimulus. Source: Blakemore and Campbell, 1969.

a multiresolution theory: use a neural representation that consists of a collection of component-images, each sensitive to a narrow band of spatial frequencies and orientations. This separation of the visual image information can be achieved by using a variety of convolution kernels, each of which emphasizes a different spatial frequency range in the image. This calculation might be implemented in the nervous system by creating neurons with a variety of receptive-field properties, much as we have found in the variety of receptive fields of linear simple cells in the visual cortex; these cells have both orientation and spatial-frequency preferences (Chapter 6). Because the individual component images are assumed to represent different spatial frequency resolutions, we say that the neural image is a **multiresolution representation**.

Multiresolution representations provide a simple framework to explain pattern adaptation (Figure 7.12). Suppose the visual system ordinarily encodes the image using a collection of shift-invariant component images whose contrast-sensitivity curves are shown on the top of Figure 7.12A. Before adaptation, each of the component images represents the square wave at an amplitude that depends on the square-wave frequency and the channel sensitivity. The bar plot at the bottom of Figure 7.12A shows the amplitude of the component-image representations to the test pattern before adaptation.

Adaptation to a low-frequency square wave suppresses sensitivity of some of the component images, as shown in the top of Figure 7.12B. Consequently, the pattern of responses to the test frequency follow-

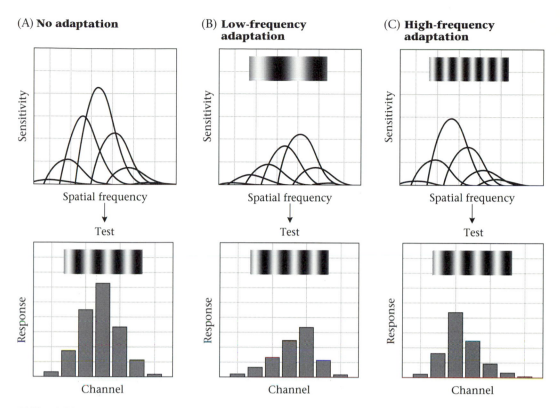

7.12   A MULTIRESOLUTION MODEL can explain certain aspects of pattern adaptation. (A) In normal viewing, the bar width is inferred from the relative responses of a collection of component-images, each responding best to a selected spatial frequency band. The spatial-frequency selectivity of each component image is shown above, and the amplitude of the component-image encoding of the test stimulus is shown in the bar graph below. (B) Following adaptation to a low-frequency stimulus (shown in inset), the sensitivity of the neurons comprising certain component images is reduced. Considering the responses of all the component images, the response to the test is similar to the unadapted response to a high-frequency target. (C) Following adaptation to a high-frequency pattern (shown in inset), the neural representation is consistent with the unadapted response to a low-frequency target.

ing adaptation changes, as shown in the bottom of Figure 7.12B. The new pattern of responses is consistent with the responses that would be caused by the unadapted response to a finer square-wave pattern. This is the explanation of the observation that, following adaptation to a low-frequency square wave, the test pattern appears to shift to a higher spatial frequency. Figure 7.12C illustrates the component-image sensitivities following adaptation to a high-frequency square wave (top) and how the amplitude of the component image responses are altered (bottom). In this case, the pattern of responses is consistent with the unadapted encoding of a lower-frequency target.

According to the multiresolution model, pattern adaptation is much like a lesion experiment. Adaptation reduces or eliminates the contribution of one set of neurons, altering the balance of activity and producing a change in the perceptual response. Following adaptation to a low-frequency target, the excitation in component images at higher spatial frequencies is relatively greater, giving the test bars a narrower appearance. Conversely, following adaptation to a high-frequency target, the excitation in component images representing low spatial frequencies is relatively greater, giving the test bars a wider appearance.

In summary, the empirical observations using pattern adaptation suggest that square-wave or sinusoidal adapting patterns only influence the contrast sensitivity of patterns of roughly the same spatial frequency. This observation suggests that the component images might be organized at multiple spatial resolutions.

Pattern Discrimination and Masking

There are several other experimental observations, in addition to pattern adaptation, that can be used to support multiresolution representations for human perception. Historically, one of the most important papers on this point was Campbell and Robson's (1968) study, in which they made detection and discrimination measurements using square-wave gratings and other periodic spatial patterns.

Square waves, like all periodic stimuli, can be expressed as the weighted sum of sinusoidal components using the discrete Fourier series. A square wave, $sq(x)$, that oscillates between $+1$ and -1 with a frequency of f, can be expressed in terms of sinusoidal components as

$$sq(x) = \frac{4}{\pi} \sum_{n=0}^{\infty} \frac{1}{2n+1} \sin(2\pi(2n+1)fx) \qquad (7.9)$$

A square wave at frequency f is equal to the sum of a series of sinusoids at the odd-numbered frequencies, f, $3f$, $5f$, and so forth. The amplitude of the sinusoids declines with increasing frequency; the amplitude of the $3f$ sinusoid is one-third the amplitude of the component at f, the amplitude of the $5f$ sinusoid is one-fifth, and so forth. When the overall contrast of the square wave is very low, the amplitude of the higher-order terms is extremely small and they can be ignored. At low square-wave contrasts, only one or two sinusoidal terms are necessary to generate a pattern that is very similar in appearance to the true square wave. For low-contrast values, then, the square-wave pattern can be well approximated by the pattern

$$sq(x) \approx \frac{4}{\pi} \left[\sin(2\pi fx) + \frac{1}{3}\sin(2\pi(3f)x) + \frac{1}{5}\sin(2\pi(5f)x) \right] (7.10)$$

Campbell and Robson used square waves (and other periodic patterns) to test the multiresolution hypothesis in several ways. First, they measured the smallest contrast level at which observers could detect the square-wave grating. Notice that the amplitude of the lowest-frequency

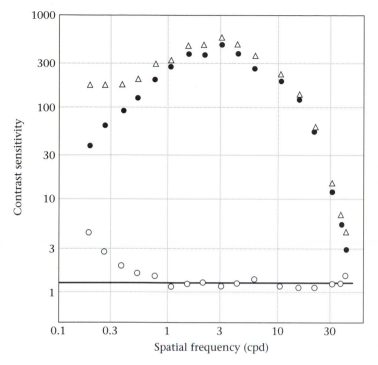

7.13 CONTRAST SENSITIVITY MEASURED USING SQUARE-WAVE GRATINGS greater than 1 cpd can be predicted from the contrast of the square-wave fundamental frequency. The open triangles and filled circles show contrast sensitivity to square waves and sine waves, respectively. The open circles show the ratio of contrast sensitivities at each spatial frequency. The solid line is drawn at a value of $4/\pi \approx 1.273$, the amplitude of a square-wave fundamental in a unit-contrast square wave. Source: Campbell and Robson, 1968.

component, which is called the **fundamental**, is $4/\pi$. Since the fundamental has the largest contrast, and since for patterns above 1 cpd sensitivity begins to decrease, Campbell and Robson argued that the neurons whose receptive-field size is well-matched to the fundamental component will signal the presence of the square wave first. If this is the most important term in defining the visibility of the square wave, then the threshold contrast of the square wave should be $4/\pi$ times the threshold contrast of a sinusoidal grating at the same frequency. The data in Figure 7.13 show contrast-sensitivity functions to both sinusoidal and square-wave targets, and the ratios of the contrast sensitivities. As predicted for patterns above 1 cpd, the ratio of contrasts at detection threshold is $1.28 \approx 4/\pi$.[6]

In addition to detection thresholds, Campbell and Robson also measured how well observers can discriminate between square waves and sinusoids. In these experiments, observers were presented with a square wave and a sine wave at frequency f. The two patterns were set in a contrast ratio of $4/\pi$, insuring that the fundamental component of the square wave and the sinusoid had equal contrast. The observers

---

[6] Campbell and Robson's square-wave detection experiment is a special case of the test-mixture experiment reviewed above. The results show that the $3f$ and higher-frequency components do not help the observer detect the square-wave grating. The more general question of how different frequency components combine is answered by test-mixture experiments, such as those performed by Graham and Nachmias (1971), in which the relative contrasts of all the components are varied freely.

adjusted the contrast of the two patterns, maintaining this fixed contrast ratio, until the square wave and sinusoid were barely discriminable. Since the contrast of the square-wave fundamental was held equal to the contrast of the sinusoid, the stimuli could only be discriminated based on the frequency components at $3f$ and higher.

Campbell and Robson found that observers discriminated between the sinusoid and the square wave when the contrast in the third harmonic reached its own threshold level. Their conclusions are based on the measurements shown in Figure 7.14. The filled circles show the contrast-sensitivity function. The open circles show the contrast of the square wave when it is just discriminable from the sinusoid. Evidently, the square-wave contrast needed to discriminate the two patterns exceeds the contrast needed to detect the square wave. However, we can explain the increased contrast by considering the contrast in the $3f$ component of the square wave. Recall that this component has one-third the contrast of the square wave. By shifting the square-wave discrimination data (open circles) to the left by a factor of 3 for spatial frequency, and downward by a factor of 3 for contrast, we compensate for these two factors. The open triangles show the open circles shifted in this way. The open triangles align with the original contrast-sensitivity measurements. From the alignment of the shifted discrimination data with the contrast-sensitivity measurements, we can conclude that the square wave can be discriminated from the sinusoid when the $3f$ component is visible at detection threshold.

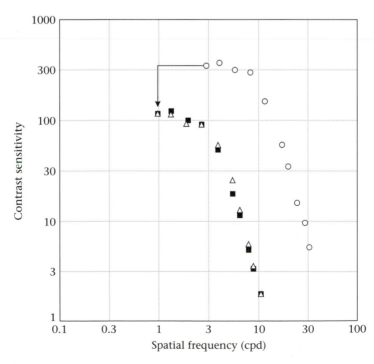

7.14 DISCRIMINATION OF SINUSOIDAL AND SQUARE-WAVE GRATINGS becomes possible when the third harmonic in the square wave reaches its own independent threshold. The open circles plot the contrast-sensitivity function. The open triangles show the contrast level at which a square wave can be discriminated from its fundamental frequency. The filled squares show the square-wave discrimination data shifted by a factor of 3 in both frequency and contrast. The alignment of the shifted curve with the contrast-sensitivity function suggests that square waves are discriminated when the third harmonic reaches its own threshold level. Source: Campbell and Robson, 1968.

Masking and Facilitation

Campbell and Robson's discrimination results are consistent with a multiresolution representation of the pattern. It is as if the fundamental and third harmonics are encoded by different component images. Because the amplitude of the fundamental component is the same in the square wave and sinusoid, the observer cannot use that information to discriminate between them. When the contrast of the third harmonic exceeds its own independent threshold, the observer can use the information and discriminate between the two patterns.

Although multiresolution representations are consistent with this result, we should ask whether the evidence is powerful. Specifically, we should ask whether the data might be explained by simpler theories. One more general hypothesis we should consider is this: observers discriminate between two spatial patterns, S and $S + \Delta S$, whenever ΔS is at its own threshold. This is the phenomenon that Campbell and Robson report when S and ΔS are low-contrast stimuli, widely separated in spatial frequency. Can subjects always discriminate S from $S + \Delta S$ when ΔS is at its own threshold? The answer is no.

In fact, the case described by Campbell and Robson is very rare. In many cases the two patterns S and $S + \Delta S$ cannot be discriminated even though ΔS, seen alone, is plainly visible. In this case, we say the stimulus S masks the stimulus ΔS. There are also cases when S and $S + \Delta S$ can be discriminated even though ΔS, seen alone, cannot be detected. In this case, we say the stimulus S facilitates the detection of ΔS. **Masking** and **facilitation** are quite common; the absence of masking and facilitation, as in the data reported by Campbell and Robson, is fairly unusual.

The images in Figure 7.15A demonstrate the phenomenon of visual masking. The pattern shown on the left is the target contrast pattern, ΔS. This contrast pattern is added into one of the masking patterns shown in the middle column. The masking pattern on the top is similar to the target in orientation, but different by a factor of 3 in spatial frequency. If you look carefully, you will see a difference between the mask alone and the mask plus the target. Specifically, near the center of the pattern several of the bars on the left appear darkened, and several bars on the right appear lightened. The second mask is similar to the target in both orientation and spatial frequency. In this case, it is harder to see the added contrast, ΔS. The third mask is similar in spatial frequency, but different in orientation. In this case, it is easy to detect the added target.

Figure 7.15B shows measurements of masking and facilitation between patterns with similar spatial frequency and the same orientation (Legge and Foley, 1980). Observers discriminated a mask, S, from a mask plus a 2-cpd sinusoidal target, $S + \Delta S$. The vertical axis measures the threshold contrast of the target needed to make the discrimination, and the horizontal axis measures the contrast of the masking stimulus

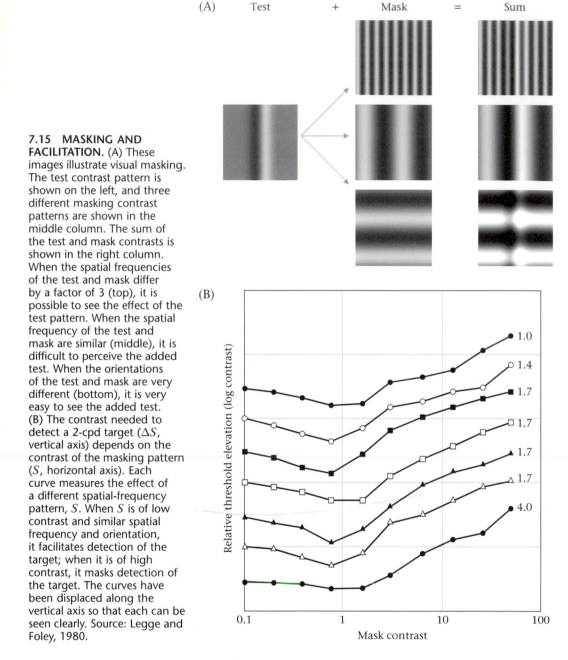

7.15 MASKING AND FACILITATION. (A) These images illustrate visual masking. The test contrast pattern is shown on the left, and three different masking contrast patterns are shown in the middle column. The sum of the test and mask contrasts is shown in the right column. When the spatial frequencies of the test and mask differ by a factor of 3 (top), it is possible to see the effect of the test pattern. When the spatial frequency of the test and mask are similar (middle), it is difficult to perceive the added test. When the orientations of the test and mask are very different (bottom), it is very easy to see the added test. (B) The contrast needed to detect a 2-cpd target (ΔS, vertical axis) depends on the contrast of the masking pattern (S, horizontal axis). Each curve measures the effect of a different spatial-frequency pattern, S. When S is of low contrast and similar spatial frequency and orientation, it facilitates detection of the target; when it is of high contrast, it masks detection of the target. The curves have been displaced along the vertical axis so that each can be seen clearly. Source: Legge and Foley, 1980.

S. The different curves show results for masks of various spatial frequencies. In general, the presence of S facilitates detection at low contrasts and masks detection at high contrasts. When the spatial frequencies of ΔS and S differ by a factor of 2, the amount of facilitation is small, though there is still considerable masking. Other experimental measurements show that when the spatial frequencies of the test and mask differ by a factor of 3, the effect of masking is reduced (DeValois, 1977a, b; Wilson et al., 1983). We will discuss the effect of orientation on masking later in this chapter.

The implications of these experiments for multiresolution models can be summarized in two parts. First, Campbell and Robson's data show no facilitation or masking when S and ΔS are low-contrast and widely separated in spatial frequency. Second, the Legge and Foley data show that for many stimulus pairs more similar in spatial frequency, S influences the visibility of an increment ΔS. Taken together, these results are consistent with the idea that stimuli with widely different spatial frequencies are encoded by different component images.

The Conceptual Advantage of Multiresolution Theories

Today, many different disciplines represent images using the multiresolution format; that is, by separating the original data into a collection of component images that differ mainly in their peak spatial-frequency selectivity. The multiresolution representation has opened up a large set of research issues, and I will discuss several of these in Chapter 8. While the behavioral evidence for multiresolution is interesting, it is hardly enough to explain why multiresolution hypotheses have led to something of a revolution in vision science. Rather, I think that it is the conceptual advantages of multiresolution representations, described below, that have made them an important part of vision science.

To understand these conceptual advantages, consider two problems that arise when theorists abandon the simple shift-invariance hypothesis. First, the set of possible encoding functions, even just linear encoding functions, becomes enormous. How can one choose among all of the possible linear transformations? Second, without shift-invariance, the theorist loses considerable predictive power, since many important derivations we have made depend on shift-invariance. For example, without shift-invariance we cannot derive the same quantitative prediction concerning the test-mixture threshold of a pair of sinusoids (Equation 7.8).

Simply abandoning shift-invariance opens up the set of possible encodings too far; theorists need some method of organizing their choices among the set of possible linear encodings. The multiresolution structure helps to organize the theorist's choices, because it provides some guidelines about how to specify the properties of the collection of shift-invariant calculations. The multiresolution organization helps the theorist reason and describe the properties of the linear encoding.

Even though multiresolution theories offer a general organizational scheme for the linear encoding, they still permit considerable flexibility in designing the properties of the component images. This flexibility is used to create component images whose response properties are analogous to the receptive field properties of different populations of cortical neurons. For example, orientation selectivity is an important property of many cortical neurons in area V1 (see Chapter 5). A simple shift-invariant theory, containing only a single convolution kernel, cannot represent orientation selectivity because if the convolution kernel is orientation selective, then the theory predicts that observer must be more sensitive to stimuli in that orientation. Since observers are not more sensitive to stimuli in one orientation than any other, oriented kernels are inappropriate for a single-resolution model. But it is possible to use orientation selective convolution kernels in multiresolution theories. As long as the collection of kernels at each resolution encodes all orientations, the model does not predict that sensitivity is better in any particular direction. For this reason, some theorists argue that there is a closer connection between the multiresolution theories and the cortical representation of pattern information.

The complexity of the calculations is an important challenge in developing multiresolution models of human pattern sensitivity. Figure 7.16 is an overview of a fairly simple multiresolution model de-

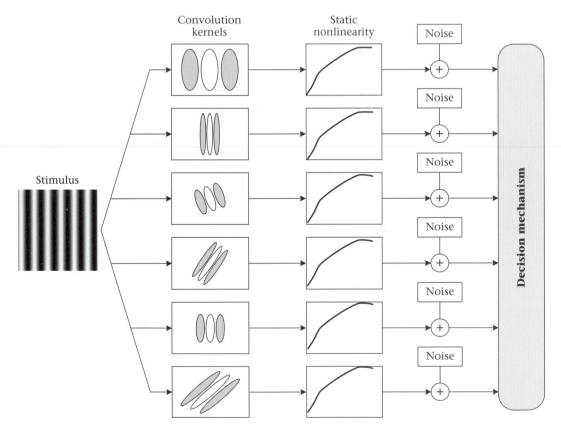

7.16 A MULTIRESOLUTION MODEL OF SPATIAL PATTERN SENSITIVITY. The stimulus is convolved with a collection of spatial filters with different peak spatial-frequency sensitivity. The filter outputs are modified by a nonlinear compression, noise is added, and the result is combined into a neural image. Source: Spillman and Werner, 1990.

scribed by Wilson and Regan (1984; see also Foley and Legge, 1981; Watson, 1983; Wilson and Gelb, 1984; Watt and Morgan, 1985). The initial image is transformed linearly into a neural image comprising a set of component images. In a recent implementation of this model, Wilson and Regan (1984) suggest that the neural image consists of 48 component images, organized by six spatial scales and eight orientations (i.e., all scales at all orientations). Each component image is followed by a static nonlinearity that is a modification of the vector-length measure. To see the development of an even more extensive model, the reader should consult the work by Watson and his colleagues (e.g., Watson, 1983; Watson and Ahumada, 1989). They have developed a substantially larger multiresolution model, using very sophisticated assumptions concerning the observer's internal noise and decision-making capabilities.

It is difficult to reason about the performance of these multiresolution models from first principles (but see Nielsen and Wandell, 1988; Bowne, 1990). Consequently, most of the predictions from these models are derived using computer simulation. Analyzing the model properties closely could easily fill up a book; in fact, Graham (1989) has completed an authoritative account of the present status of work in this area.

Challenges to Multiresolution Theory

Multiresolution theories are the main tool that theorists use to reason about pattern sensitivity. As we reviewed in the preceding section, multiresolution representations have many useful features, and they can be used to explain several important experimental results. There are, however, a number of empirical challenges to the multiresolution theories. In this section, I will describe a few of the measurements that represent a challenge to multiresolution theories of human pattern sensitivity. As you will see, many of these challenges derive from the same source as challenges to a shift-invariant theory: mixture experiments.

Pattern Adaptation to Mixtures

If we are to use pattern adaptation to justify multiresolution theories, then we should spend a little more time studying the general properties of pattern-adaptation measurements. Perhaps the first step we should take is to extend the pattern-adaptation measurements from simple sinusoids to more general patterns consisting of the mixture of two patterns.

Nachmias et al. (1973) performed a pattern-adaptation experiment using individual sinusoidal stimuli and their mixtures as adapting stimuli. The question they pose, as in all mixture experiments, is whether we can use the individual measurements to predict the behavioral performance in response to the sum of the stimuli.

The results of their measurements are shown in Figure 7.17. Each curve in the figure represents threshold elevation of sinusoidal test gratings at different spatial frequencies. The solid curve measures threshold elevation when the adapting stimulus was a 3-cpd sinusoidal grating. Confirming Blakemore and Campbell (1969), there is considerable threshold elevation at 3 cpd and less adaptation at both higher and lower spatial frequencies. The dashed curve measures threshold elevation when the adapting field was a 9-cpd grating. For historical reasons, the contrast of this grating was one-third the contrast of the grating at the fundamental. Even at this reduced contrast, the 9-cpd grating also causes a significant threshold elevation for 9-cpd test stimuli.

The dot-dash line shows the threshold elevation following adaptation to the mixture of the two adapting stimuli. For this observer, adaptation to the mixture shows no threshold elevation to test gratings at 9 cpd. For all of the observers in this study, the threshold elevation at 9 cpd following adaptation to the mixture is smaller than the threshold elevation following adaptation to the 3-cpd adapting stimulus. The mixture of 3- and 9-cpd stimuli is *less* potent in terms of threshold elevation than a 9-cpd stimulus alone.

This result is difficult to reconcile with the simple interpretation of adaptation and spatial frequency channels in Figure 7.12. If the adaptation to 3 cpd stimulates a different set of neurons from adaptation to 9 cpd, then why should adapting to 3-cpd and 9-cpd stimuli improve sensitivity at 3 cpd? I am unaware of any explanations of this phenomenon that also preserve the basic logical structure of the multiresolution representations.

The results of these mixture experiments should motivate us to rethink the basic mechanisms of pattern adaptation. If we plan to use this experimental method to provide support for a notion as significant as

7.17 PATTERN ADAPTATION MIXTURE EXPERIMENTS. These curves measures log threshold contrast elevation at various test frequencies following adaptation. The curves show the results following adaptation to a 3-cpd sinusoid (solid line), a 9-cpd sinusoid (dashed line), and their sum (dot-dash line). Threshold elevation following adaptation to the sum is smaller than threshold elevation following adaptation to the individual components. Source: Nachmias et al., 1973.

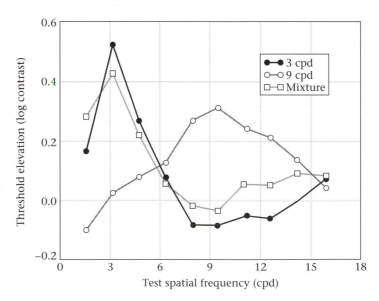

multiresolution representation of pattern, then we should understand the adaptation phenomenon. Figure 7.18 illustrates one of the difficulties we face when we try to integrate results from detection and adaptation experiments. When we group results from detection and adaptation experiments, we assume implicitly that the visual mechanisms that limit detection are the same as those that alter visual sensitivity following pattern adaptation. But behavioral measurements provide no direct evidence that the neurons that limit sensitivity are the same as those that underlie adaptation.

The diagram in Figure 7.18 illustrates one way in which this assumption may fail. Suppose that neurons indicated as "Group T" are located early in the visual pathways and that these neurons are noisy and have low contrast gain. If these are the least reliable neurons in the pathway, then the sensitivity may be limited by their properties. In that case, we can improve the observer's detection performance by testing with stimuli that are well matched to response properties of the Group T neurons.

We have assumed that the effects of pattern adaptation are due to neural fatigue caused by strong stimulus excitation. Because the Group T neurons have relatively low gain, they will not respond very strongly

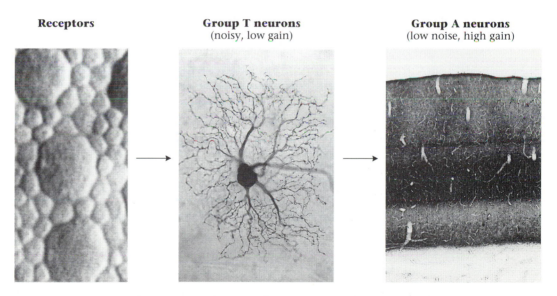

Receptors   **Group T neurons**   **Group A neurons**
                (noisy, low gain)   (low noise, high gain)

7.18   THE NEURONS THAT LIMIT DETECTION AND THOSE THAT CAUSE PATTERN ADAPTATION may not be the same. For example, one group of neurons (Group T) may be noisy and have low contrast gain. Because of their noise properties, these neurons would limit detection threshold. Neurons in a second population (Group A) may integrate the responses of the first group of neurons and have high contrast gain. Because of their high gain, this group of neurons may fatigue easily and be the neural basis of pattern adaptation. If the neural units that limit these two types of behavioral responses are different, then the spatial receptive fields of neurons that are inferred from detection and pattern-adaptation experiments may well be different. Sources: Left, courtesy of Christine Curcio; center, from Yamashita and Wässle, 1991; right, courtesy of Jennifer Lund.

to most stimuli, and consequently they may not be susceptible to pattern adaptation. Instead, it may be that another group of neurons, "Group A" neurons, are the ones most influenced by the adapting pattern. I have shown these neurons in Figure 7.18 at a later stage in the visual pathways. The spatial properties of the pattern-adaptation experiment (for example, the way test sensitivity varies with the spatial properties of the adapting pattern) may be due to the spatial receptive-field properties of the Group A neurons. Group T and Group A neurons may have quite different spatial receptive fields.[7]

From this analysis, it should be clear that the spatial properties of the neural encoding derived from pattern adaptation may differ from the spatial properties of the neural encoding derived from detection tasks. To argue that the mechanisms limiting detection and mediating pattern adaptation are the same, we must find behavioral experimental measurements that support this point. In that case, we can piece together the results from detection and pattern adaptation to infer the organization within multiresolution models.

Masking with Mixtures

In Campbell and Robson's (1968) discrimination experiment, the observer was asked to distinguish between two stimuli S and $S + \Delta S$, where S and ΔS effectively were sinusoidal patterns. Campbell and Robson found that when S and ΔS were sinusoidal stimuli at well-separated spatial frequencies the two patterns were discriminable when ΔS was at its own threshold. In reviewing their experiments we considered how masking depends on the relative spatial frequency of the test and masking patterns (see Figure 7.15).

The data in Figure 7.19 show how masking depends on the relative orientation of the target and masker (Phillips and Wilson, 1984). In this study, the masker S and test ΔS were at the same spatial frequency. Phillips and Wilson measured the contrast needed in the test to discriminate $S + \Delta S$ from S for various orientations of the masker. The horizontal axis in Figure 7.19 measures the orientation of the masking stimulus, S. The vertical axis measures the threshold elevation of the test. As the difference in orientation between the test stimulus ΔS and masking stimulus S increases, the masking effect decreases. In this data set, when the orientation difference exceeds 40 degrees, $S + \Delta S$ can be discriminated from S when ΔS is at its own threshold level.

From these measurements, one might suspect that one-dimensional contrast patterns separated in orientation by 40 degrees are encoded by separate neurons. Experimental results like these might be used to deter-

---

[7] You should also consider the possibility that the basic mechanism of neural fatigue is not the main source of pattern adaptation. Recently, Barlow and Foldiak (1989) have put forward an entirely different explanation of pattern adaptation that is based on learning principles, not on neural fatigue. While the work on this topic is too preliminary to include in this volume, I think this line of research has great potential for clarifying many visual phenomena.

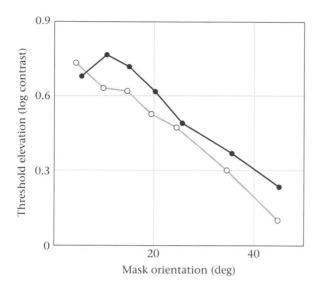

7.19 ORIENTATION TUNING IN THE MASKING EXPERIMENT. Threshold elevation to a 2-cpd test as a function of the orientation of a 2-cpd masking stimulus for two observers. The data include only maskers with positive orientations since masking is symmetric with respect to the orientation of the masking stimulus. Source: Phillips and Wilson, 1984.

mine the orientation-selectivity properties of convolution kernels used in multiresolution models.

Results from test-mixture experiments based on visual masking call the validity of this conclusion into question. Derrington and Henning (1989) report mixture experiments in which they measured threshold elevation using two separate masking patterns and their mixture. The individual masking patterns were 3-cpd sinusoidal gratings; one grating was oriented at +67.5 degrees and the other at −67.5 degrees relative to vertical. They measured the effect of these masking patterns on a variety of vertically oriented sinusoidal gratings.

If the two masking stimuli are represented by neurons that are different from those that represent the vertical test patterns, then the superposition of these two masking stimuli should not influence the target visibility. The data in Figure 7.20 show that this is not the case. The mixture of the two masking patterns is a potent mask even though each alone fails to have any effect.[8]

Multiresolution Theory: Current Status

The multiresolution representations are a very important theoretical tool. They help us think about the general problem of pattern sensitivity, and they provide a framework for organizing computational models of pattern sensitivity and other pattern-related tasks. There is some evidence that these representations are an important part of the human visual pathways. But there is a bewildering array of experimental methods, ranging from detection to pattern adaptation to masking, whose

---

[8] Similar difficulties in interpreting the effects of masking, but with respect to mixtures of sinusoidal gratings, have been studied by Nachmias and Rogowitz (1983) and Perkins and Landy (1991).

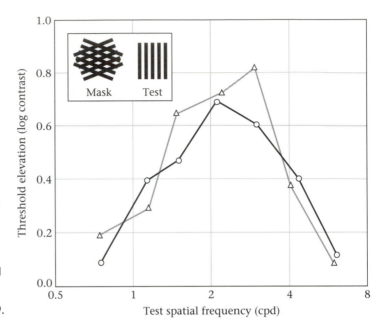

7.20 MASKING MIXTURE EXPERIMENTS. When a test and masking grating are separated in orientation by 67.5 degrees, the masker has no influence on the visibility of the test. But the combination of two masking gratings at 67.5 degrees, neither of which alone has any effect, acts as a powerful masker. The solid and shaded lines show results from two different subjects. Source: Derrington and Henning, 1989.

results are inconsistent with the central notions of multiresolution representations. As we have seen, mixture experiments using pattern adaptation and masking are difficult to understand if we believe that components of the image associated with spatial frequency and orientation bands are encoded by independent sets of neurons.

The conflicting pattern of experimental results show us that we have yet to achieve a complete understanding of the basic neural processes that cause adaptation and masking. Also, we do not understand how these neural processes are related to the neural processes that limit pattern sensitivity. Achieving this understanding is important because these experiments provide the key results that support multiresolution representations. Perhaps, once we understand the properties of these separate experimental methods more fully, we will understand the role of multiresolution representations and find a way to make sense of the complete set of experimental findings. Up to this point, I think you should see that we are well under way in understanding these issues, but many questions remain unanswered.

Pattern Sensitivity and Other Viewing Parameters

Next, we will review how pattern sensitivity depends on other aspects of the viewing conditions, such as the mean illumination level, the temporal parameters of the stimulus, and the wavelength properties of the pattern. In each of these cases, we will use some form of the contrast-sensitivity function as a summary of the observer's behavior.

In the remainder of this chapter, the contrast-sensitivity function plays a role that differs from the way we have used it up to now. To this point, I have emphasized the special role of the contrast-sensitivity function in linear-systems theories. If we understand the structure of the data well enough, then the contrast-sensitivity function can be used to predict sensitivity to many other different patterns. A clear example of this is Schade's use of the contrast-sensitivity function: if visual sensitivity is limited by a shift-invariant neural image, then we can use the contrast-sensitivity function to predict sensitivity to any other pattern.

We do not have yet a complete theory that permits us to use the contrast-sensitivity function to characterize behavior generally. My purpose in continuing to treat pattern sensitivity in terms of the contrast-sensitivity function now is that it serves as a summary measure of visual pattern sensitivity. Hence, in the remainder of this chapter, we will not look at the contrast-sensitivity function as a complete description of the observer's pattern sensitivity. Rather, we will use it as a descriptive tool to help us learn something about the general pattern sensitivity of the visual system.

Part of the reason for standardizing on the contrast-sensitivity function is that the measure is used widely in both physiology and psychophysics. Hence, behavioral measurements of the contrast-sensitivity function can provide us with a measure that we can compare with the neural response at different points in the visual pathway. If a particular class of neurons, say, retinal ganglion cells, limits visual sensitivity, we should expect behavioral contrast-sensitivity curves and neural contrast-sensitivity curves to covary as we change the experimental conditions.

Light Adaptation

Figure 7.21 shows that the contrast-sensitivity function changes when it is measured at different mean background intensities. The curve in the lower left shows a contrast-sensitivity function measured at a low mean luminance level (9×10^{-4} Trolands), when rods dominate vision.[9] Under these conditions the contrast sensitivity function peaks at 1–3 cpd and the curve is lowpass rather than bandpass. The curve on the upper right shows a contrast-sensitivity function measured on a bright photopic background, one million times more intense. Under these conditions the peak of the contrast-sensitivity function is near 6–8 cpd, and the shape of the curve is bandpass. At mean background intensities higher than 1,000 Trolands, the contrast-sensitivity function remains unchanged (Westheimer, 1960; van Nes and Bouman, 1967).

The change in the shape of the contrast-sensitivity function is consistent with a few simple imaging principles. The first principle concerns the importance of achieving an adequate signal under the

[9] The Troland (Td) is a unit of measurement that represents the intensity of light in the retinal image. To measure in units of Troland it is necessary to correct for the pupil diameter. One Troland is produced on the retina when the eye is looking at a surface of 1 cd/m^2 through a pupil of area 1 mm^2.

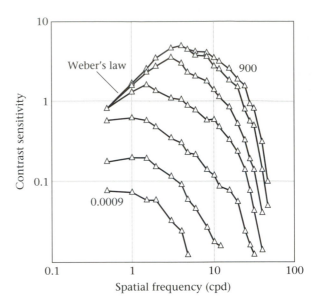

7.21 HUMAN CONTRAST SENSITIVITY VARIES WITH MEAN FIELD LUMINANCE.
Each curve shows a contrast-sensitivity function at a different mean field luminance level ranging from 9×10^{-4} Trolands to 9×10^{2} Trolands, increasing by a factor of ten from curve to curve. The stimulus consisted of monochromatic light at 525 nm. At the lowest level, under scotopic conditions, the contrast-sensitivity function is lowpass and peaks near 1 cpd. On intense photopic backgrounds the curve is bandpass and peaks near 8 cpd. Above these mean background levels, the contrast-sensitivity function remains constant. Source: van Nes and Bouman, 1967.

ambient viewing conditions. At very low light levels, the observer needs to integrate light across the retina in order to achieve a reliable signal. If an observer must spatially average the light signal to obtain a reliable signal, then the observer cannot also resolve high spatial frequencies. Consequently, under dim, scotopic conditions observers should have poor sensitivity to high spatial frequencies, as they do. On more intense backgrounds, when quanta are plentiful, observers can integrate information over smaller spatial regions, and spatial-frequency resolution improves.

The second principle concerns the importance of contrast, rather than absolute intensity, for visual processing. Figure 7.21 shows that contrast sensitivity of low-spatial-frequency patterns (below 1 cpd) rises with mean luminance and then becomes constant. The range in which contrast sensitivity becomes constant is called the Weber's law regime. For low-spatial-frequency patterns, Weber's law is a good description of the results. At higher spatial frequencies, contrast sensitivity continues to rise with the mean luminance. For these patterns Weber's law is not a precise description of behavioral sensitivity.

Even though Weber's law is imprecise, it does contain a kernel of truth. Consider the overall dynamic ranges we are measuring. The background intensities used in these experiments vary by a factor of one million (i.e., six orders of magnitude). Yet, the contrast sensitivity generally varies by only a factor of 20 or so (only one order of magnitude), while sensitivity to absolute light level varies by four or five orders of magnitude. The pattern of results suggests that the visual system preserves contrast sensitivity, as suggested by Weber's law, rather than absolute intensity. The visual system succeeds quite well at preserving contrast sensitivity at low spatial frequencies, and it comes close at high spatial frequencies. The significance of contrast rather than absolute intensity for vision confirms the general view we have adopted, beginning with measurements of contrast sensitivity in retinal ganglion cells and cat behavior described in Chapter 5.

Spatiotemporal Contrast Sensitivity

Figure 7.4 showed several contrast-sensitivity functions measured using contrast-reversing sinusoids. Those data illustrate how the contrast-sensitivity function varies when we measure at a few different temporal frequencies. Figure 7.22 contains a surface plot that represents how spatial contrast-sensitivity functions vary when we measure at many different temporal frequencies. One axis of the graph shows the spatial frequency of the test pattern; a second axis shows the test pattern's temporal frequency. The height of the surface represents the observer's contrast sensitivity. The surface represents the observer's **spatiotemporal**

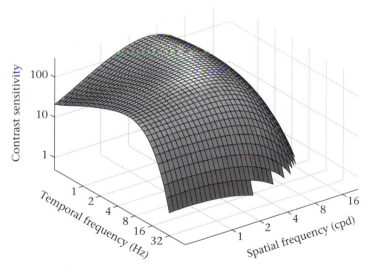

7.22 HUMAN SPATIOTEMPORAL CONTRAST-SENSITIVITY FUNCTION. The two lower axes represent the spatial and temporal frequencies of a contrast-reversing pattern; the vertical axis represents the observer's contrast sensitivity to each of the contrast-reversing patterns. The data used to estimate this surface were made on a mean background luminance of 1,000 Trolands. Curves running parallel to the spatial-frequency axis define a set of spatial contrast-sensitivity functions measured at different temporal frequencies (cf. Figure 7.4). Curves running parallel to the temporal-frequency axis represent the temporal contrast sensitivity measured at different spatial frequencies. Human spatiotemporal contrast sensitivity is not space–time separable. Source: Kelly, 1966, 1979a, b.

contrast-sensitivity function. This single surface represents a large range of spatial and temporal contrast-sensitivity functions. Paths through the surface running parallel to the spatial frequency axis represent the spatial contrast-sensitivity function; paths through the surface running parallel to the temporal frequency axis represent temporal contrast-sensitivity functions. Kelly (1979a, b) derived the analytical curve that yields the surface shape from an extensive set of psychophysical measurements.

If the spatial contrast-sensitivity functions had the same shape up to a scale factor, and similarly for the temporal contrast-sensitivity functions, we would say that human spatiotemporal contrast sensitivity is space–time separable.[10] From the shape of the contrast-sensitivity surface, it is apparent that the spatial contrast-sensitivity curves have different shapes when measured at different temporal frequencies (cf. Figure 7.4). Hence, human contrast sensitivity is not space–time separable (Kelly and Burbeck, 1984).

There are several considerations that make space–time separability an important property. First, in Chapter 5, I explained that only space–time separable systems have unique spatial and temporal sensitivity functions. When a system is not separable, it does not have a unique contrast-sensitivity function; rather it has a different function for each temporal measurement condition.

Second, space–time separability is significant because it simplifies computations and representations. For example, suppose we want to represent the spatiotemporal contrast-sensitivity function at $N_s = 60$ spatial and $N_t = 60$ temporal frequencies. If the contrast-sensitivity function is not separable, we may need to store as many as $N_s \times N_t = 3,600$ values of the sensitivity function. But, if the function is space–time separable, we need to represent only the the spatial contrast-sensitivity function and the temporal contrast-sensitivity function ($N_s \times N_t = 120$). Sensitivity to any space–time pattern can be calculated from the products of these two functions.

While the observer's behavior as a whole is not space–time separable, it is not necessary that we forgo all of the advantages of space–time separability. We may be able to describe the observer's performance as if it depends on the combination of a few space–time-separable mechanisms.[11] We first saw this approach in Chapter 5 when we studied the receptive field of retinal ganglion cells. Although their receptive fields are not space–time separable, we could model them as comprising two space–time separable components, namely, the center and surround.

Kelly (1971, 1979a, b; Kelly and Burbeck, 1984) has modeled the human spatiotemporal contrast-sensitivity function as if visual sensitivity is limited by contributions from two space–time separable components. This description of contrast sensitivity is a single-resolution description,

---

[10] See Chapter 5 for a discussion of space–time separability of receptive fields.
[11] Indeed, it is possible to show this is always a theoretical possibility. The result follows from an important representation in linear algebra called the *singular value decomposition*.

much like Schade's. The convolution kernel of the system is composed of a central and a surround region, much like a difference of a Gaussian, in which the two components are each space–time separable. When the two components are summed, as for retinal ganglion cells, the resulting convolution is not separable. Using suitable parameters for the Gaussians and temporal parameters, it is possible to approximate the contrast-sensitivity surface by computing the output of the convolution kernel. This single-resolution convolution kernel provides a convenient method for computing the surface, but as we have seen in other parts of this chapter the single-resolution system does not generalize well to predict sensitivity to other space–time patterns formed by the mixture of harmonic functions.

Temporal Sensitivity and Mean Luminance

The **temporal contrast-sensitivity function** measures sensitivity to temporal sinusoidal variations in the stimulus contrast. Figure 7.23A shows measurements of the temporal contrast-sensitivity function at a variety of mean background intensities.

First, consider how contrast sensitivity to the lowest temporal frequencies varies with background intensity. At the very lowest back-

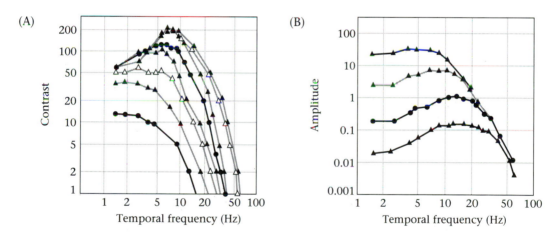

7.23 HUMAN TEMPORAL CONTRAST SENSITIVITY measured at various mean background illuminance levels. (A) Temporal contrast sensitivity. The spatial pattern was a 2-degree disk presented on a large background. Each curve measures contrast sensitivity (vertical axis) as a function of temporal frequency (horizontal axis). The curves show measurements on a variety of backgrounds. In sequence from lowest curve to highest, the mean luminance was 0.375, 1, 3.75, 10, 37.5, 100, 1,000, and 10,000 Trolands. Once the background illumination reaches roughly 5 Trolands, contrast sensitivity to low temporal frequencies remains constant, consistent with Weber's law. (B) Temporal amplitude sensitivity. The spatial pattern was a 60-degree disk. Each curve measures the threshold amplitude, not contrast, as a function of temporal frequency. The mean background levels are 0.85, 7.1, 8.5, and 850 Trolands. Notice that at high temporal frequencies the threshold amplitude appears to fall along a single curve, independent of the mean background level. This convergence is consistent with a purely linear response, involving no light adaptation, for high-temporal-frequency stimuli. Sources: A, de Lange, 1958; B, Kelly, 1961.

ground levels, contrast sensitivity increases with mean luminance. Once the mean background luminance reaches 5 Trolands, contrast sensitivity to low frequencies changes by less than a factor of 2 while the background intensity changes over a factor of 100. For low temporal frequencies, contrast sensitivity remains relatively constant across changes in the mean background intensity. This is the form of light adaptation called Weber's law.

Second, consider the contrast sensitivity at high temporal frequencies. For these tests, contrast sensitivity increases systematically at all background levels, a deviation from Weber's law. The nature of the deviation can be clarified by replotting the data as shown in Figure 7.23B where sensitivity is plotted as a function of the *amplitude* of the high-frequency flicker, not contrast (which is the amplitude divided by the mean level). When plotted as a function of amplitude, the temporal flicker sensitivity curves converge at high temporal frequencies. The convergence of the functions measured at many different mean luminance levels implies that sensitivity to high-temporal-frequency signals is predicted by the amplitude of the signal, not its contrast. This is the behavior one expects from a pure linear system, without light adaptation. In this temporal frequency range, then, Weber's law does not describe the data well at all. These data show that light adaptation does not play a significant role in determining the visibility of high-temporal-frequency flicker.

Pattern–Color Sensitivity

There is a very powerful relationship between the wavelength composition of a target and our sensitivity to pattern. In Chapter 2 we reviewed one of the most important factors that relates wavelength and pattern sensitivity: the chromatic aberration of the optics. The consequences of chromatic aberration are quite significant for the organization of the entire visual pathways. For example, based on the measurements we reviewed in earlier chapters, the chromatic aberration of the lens, coupled with the wide spacing of the S-cones, implies that a signal beginning in the S-cones can only represent signals less than 3–4 cpd (cf. Figure 2.23). This compares to the basic optical and sampling limit of nearly 50 cpd for signals initiated by a mixture of L- and M-cones. The consequences of these neural limitations and others can be measured easily in people's ability to detect, discriminate, and perceive colored patterns: people's ability to resolve short-wavelength patterns is very poor (Williams, 1986).

While it is easy to understand some of the relationship between pattern and color in terms of the optics and the cone mosaic, the limitations that relate color and pattern are best understood by thinking about the neural pathways that encode color, rather than the cones. A great deal of physiological and behavioral evidence (see Chapters 6 and 9) demonstrates that we perceive color via neural pathways that combine the signals from the three cone classes. One pathway carries the sum of the cone signals, while other pathways, called **color opponent-pathways**, carry signals representing the difference between cone signals. Signals are represented on these pathways at very different spatial resolution (Noorlander and Koenderink, 1983; Mullen, 1985; Poirson and Wandell, 1993; Sekiguchi et al., 1993b).

High-spatial-frequency signals (20–60 cpd) appear to excite only the pathway formed by summing the cone signals. We experience these patterns as light–dark modulations around the mean luminance. Spatial frequency patterns below 12 cpd can excite a pathway that encodes the difference between L and M signals. Only the lowest spatial frequencies excite the third pathway, a pathway that includes the S-cones.

These effects have been roughly understood for many years. For example, the color television broadcast system that is transmitted into many homes is organized into three color signals that correspond to a light–dark signal and two color-difference signals. Only the light–dark signal includes high-spatial-frequency information about the image; the two color channels represent only low-spatial-frequency information. This representation is very efficient for transmission, since leaving out high spatial frequencies in two of the signals permits a large compression in the bandwidth of the signal. Despite the missing spatial-frequency information, the broadcast images do not appear spatially blurred. The reason is that the high-spatial-frequency color information that is omitted in the transmission is not ordinarily perceived.

The color pathways also differ in their temporal sensitivity. Perhaps the most important observation is based on the **flicker photometry experiment**. In this experimental procedure, a pair of test lights alternate with one another. When the lights are alternated slowly the pattern appears to change between the colors of the two lights. When the lights alternate rapidly, observers fail to see the color modulation, and all differences appear as a light–dark modulation upon a steady colored background. Our temporal resolution for distinguishing blue–yellow flicker is poorest, that for red–green is in the middle, and that for light–dark is best.

The relationship between spatial resolution and temporal resolution suggests a hypothesis that we considered in Chapter 3: namely, that spatial and temporal resolution covary because they are both related through the rigid motion of objects. If the most important source of temporal variation in the image is due to motions of the eye or motions of an object, temporal-frequency and spatial-frequency resolution should covary. At a single velocity, the motion of a low-spatial-frequency image produces a slower temporal variation than motion of a high-spatial-frequency image. Hence, in those wavelength bands where only low spatial frequencies are imaged, the visual system may not require high-temporal-frequency resolution.

I have summarized the covariation of color, space, and time in Color Plate 3. The image represents how color appearance varies across different spatiotemporal frequency ranges. We are trichromatic only in a relatively small range of low spatial and temporal frequencies represented near the origin of the figure. As the spatial or temporal frequency increases we fail to see blue–yellow variation, and vision becomes dichromatic. At the higher spatial and temporal frequencies we are monochromatic, and we see only light–dark variation.

Retinal Eccentricity

The contrast-sensitivity measurements we have reviewed were all made using small patches of sinusoidal grating presented within the central few degrees of the visual field. As one measures contrast sensitivity at increasingly peripheral locations in the visual field, sensitivity decreases.[12] There are a number of neural factors that conspire to reduce both absolute sensitivity and spatial resolution. The density of the cone mosaic falls off rapidly as a function of visual eccentricity, so that there are fewer sensors available to encode the signal. The retinal ganglion cell density falls as well, as does the amount of cortical area devoted to representing the periphery. Approximately half of primary visual cortex represents only the central 10 degrees of the visual field (314 square degrees), while the remaining half of visual cortex must represent the rest of the visual field, which extends to a radius of 80 degrees (20,000 square degrees; see Chapters 5 and 6).

Figure 7.24A shows a set of contrast-sensitivity functions measured using a small grating patch at several different visual eccentricities. The top curve shows the observer's contrast sensitivity in the fovea. The observer's peak contrast sensitivity is 100 for gratings near 5–8 cpd, meaning that the observer can detect these at 1-percent contrast. In the fovea, the observer can resolve gratings as fine as 40–60 cpd. When the same stimulus is used to make measurements in the visual periphery, observers become less sensitive in all respects, so that stimuli 30 degrees in the periphery have a peak contrast sensitivity of 3 and an upper limit of 2 cpd.

We do not ordinarily notice this decrease in contrast sensitivity. When asked, most people believe that their spatial resolution is fairly uniform over a much wider extent of the image than just 2 degrees (their thumb joint at arms length). Yet, from the curves in Figure 7.24A, it is plain that our visual resolution is very poor by 7–10 degrees (a fist at arms length). Hence, our impression of seeing sharply over a large spatial extent must be due in part to our ability to integrate spatial information using eye movements.

Rovamo et al. (1978; Rovamo and Virsu, 1979; Virsu and Rovamo, 1979) suggested that the decrease in contrast sensitivity with eccentric viewing can be explained quantitatively by the reduced representation

---

[12] The quality of the optics does not appear to decline significantly over the first 20 degress of visual angle (Jennings and Charman, 1981).

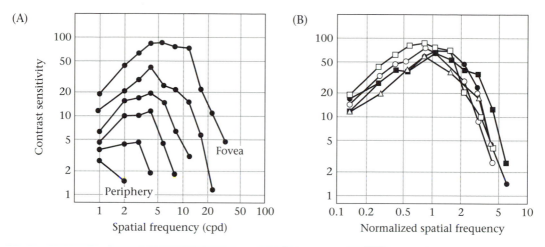

7.24 THE CONTRAST-SENSITIVITY FUNCTION VARIES WITH RETINAL ECCENTRICITY. (A) Contrast-sensitivity functions measured using a 1 degree × 2 degree grating patch at retinal eccentricities of 0, 1.5, 4, 7.5, 14, and 30 degrees are shown. Contrast sensitivity measured using this stimulus is highest in the fovea and falls dramatically with retinal eccentricity. (B) Contrast-sensitivity functions measured with the test stimulus scaled in size and spatial frequency in order to compensate roughly for the reduced cortical area devoted to different retinal eccentricities. Source: Rovamo et al., 1978.

of the visual field in the cortex. Qualitatively, the decrease in contrast sensitivity and the coarse neural representation of the periphery do parallel one another. The rough agreement between these factors is demonstrated by the results in Figure 7.24B. These contrast-sensitivity functions, like those in Figure 7.24A, were made at different retinal eccentricities. For these measurements, however, the size and spatial frequency of the grating patch were scaled to compensate for the reduced cortical representation at that retinal eccentricity. When the size and spatial frequency of the stimulus are adjusted to compensate for the reduced cortical representation, the contrast-sensitivity functions become fairly similar.

Visual performance deteriorates with eccentricity for all known spatial-acuity tasks and spatial-localization tasks, which we will review later in this chapter; however, the performance decrease as a function of retinal eccentricity varies considerably across observers and across tasks. The reduced representation of the periphery is present in all of the neural representations beginning with the photoreceptors and continuing into the central nervous system. The variance in observers' performance coupled with the wide number of neural representations with similar decrease in the peripheral representation, make it difficult to attribute the decline in performance to any single anatomical structure. The decline of acuity with eccentric viewing is an important and widespread feature of the visual system; it may not be possible to localize its cause to a single site in the visual pathways (e.g., Westheimer, 1979; Levi et al., 1985; Legge et al., 1987; Yap et al., 1987; Farrell and Desmarais, 1990).

Linking Hypotheses

We have now reviewed several instances in which the variation of behavioral contrast-sensitivity functions with stimulus conditions is similar to the variation of retinal ganglion cell responses. These correlations suggest that there is a causal relationship between the retinal ganglion cells' receptive fields and the behavioral measurements. But such a relationship is quite difficult to prove with the certainty that we would like to have. At this point, I think it is worth reviewing what we have learned about making such inferences.

Behavioral and neural theorizing supplement one another. Psychophysicists measure behavioral responses and then build theories about neural mechanisms. The properties of these theoretical mechanisms summarize the data and lead to new behavioral predictions. Neurophysiological measurements tell us about the neural activity directly; but we must theorize about how the neural activity influences behavior. Each field contributes part of the information about visual function.

In an influential chapter in his book, Brindley (1970) called hypotheses that connect measurements in the two fields **linking hypotheses**. He took a very conservative view concerning the type of experiments that could be used to reason about physiology from performance. His comments initiated a discussion that continues to this day (Teller, 1990; Westheimer, 1990). Brindley felt that the only truly secure argument connecting physiology and perception is this (p. 133):

> . . . whenever two stimuli cause physically indistinguishable signals to be sent from the sense organs to the brain, the sensations produced by these stimuli, as reported by the subject in words, symbols, or actions, must also be indistinguishable.

By stating his hypothesis clearly and forcefully, Brindley has drawn a great deal of attention to the problem of linking results between the separate disciplines. My purpose in writing this section is to question whether he may have succeeded too well; the emphasis on linking results from behavioral and physiological studies sometimes distracts us from making sure that the experimental logic within each discipline is complete.

We establish the most secure links between behavior and physiology when we first understand the separate measurements very well. For example, the relationship between the color-matching functions and photopigment sensitivities are strong because we have extensive quantitative studies, ranging over many measurement conditions, that tell us about each set of measurement conditions on their own. The color-matching experiment stands no matter what the photochemist observes, and the cone photopigment measurements stand no matter what the psychophysicist observes. Because each set of results stands on its own, we can feel confident that their relationship is a strong case for a connection between the two fields. If we require that the analysis within each discipline stands on its own, then when it comes time to join the two sets of observations we can have greater confidence in the link.

I mean to contrast the view stated here with an alternative approach in which the behaviorist uses the discovery of a particular neural response as the logical basis for a purely behavioral experiment; or conversely, the case in which a physiologist explains a set of recordings in terms of some potentially related behavioral measure. Such ideas may be useful in the background to help formulate specific experimental measurements. However, the logic of theories and experiments based on a web of interconnections from behavior to physiology often serve to entangle our thinking.

Given this standard, what should we think about the connection between behavioral contrast sensitivity and neural receptive fields? In this chapter we have found that there is a powerful theory underlying behavioral contrast-sensitivity functions. This theory is a good match to the logic of receptive-field organization we reviewed in earlier chapters. The psychophysical results based on the contrast-sensitivity function, however, do not fully support the basic theory. We cannot yet generalize from contrast-sensitivity functions to sensitivity to other stimuli. Hence, the association between receptive-field properties and contrast-sensitivity functions are far more tentative than the connection between the color-matching functions and the photopigment spectral sensitivities.

Having stated this limitation in our current understanding, I must add that I do not think we should be discouraged. The similarities between the properties of the contrast-sensitivity functions and neural receptive fields are too striking to ignore. By continuing to improve on the models for behavior and receptive fields separately, the links we forge and the quantitative comparisons we make could well turn out to form a complete model, linking behavioral pattern sensitivity and neural receptive fields.

Spatial Localization

In this section we will review how well human observers can localize the position of a target. Wulfing (1892) showed that human observers can make surprisingly fine discriminations between the positions of two objects. Observers can reliably distinguish spatial offsets between a pair of lines as small as one fifth the width of a single cone photoreceptor. Moreover, people can distinguish this spatial offset even when the objects are moving (Westheimer, 1979).

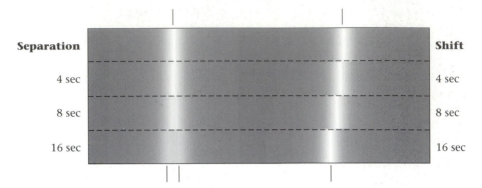

7.25 A COMPARISON OF LOCALIZATION AND SPATIAL-RESOLUTION EXPERIMENTS. In a two-line spatial-acuity experiment, the observer distinguishes between a stimulus consisting of a single line from a stimulus consisting of a pair of lines separated by a small amount. The images on the left side show the estimated retinal light distribution of a reference line and of three pairs of lines separated by increasing amounts. In a localization experiment, the observer distinguishes the position of a single line from the position of a displaced line. The images on the right side of the figure show a reference line and the estimated retinal light distribution of three offset lines.

The ability to discriminate between targets at different spatial positions is an aspect of human spatial resolution. It is important to recognize that that the ability to localize a target is a different kind of resolution from the spatial resolution we measure when we ask observers to discriminate a pattern from a uniform background.[13] The differences between the tasks are illustrated in Figure 7.25. The left side of the image in Figure 7.25 shows the estimated retinal light distributions of several stimuli a subject might be shown in a spatial resolution task. In this experiment, the subject must discriminate between the light distribution of a single line (top left) from the light distribution of a line-pair in which the two lines are separated by a small amount (bottom left). In this task, the stimuli are all centered at the same point, so there is no difference in where they are located. The right side of the image in Figure 7.25 shows the retinal light distributions of stimuli a subject might be shown in a spatial-localization task. In this experiment, the subject must discriminate the position of the retinal light distribution created by a reference line (top right) from the positions of the light distributions of a line that is offset (bottom right).

Westheimer and McKee (1977) measured observers' ability to localize a line (Figure 7.26). Subjects judged whether a line was located to the right or left of the tip of a chevron (see inset in the figure). The vertical axis of the graph measures the displacement needed to discriminate re-

[13] The terminology associated with these two types of spatial tasks can be confusing. The word *hyperacuity* refers to the fact that people localize spatial position with very high precision. Unfortunately acuity is also used to refer to the spatial-frequency sensitivity of the observer, which is a different matter. Here, I will use the term *localization* to refer to spatial resolution for position.

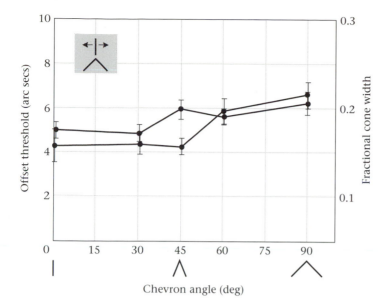

7.26 LOCALIZATION SENSITIVITY. Subjects detected whether a line was offset to the right or left of the tip of a chevron for a variety of angles of the opening of the chevron. Data from two observers are shown. Both observers could reliably report offsets as small as six seconds of arc (left vertical scale) which is one-fifth the width of a single photoreceptor (right vertical scale). Source: Westheimer and McKee, 1977.

liably when the line is offset from the middle of the chevron. This task was repeated for chevrons with various angles; for all angles, the offset thresholds are on the order of 5 seconds of arc, roughly one-fifth the width of a single cone. Performance does not vary much as we change the stimulus. This suggests that localization performance is robust with respect to spatial manipulations of the target. This very fine localization applies to many different kinds of stimuli, including the relative positions of a pair of vertical lines, moving lines, and many other targets (Westheimer, 1979).

At first, it seems surprising to learn that we can localize targets at a finer resolution than the spacing of the cone mosaic. We know that the sampling grid determined by the cone mosaic imposes a fundamental limit on spatial pattern resolution through the phenomenon of aliasing (see Chapter 3). Why should the cone mosaic not also impose a limitation on our ability to localize position?

In fact, a coarse sampling grid does not eliminate the possibility of localizing a target precisely. The physical principles we can use to achieve fine spatial localization on a coarse sampling grid are illustrated in Figure 7.27. The main portion of the figure shows the pattern of cone absorptions we expect in response to a reference line centered over a cone and a line that is displaced to the right by 12 seconds of arc. The separation between the tick marks on the horizontal axis are set at 30 seconds, the size of an individual cone. The values were calculated using Westheimer's optical linespread function (Chapter 2).

Because the offset is very small compared to the sampling, the same cones respond to the reference line and the offset line. It follows that the identity of the cones cannot be used to estimate the locations of the

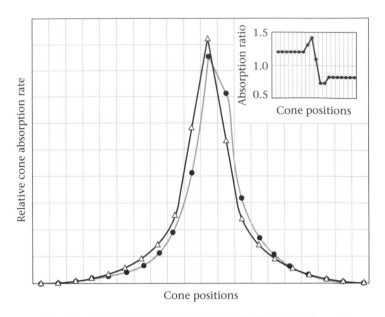

7.27 A PHYSICAL BASIS FOR LOCALIZATION IN LOCALIZATION TASKS. The points in the main graph show the estimated rate of light absorption by foveal cones in response to a fine line stimulus. The open triangles show absorptions to a reference line and the filled circles show the absorptions to a line offset by 12 seconds of arc. The grid lines on the horizontal axis are separated by the width of a single cone. The solid and shaded lines linearly connect the estimated absorption rates. The inset shows the ratio of cone absorptions from the reference line and the displaced line at each cone position. The graph shows that a 12-second shift (roughly one-third the width of a photoreceptor) changes the cone absorption rate by as much as 50 percent. This information can be used to localize the position of the line at a resolution that is substantially finer than the separation between cones.

two lines. Although the same cones respond to the two lines, the spatial pattern of cone absorptions when the lines are in these two positions is quite different. The inset to Figure 7.27 shows the ratio of the cone absorptions to the two different lines. A small spatial shift of 12 seconds of arc causes a 50-percent change in the absorption rate at an individual cone. Hence, the spatial pattern of absorption rates is a reliable signal that can be interpreted to infer the line position at a resolution finer than the spacing of the cone mosaic.

Notice that the optical blurring of the light distribution is essential if we wish to localize the line at positions finer than the sampling grid. Were there no optical blurring, the image of a line would fall within the width of a photoreceptor, and spatial displacements less than the width of a photoreceptor would not be detectable. Optical blur, which seems like a nuisance when we consider spatial resolution of contrast patterns, is a help when we consider spatial resolution in terms of localizing targets.

Our ability to localize the position of edges and lines is very robust with respect to various stimulus manipulations. If we vary the target contrast, set the display into motion, or flash the display briefly, performance remains excellent. Since performance is robust with respect to these experimental manipulations, it is clear that the simple calculation shown in Figure 7.27 is only a demonstration of how localization is possible; the visual system must use a much more sophisticated method to calculate position. Eye movements during examination of a static display, or tracking errors during examination of a visual display, will make it impossible to compare the outputs of a single small set of cones. Rather, people must be capable of estimating the position at fine precision even though the precise identity of the cones mediating the signal varies. Although we have some basic principles to work from, how we estimate the relative position of moving targets using active eyes remains an important challenge for study.

Summary

Theories of human pattern sensitivity are organized around a few basic principles. In the earliest and simplest theories, the visibility of different types of test patterns was explained by the properties of a single shift-invariant linear system. This type of theory is simple for computation and also parallels nicely our understanding of the initial encoding of light by retinal nerve cells in certain visual streams. The convolution kernel of the shift-invariant linear system and the neural receptive field play analogous roles and provide a natural basis for comparison of behavioral and physiological data. By using common experimental measures, such as contrast-sensitivity functions, the properties of neural mechanisms and behavioral theories can be compared directly.

While certain aspects of single-resolution theories provide a reasonable description of human pattern sensitivity, they fail a number of direct empirical tests. Consequently, theorists have tried to assemble new theories in which the pattern representation is based on a collection of shift-invariant representations, not just a single one. This idea parallels the physiological notion that the visual system contains a set of visual streams. The more complex modern theories must specify a larger number of convolution kernels (receptive fields). To keep these organized, and to parallel some of the properties of cortical receptive fields, theorists generally choose convolution kernels that respond best to restricted bands of spatial frequency and to restricted stimulus orientations. These theories can predict more experimental results, but there remain many computational and experimental challenges before we will have a complete satisfactory theory of pattern sensitivity.

Because human vision constantly adapts to new viewing conditions, human pattern sensitivity cannot be described by a single pattern-sensitivity function. Pattern sensitivity covaries with the temporal properties of the test stimulus, the mean background level, and with the wavelength composition of the stimulus. Thus, a general specification of human pattern sensitivity must take all of these factors into account.

Behavioral experiments show that people are also exquisitely sensitive to the spatial location of targets. Observers can localize test stimuli to a resolution that is considerably finer than the spacing of the cone mosaic. The ability to localize is quite robust, surviving many different stimulus manipulations. The principles of how one might localize to a very fine resolution are clear, but the methods that the visual pathways use to acquire the necessary information remain to be determined.

Exercises

1. Use a computer program, such as MATLAB or Mathematica, and experiment with vector-length calculations:

    (a) Define a discrete representation of a one-dimensional sinusoidal stimulus. Using a range of locations for x from 0 to 1 degree, and 64 sample values, create two sinusoidal patterns, s_1 and s_3.

    (b) Compute the contrast patterns $s_1 + s_3$ and $s_1 - s_3$. Plot them and compare the deviations around zero.

    (c) Compute the squared vector-length of a vector s_1 using a matrix multiplication of the form $s_1^T s_1$.

    (d) Show that a shift-invariant, vector-length calculation predicts that the visibility of the pattern $\sin(2\pi f x) + \sin(2\pi(3f)x)$ is the same as the visibility of $\sin(2\pi f x) - \sin(2\pi(3f)x)$.

    (e) Show that a shift-invariant, vector-length calculation predicts that the visibility of the pattern $\sin(2\pi f x) + \sin(2\pi(3f)x)$ is the same as the visibility of $\cos(2\pi f x) + \cos(2\pi(3f)x)$.

2. Answer these questions about shift-invariant vector-length calculations.

    (a) Consider the two stimulus contrast patterns, $\cos(2\pi f x)$ and $\cos(2\pi(3f)x)$. Suppose that the contrast threshold for the sinusoid alone is C_f and that the contrast threshold for the cosinusoid alone is C_{3f}. Compute the predicted contrast threshold for the mixture $\cos(2\pi f x) + \cos(2\pi(3f)x)$ according to a shift-invariant, vector-length theory.

    (b) What will the contrast threshold be for $\sin(2\pi f x)$?

    (c) What will the contrast threshold be for $\sin(2\pi f x) + \cos(2\pi(3f)x)$?

    (d) Suppose that we have a one-degree wide monitor region that has 32 lines. Using the Fourier series, we can describe a contrast pattern of a line as the sum of a set of 32 cosinusoids of equal amplitude and frequencies of $0, 1, \ldots, 31$ cpd. Assume that you know the visual sensitivity to each of these cosinusoids (call them s_i). Use the shift invariant, vector-length theory to predict when the contrast line will be visible.

3. Answer these questions about texture and spatial frequency.

    (a) Suppose that we are looking at a texture pattern on a wall. As we walk toward the wall, the spatial-frequency content of the image incident at our cornea changes. Describe the nature of the change in amplitude of the different spatial-frequency components.

    (b) Describe the nature of the change of the phase components of the image.

    (c) There are many instances in which we would like to predict whether one image is a good replica of another. There is a field of engineering in which individuals have developed *image-quality metrics* to compute whether small differences will be perceptible, and if so how perceptible. Consider only the problems of black and white images and describe what image formation factors you think should be included in an image-quality metric?

(d) How would you incorporate the human contrast-sensitivity function into an image quality metric?

(e) Many investigators do not use the human contrast-sensitivity function to evaluate the quality of the reproduction. Instead they evaluate the error of the replication by computing the mean squared error between the original and the replica. Can you devise a thought experiment to illustrate when this procedure will surely fail?

(f) For many images, the mean squared error between the original and the replica performs reasonably well as a predictor of the perceptual difference between the image and its replica. Can you explain what factors might make this so?

4. Answer these questions about light adaptation.

(a) Design a set of stimuli and experimental procedure for measuring the contrast-sensitivity function by signals initiated in the L-cone mosaic. What will be the main difficulties in creating the stimuli? What about for the S-cone mosaic?

(b) The experiments we reviewed in this chapter were based mainly on backgrounds and targets that appear light–dark. Suppose that we adjust the color of the background light such that the L-cones are adapted to a much higher level of illumination than the S-cones. What do you think will happen to the contrast-sensitivity function measured with a light–dark modulation? What do you think will happen to the contrast-sensitivity function measured with a colored target?

(c) Why should contrast sensitivity, rather than absolute light sensitivity, be a key visual variable preserved by adaptation?

(d) As the mean background intensity increases, people can perceive increasingly rapid flicker. What imaging principles does this illustrate?

5. Answer these questions about wavelength and pattern.

(a) Chromatic aberration reduces spatial resolution in the short-wavelength portion of the spectrum. Does this mean that a blue–yellow neural pathway must have poor spatial resolution?

(b) Define pattern–color separability.

(c) Suppose that pattern–color separability is a desirable feature of a opponent-color pathway. How would you create a blue–yellow neural signal that is pattern–color separable?

(d) Suppose that pattern–color separability is not important and that only spatial resolution is valuable. Describe how you would create a blue–yellow neural signal.

6. Answer these questions about the physical basis for localization.

(a) Is there any reason that localization would improve if the human cones were spaced more finely?

(b) How well should we be able to localize using only the signals from the S-cone mosaic?

(c) Is there any reason that localization would deteriorate if the human cones were spaced more coarsely? What effect would broadening (narrowing) the linespread function have on localization?

8

Multiresolution Image Representations

Our review of the organization of neural and behavioral data has led us to several specific hypotheses about how the visual system represents pattern information. Neural evidence suggests that visual information is segregated into a number of different visual streams that are specialized for different tasks. Behavioral evidence suggests that, within the streams that are specialized for pattern sensitivity, information is further organized by local orientation and spatial scale and color. All of the evidence we have reviewed to this point suggests that image contrast, rather than image intensity, is the key variable represented by the visual pathways.

We will spend this chapter mainly just thinking about how these and other organizational principles might be relevant to solving various visual tasks. In addition to the intrinsic and practical interest of solving visual problems, finding principled solutions for visual tasks can also be helpful in understanding and interpreting the organization of the human visual pathways.

Which tasks should we consider? There are many types of visual problems; only some of these have to do with tasks that are essential for human vision. One approach to thinking about visual algorithms is to adopt a general approach to vision, sometimes called **computational vision**, in which we do not restrict our thinking to those problems that are important for human vision. Instead, we open our minds to visual algorithms that may have no biological counterpart.

In this book, however, I will restrict our analysis to the subset of algorithms that is related to human vision. While this is not the broadest possible class, it is a very important one because there are many potential applications for visual algorithms that emulate human performance. For example, suppose a person wants to search through a database of images to find images with "red vehicles." To assist the person, the computer program must have some algorithmic representation related to human vision; after all, the words "red" and "vehicle" are defined by human perception. This is but one example from the set of computer vision algorithms that can serve to augment the human ability to manipulate, analyze, search, and create images. These algorithms will be of tremendous importance over the next few decades.

There is a second reason for paying special attention to visual problems related to human vision. Many investigators have argued that studying the visual pathways and visual behavior is an efficient method for discovering novel algorithms for computational vision. The idea is that by studying the specific properties of a successful visual system, we will be led to an understanding of the general design principles of computational vision. This process is analogous to the idea of **reverse-engineering** that is frequently used to improve instrument design in manufacturing. This view has been suggested by many authors, but Marr (1982) has argued particularly forcefully that biology is a good source of ideas for engineering design. I have never been persuaded by this argument; it seems to me that reverse-engineering methods are most successful when one understands the fundamental principles and only wishes to improve the implementation. It is very difficult to analyze how a system works from the implementation unless one already has a set of general principles as a guide. I think engineering algorithms have done more for understanding neuroscience than neuroscience has done for engineering algorithms.

Whichever way the benefits flow, from neuroscience to engineering or the other way around, just the presence of a flow is a good reason for the vision scientist and imaging engineer to be familiar with biological, behavioral, and computational issues. In the remainder of this book, we will spend more time engaged in thinking about computational issues related to human vision. In this chapter I will describe ideas and algorithms related to multiresolution image representations. In the following chapters I will describe work on color appearance, motion, and seeing. Algorithms for all of these topics continue be an important part of vision science and engineering.

Efficient Image Representations

In this chapter we will consider several different multiresolution representations. Multiresolution representations have been used as part of a variety of visual algorithms ranging from image segmentation to stereo depth and motion (e.g., Burt, 1988; Vetterli and Meten, 1992). To unify the introduction of these various representations, however, I will introduce them all by considering how they solve a single engineering problem: efficient storage of image information.

Efficient image representations are important for systems with finite resources, which is to say all visual systems. No matter how much computer memory or how many visual neurons we have, we can always perform better computations, transmit more information, or store higher quality images if we use efficient storage algorithms. If we fail to consider efficiency, then we waste resources that could improve performance.

Image-compression algorithms transform image data from one representation to a new one that requires less storage space. To evaluate the efficiency of a compression algorithm, we need some way to describe the amount of space required to store an image. The most common way to measure the amount of storage space necessary to encode an image is to count the total number of bytes used to represent the image.[1] Color images acquired from cameras or scanners, or color images that are about to be displayed on a monitor, are represented in terms of the intensities at a set of picture locations called **pixels**. The color data are represented in three color bands, usually called the red, green, and blue bands. We can compute the number of bytes of data represented in a single image fairly easily. Suppose we have a modest-size image of 512 rows and 512 columns and that each color band represents intensity using one byte. The image representation within a single color band requires $512 \times 512 \times 3$ bytes of data, or approximately 0.75 megabytes of data. If we have an image comprising 1,024 rows and columns, we will require 3.0 megabytes to represent the image. In a movie clip, in which we update the image 60 times a second, the numbers grow at an alarming rate; one minute requires 10 gigabytes of information, and one hour requires 600 gigabytes.

Notice that color image encoding already involves a significant amount of image compression that is made possible by the special characteristics of human vision. The physical signal consists of light with energy at many wavelengths (i.e., a complete spectral power distribution). The image data, however, do not encode the complete spectral power distribution of the displayed or acquired color signal. The data represent only three color bands, a very compressed representation of the image. The results of the color-matching experiment justify the compression of information (see Chapter 4). This part of compression is so well understood that it is rarely mentioned explicitly in discussions of image compression.

In addition to color trichromacy, two main factors permit us to compress images with little loss of quality. First, adjacent pixels in natural images tend to have similar intensity levels. We say that there is considerable **spatial redundancy** in these images. This redundancy is

---

[1] A bit is a single **binary digit**, that is, 0 or 1. A byte is 8 bits and represents 256 levels (2^8). A megabyte is 10^6 bytes, while a gigabyte is 10^9 bytes.

part of the signal, and it may be removed without any loss of information in order to obtain more efficient representations. Second, we know that human spatial resolution to certain spatial patterns is very poor (see Chapters 2 and 7). People have very poor spatial resolution to short-wavelength light, and only limited spatial resolution for colored patterns in general. Representing this information in the stored image is unnecessary because the receiver (that is, the visual system) cannot detect it. By eliminating this information, we improve the efficiency of the image representation.

In this chapter we will consider efficient encoding algorithms of monochrome images, spending most of our time on issues of intensity and spatial redundancy. In Chapter 9, which is devoted to color broadly, we will again touch on some of the issues of color image representation.

Intensity Redundancy in Image Data

Suppose that we have an image we wish to encode efficiently, such as the image in Figure 8.1A. The camera I used to acquire this image codes up to 256 different intensity levels (8 bits). You might imagine, therefore, that this is an 8-bit image. To see why that is not the case, look at the distribution of pixel levels in the image.

In Figure 8.1B I have plotted the number of points in the image at each of the 256 intensity levels the device can represent. This graph is called the image's **intensity histogram**. The histogram shows that inten-

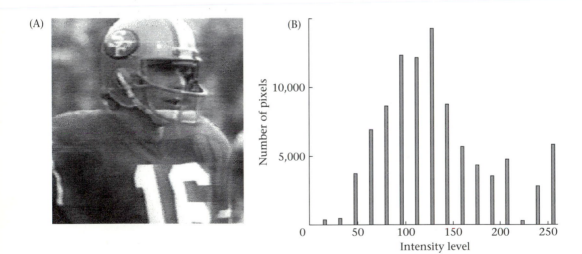

8.1 THE DISTRIBUTION OF IMAGE INTENSITIES is an important factor in obtaining an efficient image representation. (A) This image was acquired by a device capable of reproducing 256 gray levels, but the image data consists of only 16 different gray levels. (B) The histogram shows the gray levels used to code the image (A). Device properties limit the gray-level resolution; they do not enforce a resolution.

sity level 128 occurs most frequently and only a few other levels occur at all.

Although the device used to acquire this image could potentially represent 256 different intensity levels, the image itself does not contain this many levels. We do not need to represent the data at the device resolution, but only at the intrinsic resolution of the image, which is considerably smaller. Since the image in Figure 8.1A contains 16 levels, not 256, we can represent it using 4 bits per image point rather than the 8-bit resolution the device can manage. This saves us a factor of two in storage space.

The first savings in efficiency is easy to understand; we must not allocate storage space to intensity levels that do not occur in the image. We can refine this idea by taking advantage of the fact that the different intensity levels do not occur with equal frequency. Consider one method to take advantage of the fact that some intensity levels are more likely than others. Assign the 1-bit sequence, 1, to code level 128. Encode the other levels using a 5-bit sequence that starts with a zero, say $0xxxx$, where $xxxx$ is the original 4-bit code. For example, the level 5 is coded by the 5-bit sequence 00101. We can unambiguously decode an input stream as follows. When the first bit is a 1, then the current value is 128. When the first bit is a zero, read four more bits to define the intensity level at that pixel.

Suppose that the intensity level 128 had occupied 60 percent of the pixels. Our encoding scheme reduces the space devoted to coding these pixels from 4 bits to 1 bit, saving 3 bits at 60 percent of the locations. The encoding method costs us 1 bit of storage for 40 percent of the pixels. The average savings across the entire image is $0.6 \times 3 - 0.4 \times 1 = 1.2$ bits per pixel. Using these very simple rules, we have reduced our storage requirements to 2.8 bits per pixel.

The example I have provided here is very simple; many more elaborate and efficient algorithms exist for taking advantage of the redundancies in a data set. In general, the more we know about the input distribution, the better we can do at designing efficient codes. A great deal of thought has been devoted to the question of designing efficient coding strategies for single images and also for various classes of images such as business documents and natural images.

Spatial Redundancy in Image Data

Normally, intensity histograms of natural images do not exhibit such a coarse, discrete distribution as the example in Figure 8.1. In natural images, intensity distributions range across many intensity levels, and strategies that rely only on intensity redundancy do not save much storage space.

But there are spatial redundancies in natural images, and we can use the same general encoding principles we have been discussing to take advantage of these redundancies as well. Specifically, certain spatial patterns of pixel intensities are much more likely than others. There are various formal and informal ways to convince oneself of the existence of these spatial redundancies. First, consider the image in Figure 8.2. This figure contains a picture of Professor Horace Barlow, an eminent vision scientist. A few of the pixel intensities have been set randomly to a new intensity value. Kersten (1987) has shown that naive observers are quite good at adjusting the intensity of these pixels back to their original intensity. With 1 percent of the pixels deleted, observers correct the pixel intensity to its original value nearly 80 percent of the time. Even with 40 percent of the pixels deleted, observers set the proper intensity level more than half the time.

Second, we can measure the spatial redundancy in natural images by comparing intensities at neighboring pixels. Figure 8.3A shows the pixel intensities from the image shown in the center of the figure. Measured one at a time, the pixel intensities are distributed across many values and do not contain a great deal of redundancy. Figure 8.3B shows an **image cross-correlogram** that measures the intensity of a pixel, $p(x, y)$, on the horizontal axis and the intensity of its neighboring pixel, $p(x, y + 1)$, on the vertical axis. Because adjacent pixels tend to have the same intensity level, the points in the cross-correlogram cluster near the identity line. Because the intensity of one pixel tells us a great deal about the probable intensity level of an adjacent pixel, we know that the pixel intensity levels are redundant.

We can improve the efficiency of the image representation by removing this spatial redundancy. One way of removing the redundancy is to transform the image representation. For example, instead of coding the intensities of the two pixels at adjacent locations independently, we can code one pixel level, $p(x, y)$ and the difference between the ad-

8.2 EXPERIMENTAL MEASUREMENT OF SPATIAL REDUNDANCY IN AN IMAGE. The image shows Professor Horace Barlow; random noise has been added to the picture. Subjects were asked to adjust the intensity of the noisy pixels to the level they thought must have been present in the original image. Subjects are very accurate at this task, using the information present in nearby pixels. This is an experimental demonstration that people can take advantage of the spatial redundancy in image data. Source: Kersten, 1987.

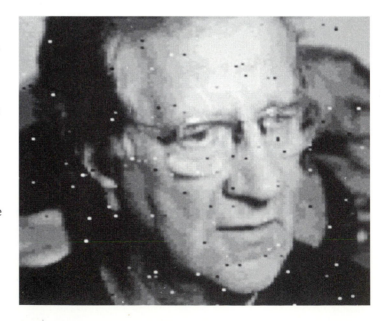

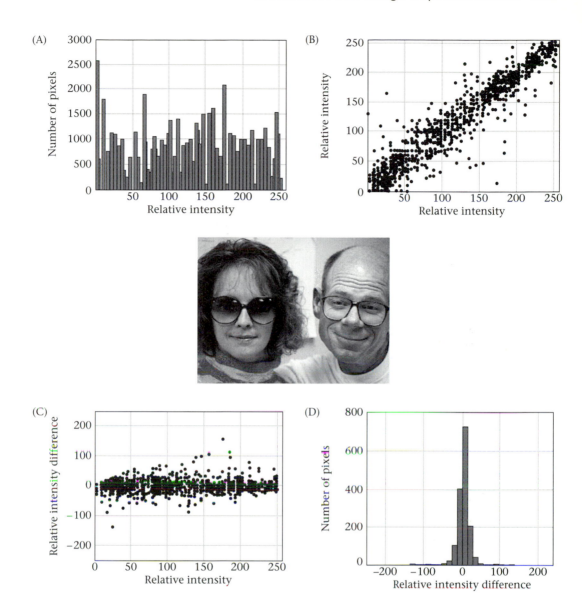

8.3 COMPUTATIONAL MEASUREMENT OF SPATIAL REDUNDANCIES IN A NATURAL IMAGE. The natural image used for these computations is shown in the middle. (A) The image intensity histogram shows the distribution of image intensities. (B) A correlogram of the intensity of a pixel located at position (x, y) and the intensity of a pixel located at position $(x, y + 1)$. (C) A correlogram of the intensity of a pixel located at position (x, y) and the intensity difference between it and the adjacent pixel at $(x, y + 1)$. (D) A histogram of the intensity differences showing that they are concentrated near the zero level.

jacent pixel values, $p(x, y + 1) - p(x, y)$. This pair of values preserves the image information since we can recover the original from $p(x, y)$ and $p(x, y + 1) - p(x, y)$ by simple subtraction. This type of procedure is known as **lossless compression**.

After transforming the data, the number of bits needed to code $p(x, y)$ is unchanged. But the difference, $p(x, y + 1) - p(x, y)$, can fall in a larger range, anywhere between 255 and −255 so that we may need as many as 9 bits to store this value. In principle, requiring an additional bit is worse, but in practice the difference between most adjacent pixels is quite small. This point is illustrated by the cross-correlogram of the transformed values shown in Figure 8.3C. The horizontal axis measures the pixel intensity $p(x, y)$, and the vertical axis measures the difference value, $p(x, y + 1) - p(x, y)$. First, notice that most of the values of the intensity difference cluster near zero. Second, notice that there is virtually no correlation between the transformed values; knowing the value of $p(x, y)$ does not help us know the value of the difference.

To build an efficient representation, we can use the same strategy I outlined in the previous section. We use a short code (say, 5 bits) to encode the small difference values that occur frequently. We use a longer code (say, 10 bits) to encode the rarely occurring large values. Because most of the pixel differences are small, the representation will be more efficient.[2]

Decorrelating Transformations

We can divide the image-compression strategies I have discussed into two parts. First, we linearly transformed the image intensities to a new representation by a linear transformation. The linear transformation computes $p(x, y)$ and $p(x, y) - p(x, y + 1)$ from $p(x, y)$ and $p(x, y + 1)$. The matrix form of this transformation is simply

$$\begin{pmatrix} p(x, y) \\ p(x, y + 1) - p(x, y) \end{pmatrix} = \begin{pmatrix} 1 & 0 \\ -1 & 1 \end{pmatrix} \begin{pmatrix} p(x, y) \\ p(x, y + 1) \end{pmatrix} \quad (8.1)$$

We apply the linear transformation because the correlation of the transformed values is much smaller than the correlation in the original representation.

Second, we find a more efficient representation of the transformed representation. Because we have removed the correlation, in natural images the variation of the transformed values will be smaller than the variation of the original pixel intensities. Hence we will be able to encode the transformed data more efficiently than the original data.

From our example, we can identify a key property of the linear transformation that is essential for achieving efficient coding. The new transformation should convert the data to **decorrelated values**. Values

[2] We could improve even this coding strategy in many different ways. For example, after the first pair of pixels we never need to encode an absolute pixel level; we can always encode only differences between adjacent pixels. This is called differential pulse code modulation, or DPCM. Or, we could consider the pair of pixels as a vector, calculate the frequency distribution of all possible vectors, and build an efficient code for communicating the values of these vectors. This is called vector quantization, or VQ. All of these methods trade on the fact that natural images are more likely to contain some spatial patterns than others.

are decorrelated when we gain no advantage in predicting one value from knowing the other. It should seem intuitive that decorrelation is an important part of efficiency: if we can predict one value from the another, there is no reason to encode both. Generalizing this idea, if we can approximately predict one value from another, we can achieve some efficiencies in our representation. In our example we found that the value $p(x, y)$ is a good predictor of the value $p(x, y + 1)$. Hence, it is efficient to predict that $p(x, y + 1)$ is equal to $p(x, y)$ and to encode only the error in our prediction. If we have a good predictor (i.e., high correlation) the prediction error will span a smaller range than the data value. Hence, the error can be encoded using fewer bits, and we can save storage space.

The transformation in Equation 8.1 does yield a pair of approximately decorrelated values. To make the example simple, I chose a simple linear transformation. We might ask how we might find a decorrelating linear transformation in general. When the set of images we will have to encode is known precisely, then the best linear transformation for lossless image compression can be found using a matrix decomposition called the **singular value decomposition**. The singular value decomposition defines a linear transformation from the data to a new representation with statistically independent values that are concentrated over smaller and smaller ranges. This representation is just what we seek for efficient image-encoding. The singular value decomposition is at the heart of principal-components analysis and goes by many other names including the Karhunen-Loeve transform and the Hoteling transform. The singular value decomposition may be the most important technique in linear algebra.

In practice, however, the image population is not known precisely. Nor are the image statistics for the set of natural images known precisely. As a result, the singular value decomposition has no ready application to image compression. As a practical matter, then, selecting a good initial linear transformation remains an engineering skill acquired by experience with algorithm design.

Lossy Compression

To this point, we have reviewed compression methods that transform the original data with no loss of information. Ordinarily, we can achieve savings of a factor of 2 or 3 based on lossless compression methods, though this number is strongly image-dependent.

If we are willing to tolerate some difference between the original image and the stored copy, then we can develop schemes that save considerably more space. Transformations that lose information are called **lossy compression** methods. Using only three sensor responses to represent color information is the most successful example of a perceptually lossless encoding. We cannot recover the original wavelength representation from the encoded signal. Still, we use this lossy representation because we know from the color-matching experiment that when done perfectly there should be no difference between the perceived image and the original image (see Chapter 4).

Lossy compression is inappropriate for many types of applications, such as storing bank records. But, some amount of image distortion is acceptable for many applications. It is possible to build lossy image-compression algorithms for which the difference between the original and stored image is barely perceptible, and yet the savings in storage space can be as large as a factor of 5 or 10. Users often judge the efficiency to be worth the image distortion. In cases when the image distortion is not visible, some authors refer to the compression as **perceptually lossless**.

As we reviewed in earlier chapters, the human visual system is very sensitive to some patterns and wavelengths but far less sensitive to others. Perceptually lossless encoding methods are designed to exploit these differences in human visual sensitivity. These schemes allocate more storage space to represent highly visible patterns and less storage space to represent poorly visible patterns (Watson and Ahumada, 1989; Watson, 1990).

Perceptually lossless image-encoding algorithms follow a logic that has much in common with the lossless encoding algorithms. First, the image data are transformed to a new set of values, using a linear transformation. The transformed values are intended to represent **perceptually decorrelated features** (see below). Second, the algorithm allocates different amounts of precision to these transformed values. In this case, the precision allocated to each transformed value depends on the visual salience of the feature the value represents; hence, salient features are allocated more storage space than barely visible features. It is at this point in the process that lossy algorithms differ from lossless algorithms. Lossless algorithms allocate enough storage so that the transformed values are represented perfectly, yet due to the decorrelation they still achieve some savings. Lossy algorithms do not allocate enough storage to represent all of the initial information; the image cannot be reconstructed perfectly from the compressed representation. The lossy algorithm is designed, however, so that the lost information would not have been visible anyway. Thus, the new picture will require less storage and will still look like the original image.[3]

Perceptually Decorrelated Features

In the overview of perceptually lossless compression algorithms, I used —but did not define—the phrase "perceptually decorrelated features." The notion of a "perceptual feature" is used widely in a very loose way to describe important image properties, but there is no consensus on

---

[3] In practice, lossy and lossless compression are concatenated to compress image data. First a lossy compression algorithm is applied, followed by a lossless algorithm.

the specific image features that comprise the perceptual features. In the context of image compression, however, there is a very useful operational definition of image feature. We can define it in terms of the linear transformation used to decorrelate the image data.

Suppose we represent the original image as a list of intensities, i_x, one intensity for each pixel in the image. We then apply a linear transformation to the image data to yield a new vector of **transform coefficients**, **t** (as in Equation 8.1):

$$
\begin{pmatrix} t_1 \\ t_2 \\ \vdots \\ t_{N-1} \\ t_N \end{pmatrix} = \begin{pmatrix} \text{Decorrelating} \\ \text{transform} \end{pmatrix} \begin{pmatrix} i_1 \\ i_2 \\ \vdots \\ i_{N-1} \\ i_N \end{pmatrix}
$$

Each transformation coefficient represents something about the contents of the input image. We can call the image information represented by each transform coefficient an **image feature**. According to this definition, we can compute the image features from vectors of transform coefficients that are zero except at one entry. For example, we can compute the image feature associated with the first transform coefficient by solving the linear equation

$$
\begin{pmatrix} 1 \\ 0 \\ \vdots \\ 0 \\ 0 \end{pmatrix} = \begin{pmatrix} \text{Decorrelating} \\ \text{transform} \end{pmatrix} \begin{pmatrix} i_1 \\ i_2 \\ \vdots \\ i_{N-1} \\ i_N \end{pmatrix}
$$

We call the image vector that solves this linear equation the image feature represented by the first transform coefficient. We can find the image features associated with each of the transform coefficients, in turn, and thus find all of the features associated with a particular decorrelating transform.[4]

Next, we must define what we mean by "perceptually decorrelated" image features. We can use Kersten's (1987) experiment to provide an operational definition. In that experiment subjects adjusted the intensity of certain pixels to estimate the intensity level in the original image. Kersten found that observers inferred the intensity levels of individual pixels quite successfully and that observers perceived a great deal of correlation when comparing individual pixels. We can conclude that pixels are a poor choice to serve as decorrelated features.

---

[4] Notice that taken together these features comprise the columns of the right inverse of the decorrelating transform.

Now, suppose we perform a variant of Kersten's experiment. Instead of randomly perturbing pixel values in the image, suppose that we perturb the values of the transform coefficients. And, suppose we ask subjects to adjust the transform coefficient levels to reproduce the original image. This experiment is the same as Kersten's task except we use the transform coefficients, rather than individual pixels, to control image features.

We concluded that individual pixels do *not* represent perceptually decorrelated features because subjects performed very well. We will conclude that a set of transform coefficients represent decorrelated features only if subjects perform poorly. When knowing all the transform coefficients but one does not help the subject set the level of an unknown coefficient, we will say the features represented by the transformation are perceptually independent. I am unaware of perceptual studies analogous to Kersten's that test for the perceptual independence of image features, but in principle, these experiments offer a means of evaluating the independence of features implicit in different compression algorithms.

The important compression step in perceptually lossless algorithms occurs when we use different numbers of bits to represent the transform coefficients. To decide on the number of bits allocated to a transform coefficient, we consider the visual sensitivity of the image feature represented by that coefficient. Because visual sensitivity to some image features is very poor, we can use very few bits to represent these features with very little degradation in the image appearance. This permits us to achieve very compact representations of image data. By saving information at the level of image features, the perceptual distortion of the image can be quite small while the efficiencies are quite large.

This compression strategy depends on the perceptual independence of the image features. If the features are not independent, then the distortions we introduce into one feature may have unwanted side effects on a second feature. If the observer is sensitive to the second feature, we will introduce unwanted distortions. Hence, discovering a set of image features that are perceptually independent is an important part of the design of a perceptually lossless image representation. If distortions of some features have unwanted effects on the appearance of other features, that is, if the representation of a pair of features is perceptually correlated, then the linear transformation is not doing its job.

A Block Transformation: The JPEG-DCT

The Joint Photographic Experts Group (JPEG) committee of the International Standards Organization has defined an image-compression algorithm based on a linear transformation called the **discrete cosine transformation (DCT)**. Because of the widespread acceptance of this

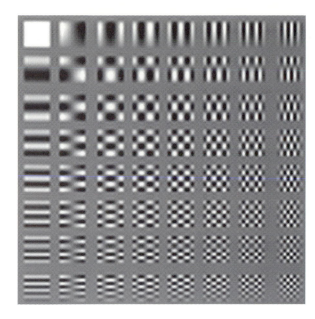

8.4 THE PERCEPTUAL FEATURES OF THE DCT. The DCT features are products of harmonic functions, $\cos(2\pi f_1 j)\cos(2\pi f_2 k)$, where j and k refer to position along the horizontal and vertical directions. These functions have both positive and negative values, and they are shown as contrast patterns varying about a constant gray background.

standard, and the existence of hardware to implement it, the JPEG-DCT compression algorithm is likely to appear on your desk and in your home within the next few years. The **JPEG-DCT compression algorithm** has a multiresolution character and bears an imprint from work in visual perception.[5]

The JPEG-DCT algorithm uses the DCT to transform the data into a set of perceptually independent features. The image features associated with the DCT are shown in Figure 8.4. The image features are all products of cosinusoids at different spatial frequencies and two orientations. Hence, the independent features implicit in the DCT are loosely analogous to a collection of oriented spatial-frequency channels. The features are not the same as the features used to model human vision since the DCT image features comprise high and low frequencies, while others contain signals with perpendicular orientations. Still, there is a rough similarity between these features and the oriented spatial frequency organization of models of human multiresolution representations; this is particularly so for the features pictured along the edges and along the diagonal in Figure 8.4, where the image features are organized along lines of increasing spatial frequency and within a single orientation.

The main steps of the JPEG-DCT algorithm are illustrated in Figure 8.5. First, the data in the original image are separated into blocks. The computational steps of the algorithm are applied separately to each

---

[5] The DCT is similar to the Fourier-series computation reviewed in Chapters 2 and Appendix A.

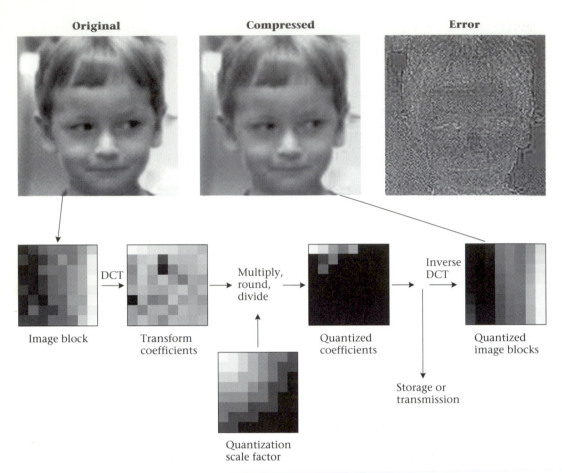

Original   **Compressed**   **Error**

DCT

Image block

Transform coefficients

Multiply, round, divide

Quantized coefficients

Inverse DCT

Quantized image blocks

Quantization scale factor

Storage or transmission

8.5   AN OUTLINE OF THE JPEG COMPRESSION ALGORITHM based on the DCT. The original image is divided into a set of nonoverlapping square blocks, usually 8 × 8 pixels. The image data are transformed using the DCT to a new set of coefficients. The transform coefficients are quantized using using a simple "multiply, round, divide" operation. The quantized coefficients are zeroed by this operation, making the image well suited for efficient lossless compression applied prior to storage or transmission. To reconstruct the image, the quantized coefficients are converted by the inverse DCT, yielding a new compressed image that approximates the original. The error in the reconstruction (i.e., the difference between the original and the reconstruction) consists mainly of high-frequency texture. The error is shown as an image on the right.

block of image data, making the algorithm well suited to parallel implementation. The image block size is usually 8 × 8 pixels, though it can be larger. Because the algorithm begins by subdividing the image into blocks, it is one of a group of algorithms called **block coding** algorithms.

Next, the data in each image block are transformed using the linear DCT. The transform coefficients for the image block are shown as an image in Figure 8.5 labeled "transform coefficients." In this image, white means a large absolute value, and black means a low absolute value. The coefficients are represented in the same order as the image features in Figure 8.4; the low-spatial-frequencies coefficients are in the upper left of the image, and the high-spatial-frequency coefficients are in the lower right.

In the next step, the transform coefficients are quantized. This is one stage of the algorithm where compression is achieved. The quantization is implemented by multiplying each transform coefficient by a scale factor between 0 and 1, rounding the result to the nearest integer, and then dividing the result by the scale factor. If the scale factor is near zero, then the rounding operation has a strong effect, and the number of coefficient quantization levels is small. The scale factors for each coefficient are shown in the image labeled "quantization scale factor." For this example, I chose factors near 1 for the low-spatial-frequency terms (top left) and factors near zero for the high-spatial-frequency terms (bottom right).

The quantized coefficients are shown in the next image. Notice that many of the quantized values are zero (black). Because there are so many zero coefficients, the quantized coefficients are very suitable for lossless compression. The JPEG-DCT algorithm includes a lossless compression algorithm applied to the quantized coefficients. This representation is used to store or transmit the image.

To reconstruct an approximation of the original image, we only need to apply the inverse of the DCT to the quantized coefficients. This yields an approximation to the original image. Because of the quantization, the reconstruction will differ from the original somewhat. Since we have removed information mainly about the high-spatial-frequency components of the image, the difference between the original and the reconstruction is an image composed mainly of fine texture. The difference image for this example is labeled "error" in Figure 8.5.

One of the most important limiting factors in compressing images arises from the separation of the original image into distinct blocks for independent processing. Pixels located at the edge of these blocks are reconstructed without any information concerning the intensity level of the pixels that are adjacent, in the next block. One of the most important visual artifacts of the reconstruction, then, is the appearance of distortions at the edges of these blocks, which are commonly called **block artifacts**. These artifacts are visible in the reconstructed image shown in Figure 8.5.

There are two aspects of the JPEG-DCT algorithm that connect it with human vision. First the algorithm uses a roughly multiresolution representation of the image data. One way to see the multiresolution character of the algorithm is to imagine grouping together the coefficients obtained from the separate image blocks. Within each block, there are 64 DCT coefficients corresponding to the 64 image features. By collecting the corresponding transform coefficients from each block, we obtain a measure of the amount of each image feature within the image blocks. Implicitly, then, the DCT coefficients define 64 images, each describing the contribution of one of the 64 image features of the

DCT. These implicit images are analogous to the collection of neural images that make up a multiresolution model of spatial vision (Chapter 7).[6]

Second, the JPEG-DCT algorithm relies on the assumption that quantization in the high-spatial-frequency coefficients does not alter the quality of the image features coded by low-spatial-frequency coefficients. If reduced resolution of the high spatial frequencies influences very visible features in the image, then the algorithm will fail. Hence, the assumption that the transform yields perceptually independent features is very important to the success of the algorithm.

The independent features in the JPEG-DCT algorithm do not conform perfectly to the multiresolution organization in models of human spatial vision. High- and low-frequency components are mixed in some of the features; components at very different orientations are also combined in a single feature. These features are desirable for efficient computation and implementation. In the next section, we will consider multiresolution computations that reflect the character of human vision a bit more closely.

Image Pyramids

Image pyramids are multiresolution image representations. Their format differs from the JPEG-DCT algorithm in several ways, perhaps the two most important being that (a) pyramid algorithms do not segment the image into blocks for processing, and (b) the pyramid multiresolution representation is more similar to the human visual representation than that of the JPEG-DCT. In fact, much of the interest in pyramid methods in image coding is born of the belief that the image-pyramid structure is well matched to the human visual encoding. This sentiment is described nicely in Pavlidis and Tanimoto's (1975) paper, one of the first on the topic (p. 104):

> It is our contention that the key to efficient picture analysis lies in a system's ability, first, to find the relevant parts of the picture quickly, and second, to ignore (not waste time with) irrelevant detail. The retina of the human eye is . . . structured so as to see a wide angle in a low-resolution ("high-level") way using peripheral vision, while simultaneously allowing high-resolution, detailed perception by the fovea.

The linear transformations used by pyramid algorithms have image features comprising periodic patterns at a variety of spatial orientations,

---

[6] There is something that may strike you as odd when you think about the JPEG representation in this way. Notice that each block contributes the same number of coefficients to represent low-frequency information as high-frequency information. Yet from the Nyquist sampling theorem (see Chapter 3), we know that we can represent the low-frequency information using many fewer samples than are needed to represent the high-frequency information. Why is this differential sampling rate not part of the JPEG representation? The reason is in part due to the block coding, and in part due to the properties of the image features.

much like human multiresolution models. Because the coefficients in the image pyramid represent data that fall mainly in separate spatial-frequency bands, it is possible to use different numbers of transform coefficients to represent the different spatial-frequency bands. Image pyramids use a small number of transform coefficients to represent the low-spatial-frequency features and many coefficients to represent the high-spatial-frequency features. It is this feature, namely, that decreasing numbers of coefficients are used to represent high to low spatial-frequency features, that invokes the name pyramid.

The Pyramid Operations: General Theory

Construction of image pyramids relies on two fundamental operations that are approximately inverses of one another. The first operation blurs and samples the input. The second operation interpolates the blurred and sampled image to estimate the original. Both operations are linear. I will describe the pyramid operations on one-dimensional signals to simplify notation; none of the principles change when we apply these methods to two-dimensional images. At the end of this section, I will illustrate how to extend the one-dimensional analysis to two-dimensional images.

Suppose we begin with a one-dimensional input vector, g_0, containing n entries. The first basic pyramid operation consists of convolving the input with a smoothing kernel and then sampling the result. The blurring and sampling go together, intuitively, because the result of blurring is to create a smoother version of the original, containing fewer high-frequency components. Since blurring removes high-frequency information, according to the sampling theorem we can represent the blurred data using fewer samples than the are needed for the original. We do this by sampling the blurred image at every other value.

As we have seen in Chapters 2 and 3, both convolution and sampling are linear operations. Therefore, we can represent each by matrix multiplication. We represent convolution by the matrix multiplication $B_0 g_0$, where the rows of B_0 contain the convolution kernel. We represent sampling by a rectangular matrix, S_0, whose entries are all zeroes and ones. The combined operation of blurring and sampling is summarized by the basic pyramid matrix $P_0 = S_0 B_0$. Multiplication of the input by P_0 yields a reduced version of the original, $g_1 = P_0 g_0$, containing only half as many entries; a matrix tableau of the blurring and sampling operator, P_0, is:

$$P_0 = \begin{pmatrix} & S_0 & \end{pmatrix} \begin{pmatrix} & B_0 & \end{pmatrix}$$

To create the image pyramid, we repeat the convolution and sampling on each resulting image. The first operation creates a reduced image from the original, g_1. To create the next level of the pyramid, we blur and sample g_1 to create g_2; then, we blur and sample g_2 to create g_3, and so forth. When the input is a one-dimensional signal, each successive level contains half as many sample values as the previous level. When the image is two-dimensional, sampling is applied to both the rows and the columns so that the next level of resolution contains only one-quarter as many sample values as the original. This repeated blurring and sampling is shown in matrix form in Figure 8.6.

The second basic pyramid operation, interpolation, serves as an inverse to the blurring and sampling operation. Blurring and sampling transforms a vector with n entries to a vector with only $n/2$ entries. While this operation does not have an exact inverse, still, we can use g_1 to make an informed guess about g_0. If there is a lot of spatial redundancy in the input signals, our guess about the original image may not be too far off the mark. Interpolation is the process of making an informed guess about the original image from the reduced image. We interpolate by selecting a matrix, call it E_0, to estimate the input. We choose the **interpolating matrix** E_0 so that in general $E_0 g_1 \approx g_0$.

We can now put together the two basic pyramid operations into a constructive sequence that we will use several times in this chapter. First, we transform the input by convolution and sampling, $g_1 = P_0 g_0$. We then form our best guess about the original using the interpolation matrix, $\hat{g}_0 = E_0 g_1 = E_0 P_0 g_0$. The estimate $\hat{g}_0$ has the same size as the original image. Finally, to preserve all of the information, we create one final image to save the error. The **error** is the difference between the true signal and the interpolated signal, $e_0 = g_0 - \hat{g}_0$. This completes construction of the first level of the pyramid.

To complete the construction of all levels of the pyramid, we apply the same sequence of operations, but now beginning with first level of the pyramid, g_1. We build a new convolution matrix, B_1; we sample using the matrix, S_1; we build $g_2 = S_1 B_1 g_1$; we interpolate g_2 using

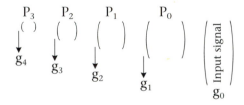

8.6 A MATRIX REPRESENTATION OF THE ONE-DIMENSIONAL PYRAMID OPERATIONS. The basic pyramid operation consists of blurring and then sampling the signal. To create a series of images at decreasing resolution, we apply the blurring and sampling operation repeatedly. Following each application of the pyramid operator, we obtain a new reduced image, g_i.

a matrix $\mathbf{E}_1$; and finally, we form the new error image $\mathbf{g}_1 - \hat{\mathbf{g}}_1$, where $\hat{\mathbf{g}}_1 = \mathbf{E}_1\mathbf{g}_2$. To construct the entire pyramid we repeat the process, reducing the number of elements at each step. We stop when we decide that the reduced image, $\mathbf{g}_n$, is small enough so that no further blurring and sampling would be useful.

The pyramid construction procedure defines three sequences of signals; the series of blurred and sampled signals whose size is continually being reduced, the interpolated signals, and the error signals. We can summarize their relationship to one another in a few simple equations. First, the reduced image at the ith level is created by applying the basic pyramid operation to the previous level:

$$\mathbf{g}_i = \mathbf{P}_{i-1}\mathbf{g}_{i-1} \tag{8.2}$$

The estimate of the image $\hat{\mathbf{g}}_i$ is created from the lower resolution representation by the calculation

$$\hat{\mathbf{g}}_i = \mathbf{E}_i\mathbf{g}_{i+1} \tag{8.3}$$

Finally, the difference between the original and the estimate is the error image,

$$\mathbf{e}_i = \mathbf{g}_i - \hat{\mathbf{g}}_i = \mathbf{g}_i - \mathbf{E}_i\mathbf{P}_i\mathbf{g}_i \tag{8.4}$$

Two different sets of these signals preserve the information in the original. One sequence consists of the original input and the sequence of **reduced signals**, $\mathbf{g}_0, \mathbf{g}_1, \mathbf{g}_2, \ldots, \mathbf{g}_n$. This sequence provides a description of the original signal at lower and lower resolution. It contains all of the data in the original image trivially, since the original image is part of the sequence. This image sequence is of interest when we display low-resolution versions of the image.

The second sequence consists of the **error signals**, $\mathbf{e}_0, \mathbf{e}_1, \ldots \mathbf{e}_{n-1}, \mathbf{g}_n$ (note that $\mathbf{g}_n$ is part of this sequence, too). Perhaps surprisingly, this sequence also contains all of the information in the original image. To prove this to yourself, notice that we can build the sequence of images, $\mathbf{g}_i$, from the error signals. The terms $\mathbf{g}_n$ and $\mathbf{e}_{n-1}$ are sufficient to permit us to construct $\mathbf{g}_{n-1}$; $\mathbf{g}_{n-1}$ and $\mathbf{e}_{n-2}$ can recover $\mathbf{g}_{n-2}$, and so forth. Ultimately, we use $\mathbf{e}_0$ and $\mathbf{g}_1$ to reconstruct the original, $\mathbf{g}_0$. This image sequence is of interest for image compression (Mallat, 1989).

Pyramids: An Example

Figure 8.7 illustrates the process of constructing a pyramid. The specific calculations used to create this example were suggested by Burt and Adelson (1983), who were perhaps the first to introduce the general notion of an image pyramid to image coding.

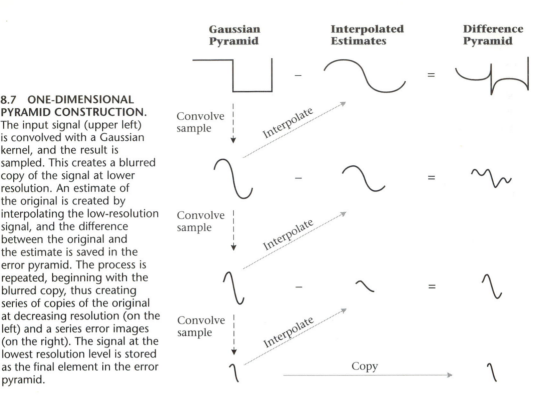

8.7 ONE-DIMENSIONAL PYRAMID CONSTRUCTION. The input signal (upper left) is convolved with a Gaussian kernel, and the result is sampled. This creates a blurred copy of the signal at lower resolution. An estimate of the original is created by interpolating the low-resolution signal, and the difference between the original and the estimate is saved in the error pyramid. The process is repeated, beginning with the blurred copy, thus creating series of copies of the original at decreasing resolution (on the left) and a series error images (on the right). The signal at the lowest resolution level is stored as the final element in the error pyramid.

The example in Figure 8.7 begins with a one-dimensional square-wave input, g_0. This signal is blurred using a Gaussian convolution kernel and then sampled at every other location; the reduced signal, g_1, is shown below. This process is then repeated to form a sequence of reduced signals. When the convolution kernel is a Gaussian function, the sequence of reduced signals is called the **Gaussian pyramid**.

To interpolate the reduced signal to a higher resolution, Burt and Adelson proposed the following ad hoc procedure. Place the data in g_1 into every other entry of a vector with the same number of entries as g_0. The procedure is called **up-sampling**; it is equivalent to multiplying the vector g_i by the transpose of the sampling matrix, S_0^T. Then, convolve the up-sampled vector with (nearly) the same Gaussian that was used to reduce the image. The Gaussian used for interpolation differs from the Gaussian used to blur the signals only in that is is multiplied by a factor of 2 to compensate for the fact that the up-sampled vector only has nonzero values at one out of every two locations. In this important example, then, the interpolation matrix is equal to 2 times the transpose of the convolution-sampling matrix,

$$E_0 = 2B_0^T S_0^T = 2P_0^T \qquad (8.5)$$

The interpolated signal, that is, the estimate of the higher-resolution signal, is shown in the middle column of Figure 8.7.

Next, we calculate the error signal, the difference between the estimate and the original. The error signals are shown on the right of Figure 8.7. The sequence of error signals forms the error pyramid. As I described above, we can reconstruct the original g_0 without error from the signals e_0 and g_1. Burt and Adelson called the error signals created by the combination of Gaussian blurring and interpolation functions the **Laplacian pyramid**.

Figure 8.8A shows the result of applying the pyramid process to a two-dimensional signal, in this case an image. The sequence of reduced images forming the Gaussian pyramid is shown on the top, with the original image on the left. These images were created by blurring the original and then representing the new data at one half the sampling rate for both the rows and the columns. Thus, in the two-dimensional case each reduced image contains only one-quarter the number of coefficients as its predecessor.[7]

The sequence of error images forming the Laplacian pyramid is shown in Figure 8.8B. Because the interpolation routine uses a smooth Gaussian function to interpolate the lower-resolution images, the large errors tend to occur near the edges in the image. And, because the images are mainly smooth (adjacent pixel intensities are correlated) most of the errors are small.[8]

Image Compression Using the Error Pyramid

From the point of view of image compression, the sequence of images in the Gaussian pyramid is not very interesting because that sequence contains the original. Rather than the use the entire sequence, we might as well just code the original. The sequence of images in the Laplacian pyramid, however, is interesting for two reasons.

First, the information represented in the Laplacian pyramid varies systematically as we descend in resolution. At the highest levels, containing the most transform coefficients, the Laplacian pyramid represents the fine spatial detail in the image. At the lowest levels, containing the fewest transform coefficients, the Laplacian pyramid represents low-spatial-resolution information. Intuitively, this is so because the error image is the difference between the original, which contains all of the fine detail, and an estimate of the original based on a slightly blurred copy. The difference between the original and an estimate from a blurred copy represents image information in the resolution band between the two levels. Thus, the Laplacian pyramid is a multiresolution representation of the original image.

Second, the values of the transform coefficients in the error images are distributed over a much smaller range than the pixel intensities in

---

[7] Therefore, in the estimation phase we multiply the interpolation matrix by a factor of 4, not 2 (i.e., $E_0 = 4P_0^T$).

[8] In order to display the error images, which have negative coefficients, the image intensities are scaled so that black is a negative value, medium gray is zero, and white is positive.

(A)

(B)

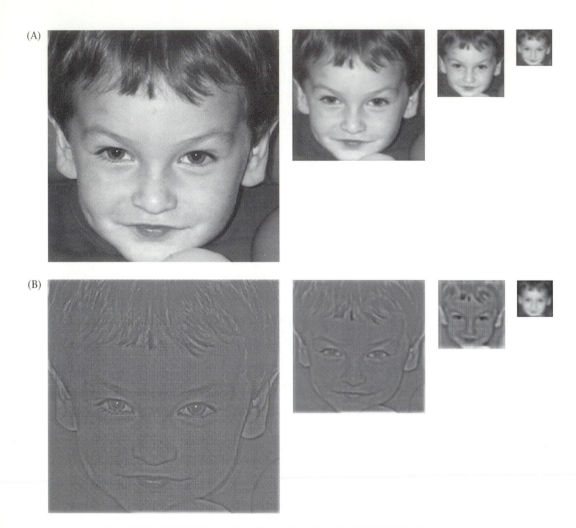

8.8 THE GAUSSIAN AND LAPLACIAN IMAGE PYRAMIDS. (A) The series of reduced images that form the Gaussian image pyramid begins with the original image, on the left. This image is blurred by a Gaussian convolution kernel and then sampled to form the image at a lower spatial resolution and size. (B) Each reduced image in the Gaussian pyramid can be used to estimate the image at a higher spatial resolution and size. The difference between the estimate and the higher-resolution image forms an error image, which in the case of Gaussian filtering is called the Laplacian pyramid. These error images can have positive or negative values, so I have shown them as contrast images in which gray represents zero error, while white and black represent positive and negative error, respectively. After Burt and Adelson, 1983.

the original image. Figure 8.9A shows intensity histograms of pixels in the first three elements of the Gaussian pyramid. These intensity histograms are broad and not well suited to the compression methods we reviewed earlier in this chapter. Figure 8.9B shows histograms of the pixel intensities in the Laplacian pyramid. The transform coefficients tend to cluster near zero, and thus they can be represented very efficiently. The reduced range of transform coefficient values in the Lapla-

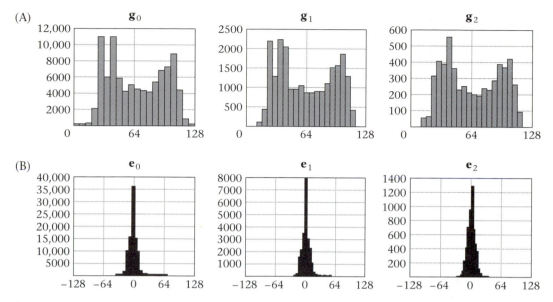

8.9 HISTOGRAMS OF THE GAUSSIAN AND LAPLACIAN PYRAMIDS. (A) The separate panels show the intensity histograms at each level of the Gaussian pyramid. The intensities are distributed across a wide range of values, making the intensities difficult to code efficiently. (B) The Laplacian pyramid coefficients are distributed over a modest range near zero and can be coded efficiently.

cian pyramid arises because of the spatial correlation in natural images. The spatial correlation permits us to do fairly well in approximating images using smooth interpolation. When the approximations are close, the errors are small, and they can be coded efficiently.

There is one obvious problem with using the images in the Laplacian pyramid as an efficient image representation: there are more coefficients in the error pyramid than pixels in the original image. When building an error pyramid from two-dimensional images, for example, we sample every other row and every other column. This forms a sequence of error images equal to 1, $1/4$, $1/16$ the size of the original; hence, the error pyramid contains 1.33 times as many coefficients as the original (see Fig. 8.8). Because of the excess of coefficients, the error image representation is called **overcomplete**. If one is interested in image compression, overcomplete representations seem to be a step in the wrong direction.

Burt and Adelson (1983) point out, however, that there is an important fact pertaining to human vision that reduces the significance of the overcompleteness: the vast majority of the the transform coefficients represent information in the highest spatial-frequency bands where people have poor visual resolution. Therefore, we can quantize these elements very severely without much loss in image quality. Quantization is the key step in image compression, so that having most of the transform coefficients represent information that can be heavily quantized is an advantage.

The ability to quantize severely many of the transform coefficients with little perceptual loss, coupled with the reduced variance of the transform coefficients, makes the Laplacian pyramid representation practical for image compression. Computing the pyramid can be more complex than the DCT, depending on the block size, but special hardware has been created for doing the computation efficiently. The pyramid representation performs about as well or slightly better than the JPEG computation based on the DCT. It is also applicable to other visual applications, as we will discuss below (Burt, 1988).

QMF's and Orthogonal Wavelets

Pyramid representations that use a Gaussian convolution kernel have many useful features, but they also have several imperfections. By examining the problematic features of Gaussian and Laplacian pyramids, we will see the rationale for using a different convolution kernel in creating image pyramids.

The first inelegant feature of the Gaussian and Laplacian pyramids is an inconsistency in the blurring and sampling operation. Suppose we had begun our analysis with the estimated image, $\hat{g}_0$, rather than g_0. From the pyramid-construction point of view, the estimate should be equivalent to the original image. It seems reasonable to expect, therefore, that the reduced image derived from $\hat{g}_0$ should be the same as the reduced image derived from g_0. We can express this condition as an equation,

$$g_1 = P_0(2P_0^T)g_1 = P_0\hat{g}_0 \qquad (8.6)$$

Equation 8.6 implies that the square matrix $P_0(2P_0^T)$ must be the identity matrix. This implies that the columns of the matrix, P_0 should be **orthogonal** to one another.[9] This is not a property of the Gaussian and Laplacian pyramid.

A second inelegant feature of the Gaussian and Laplacian pyramid is that the representation is overcomplete (i.e., there are more transform coefficients than there are pixels in the original image). The increase in the transform coefficients can be traced to the fact that we represent an image g_i with N_i pixels by a reduced signal and an error signal that contain more than N_i coefficients. For example, we represent the information in the ith level of the pyramid using the reduced image g_{i+1} and the error image e_i:

$$g_i = (2P_i^T)g_{i+1} + e_i \qquad (8.7)$$

[9] Two vectors are orthogonal when $a^Tb = 0$.

In the one-dimensional case, the error image, e_i, contains N_i transform coefficients. The reduced signal, g_{i+1}, contains $N_i/2$ coefficients. To create an efficient representation, we must represent g_i using N_i transform coefficients, not $1.5N_i$ coefficients as in the Gaussian pyramid.

The error signal and the interpolated signal are intended to code different components of the original input; the interpolated vector $\hat{g}_i = (2P_i^T)g_{i+1}$ codes a low-resolution version of the original, and e_i codes the higher-frequency terms left out by the low-resolution version. To improve the efficiency of the representation, we might require that the two terms code completely different types of information about the input. One way to interpret the phrase "completely different" is to require that the two vectors be orthogonal, that is,

$$0 = e_i^T \hat{g}_i \tag{8.8}$$

If we require that $\hat{g}_i$ and e_i be orthogonal, we can obtain significant efficiencies in our representation. By definition, we know that the interpolated image $\hat{g}_i$ is the weighted sum of the columns of P_i^T. If the error image e_i is orthogonal to the interpolated image, then the error image must be the weighted sum of a set of column vectors that are all orthogonal to the columns of P_i^T. In the (one-dimensional) Gaussian pyramid construction, P_i^T has $N_i/2$ columns. From basic linear algebra, we know that there are $(1/2)N_i$ vectors perpendicular to the columns of P_i^T. Hence, if $\hat{g}_i$ is orthogonal to e_i, we can describe both of these images using a total of only N_i transform coefficients, and the representation will no longer be overcomplete.

What conditions must be met to insure that e_i and $\hat{g}_i$ are orthogonal? By substituting Equations 8.2, 8.3 and 8.4 into Equation 8.8, we have

$$0 = e_i^T \hat{g}_i = [g_i^T(2P_i^T)P_i][(2P_i^T)P_ig_i - g_i]$$

$$= \{g_i^T(2P_i^T)[P_i(2P_i^T)]P_ig_i\} - [g_i^T(2P_i^T)P_ig_i] \tag{8.9}$$

If the rows of P_i are an orthogonal set, then by appropriate scaling we can arrange it so that $P_i(2P_i^T)$ is equal to the identity matrix. In that case, the final term in Equation 8.9 simplifies, and we have

$$e_i^T \hat{g}_i = [g_i^T(2P_i^T)P_ig_i] - [g_i^T(2P_i^T)P_ig_i] = 0 \tag{8.10}$$

thus guaranteeing that the error signal and the interpolated estimate will be orthogonal to one another. For the second time, then, we find that the orthogonality of the rows of the pyramid matrix is a useful property.

We can summarize where we stand as follows. The basic pyramid operation has several desirable features. The rows within each level of the pyramid matrices are shifted copies of one another, simplifying the calculation to nearly a convolution; the pyramid operation represents information at different resolutions, paralleling human multiresolution representations; and the rows of the pyramid matrices are localized in space, as are receptive fields, yet they are not sharply localized as the blocks used in the JPEG-DCT algorithm. Finally, from our criticisms of the error pyramid, we have added a new property we would like to have: the rows of each pyramid matrix should be an orthogonal set.

We have accumulated an extensive set of properties we would like the pyramid matrices, P_i, to satisfy. Now, one can have a wish list, but there is no guarantee that there exist any functions that satisfy all our requirements. The most difficult pair of constraints to satisfy is the combination of orthogonality and localization. For example, if we look at convolution operators alone, there are no convolutions that are simultaneously orthogonal and localized in space.

Interestingly, there exists a class of discrete-valued functions, called **quadrature mirror filters (QMF's)** that satisfy all of the properties on our wish list (Esteban and Galand, 1977; Vetterli; 1988; Simoncelli and Adelson, 1990). The QMF pair splits the input signal into two orthogonal components. One of the filters defines a convolution kernel that we use to blur the original image and obtain the reduced image. The second filter is orthogonal to the first and can be used to calculate an efficient representation of the error signal. Hence, the QMF pair splits the original signal into coefficients that define the two orthogonal terms, $\hat{g}_i$ and e_i; Each set of coefficients has only $n/2$ terms, so the new representation is an efficient pyramid representation. Figure 8.10 shows an example of a pair of QMF's. The function shown in Figure 8.10A is the convolution kernel that is used to create the reduced images, g_i.

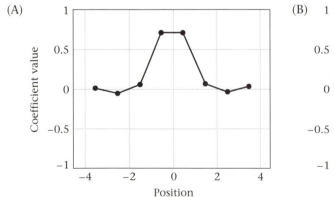
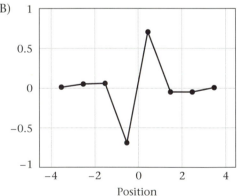

8.10 A QUADRATURE-MIRROR-FILTER PAIR. One can use these two functions as convolution kernels to construct a pyramid. Convolution with the kernel in (A) followed by sampling produces the transform coefficients in the set of reduced signals. Transformation by the kernel in (B) followed by sampling yields the transform coefficients of the error pyramid. Source: Simoncelli, 1988.

The function in Figure 8.10B is the convolution kernel needed to calculate the transform coefficients in the error pyramid directly. When the theory of these filters is developed for continuous, rather than discrete, functions the convolution kernels are called **orthogonal wavelets** (Daubechies, 1992).

The discovery of QMF's and orthogonal wavelets was a bit of a surprise. It is known that there are no nontrivial convolution kernels that are orthogonal; that is, no convolution matrix, $\mathbf{B}_i$, satisfies the property that $\mathbf{B}_i\mathbf{B}_i^{\mathrm{T}} = \mathbf{I}$. Hence, it was surprising to discover that convolution kernels do exist for the pyramid operation, which relies so heavily on convolution, and can satisfy $\mathbf{P}_i\mathbf{P}_i^{\mathrm{T}} = \mathbf{I}$.

Quadrature mirror filters and orthogonal wavelets have many fascinating properties and are an interesting area of mathematical study. They may have significant implications for compression because they remove the problem of having an overcomplete representation. But, it is not obvious that once quantization and correlation are accounted for that the savings in the number of coefficients will prove to be significant. For now, the design and evaluation of QMF's remains an active area of research in pyramid coding of image data.

Applications of Multiresolution Representations

The statistical properties of natural images make multiresolution representations efficient. Were efficiency a primary concern, the visual pathways might well have evolved to use the multiresolution format. But there is no compelling reason to think that the human visual system, with hundreds of millions of cortical neurons available to encode the outputs of a few million cone photoreceptors, was subject to very strong evolutionary pressure to achieve efficient image representations. Understanding the neural multiresolution representation may be helpful when we design image-compression algorithms, but it is unlikely that neural multiresolution representations arose to serve the goal of image compression alone.

If multiresolution representations are present in the visual pathways, what other purpose might they serve? In this section, I will speculate about how multiresolution representations may be a helpful component of several visual algorithms.

Image Blending

Imagine blending refers to methods for smoothly connecting several adjacent or overlapping images of a scene into a larger photomosaic (Milgram, 1975; Carlbom, 1994). There are several different reasons why we might study the problem of joining together several pieces of an image. For example, in practical imaging applications we may find that a camera's field of view is too small to capture the entire region of interest. In this case we would like to blend several overlapping pictures to form a complete image.

The human visual system also needs to blend images. As we saw in the early chapters of this volume, spatial acuity is very uneven across the retina. Our best visual acuity is in the fovea, and primate visual systems rely heavily on eye movements to obtain multiple images of the scene. To form a high-acuity representation of more than the central few degrees, we must gather images from a sequence of overlapping eye fixations. How can the overlapping images acquired through a series of eye movements be joined together into the single, high-resolution representation that we perceive?

Burt and Adelson (1983b) showed that multiresolution image representations offer a useful framework for blending images together. We can see some of the advantages of a multiresolution image-blending by comparing the method with a single-resolution blend. I will begin by defining a simple method of joining the two pictures, based on a single-resolution representation. Suppose we decide to join a picture on the left $L(x,y)$ and a picture on the right $R(x,y)$. We will blend the images by mixing their intensity values near the border where they join. A formal rule for blending the image data must specify how to combine the data from the two images. We do this using a blending function, call it $b(x,y)$, whose values vary between 0 and 1. To construct our single-resolution blending algorithm we form a mixture image from the weighted average

$$M(x,y) = b(x,y)L(x,y) + [1 - b(x,y)]R(x,y) \qquad (8.11)$$

Consider the performance of such a single resolution blend on the pair of simulated astronomical images in Figure 8.11. The two images were created to simulate images obtained of a starry sky. The images contain three distortions that are common amongst images that we might wish to blend.

First, the images contain two kinds of objects (stars and clouds) with very different types of spatial structure. The spatial structure of the clouds is represented mainly by low spatial frequency terms while each star is represented by spatial frequency terms at all frequencies. Second, the images have different mean intensity levels (Figure 8.11A is brighter than Figure 8.11B), perhaps due to a change in the sensitivity of the film or the ambient illumination. Third, the images are slightly shifted in the vertical direction as if the camera position had changed between the times when the two pictures were taken.

The most trivial, and rather ineffective, way of joining the two images is shown in panel C. In this case the two images are simply divided in half and joined at the dividing line. Simply abutting the two images is equivalent to choosing a function $s(x,y)$ equal to

$$b(x,y) = \begin{cases} 1 & \text{if } x < m \\ 0 & \text{otherwise} \end{cases} \qquad (8.12)$$

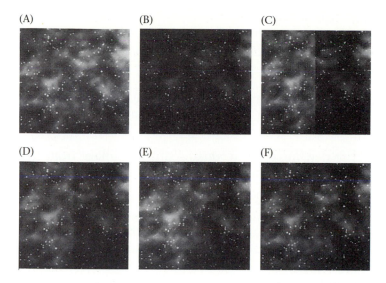

8.11   A COMPARISON OF SINGLE-RESOLUTION AND MULTIRESOLUTION IMAGE-BLENDING METHODS. The images in (A) and (B) have slightly different mean intensity levels and are translated vertically. (C) The result of abutting the right and left halves of the images; (D) spatial averaging over a small distance across the image boundary; (E) spatial averaging over a large distance across the image boundary; (F) the multiresolution blend. From Burt and Adelson, 1983.

where m is the midpoint of the image, 256 in this case. This smoothing function leads to an obvious artifact at the midpoint because of the difference in mean gray level.

We might use a less drastic blending function for $b(x, y)$. For example, we might choose a function that varied as a linear ramp over some central width of the image:

$$b(x, y) = \begin{cases} 1 & \text{if } x < m - w \\ 1 - \frac{x - m - w}{2w} & \text{if } m - w \leq x \leq m + w \\ 0 & \text{otherwise} \end{cases} \qquad (8.13)$$

Using a ramp to join the images blurs the image at the edge, as illustrated in panels D and E of Figure 8.11. In panel D the width parameter of the linear ramp, w, is fairly small. When the width is small the edge artifact remains visible. As the width is broadened, the edge artifact is removed (panel E), and elements from both images contribute to the image in the central region. At this point the vertical shift between the two images becomes apparent. If you look carefully in the central region, you will see double stars shifted vertically one above the other. Image details that are much smaller than the width of the ramp appear in the blended image, and they appear at their shifted locations. The stars are small compared to the width of the linear ramp, so the blended image contains an artifact due to the shift in the image details.

Multiresolution representations provide a natural way for combining the two images that avoids some of these artifacts. We can state the multiresolution blending method as an algorithm:

1. Form the pyramid of error images for L and R.

2. Within each level of the pyramid, average the error images with a blend function, $b(x, y)$. A simple ramp function, as in Equation 8.13 with $w = 1$, will do as the blend function.

3. Compute the new image by reconstructing the image from the blended pyramid of error images.

The image in panel F of Figure 8.11 contains the results of applying the multiresolution blend to the images. The multiresolution algorithm avoids the previous artifacts because, by averaging the two error pyramids, two images combine over different spatial regions in each of the resolution bands. Data from the low-resolution level are combined over a wide spatial region of the image, while data from the high-resolution levels are combined over a narrow spatial region of the image.

By combining low-frequency information over large spatial regions, we remove the edge artifact. By combining high-frequency information over narrow spatial regions, we reduce the artifactual doubling of the star images to a much narrower spatial region.

Burt and Adelson (1983b) also describe a method of blending images with different shapes. Figure 8.12 illustrates one of their amusing images. They combined the woman's eye shown in panel A and the hand shown in panel B into the single image shown in panel D. The method for combining images with different shapes is quite similar to the algorithm described above. Again, we begin by forming the error images e_i for each of the two images. For the complex region, however, we must find a method to define a blend function $s_i(x, y)$, appropriate for combining the data at each resolution of the pyramid over these different shapes. Burt and Adelson have a nifty solution to this problem. First build an overlay image that defines the location where the second image is to be placed over the first, as in panel C of Figure 8.12. Then, build the pyramid of reduced images, g_i, corresponding to the overlay image. Finally, use the elements of the image sequence g_i to define the blend functions for combining the images at resolution e_i.

Progressive Image Transmission

For many devices, transmitting an image from its stored representation to the viewer can take a noticeable amount of time. In some of these cases, transmission delays may hamper one's ability to perform a task. Suppose you are scanning through a database for suitable pictures to use in a drawing, or are checking a photo directory to find the name of a person who recently waved hello. You may have to look through many pictures before finding what you are looking for. If there is a consider-

(A) (B)

(C) (D)

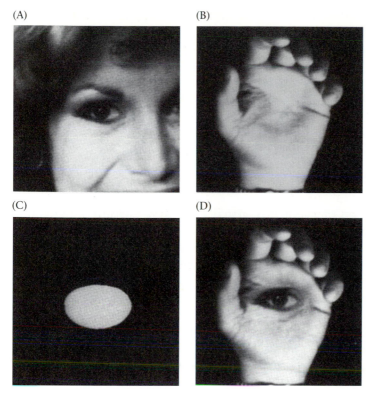

8.12 IMAGE BLENDING of two regions with arbitrary shapes. (A) An image of part of a human face. (B) An image of a human hand. (C) This binary image represents the area in panel (A) that contains the eye. The Gaussian pyramid of this binary image is used in the multiresolution blend of the hand and eye images. (D) The multiresolution blend of the hand and the eye. Source: Burt and Adelson, 1983.

able delay before you see each picture, the task may become irritating; if there is too much delay, you may simply decide not to bother.

Multiresolution image representations are natural candidates to improve the rate of image transmission and display. The reconstruction of an image from its multiresolution image proceeds through several stages. The representation stores the error images e_i and the lowest reduced image g_n. We reconstruct the original by computing a set of reduced images, g_i. These reduced images are rough approximations of the original, at reduced resolution. They are represented by fewer bits than the original image, so they can be transmitted and displayed much more quickly. We can make these low-resolution images available for the observer to see during the reconstruction process. If the observer is convinced that this image is not worth any more time, then he or she can abort the reconstruction and go on to the next image. This offers the observer a way to save considerable time.

We can expand on this use of multiresolution representations by allowing the observer to request a low-resolution reconstruction, say at level g_i, rather than a full representation at level g_0. The observer can choose a few of the low-resolution images for viewing at high resolution. Multiresolution representations are efficient because there is little wasted computation. The pyramid reconstruction method permits us to use the work invested in reconstructing the low-resolution image to reconstruct the original at full resolution.

The engineering issues that arise in progressive image transmission may be relevant to the internal workings of the human visual system. When we call up an image from memory, or sort through a list of recalled images, we may wish to see low-resolution images rather than reconstruct each image in great detail. If the images are stored using a multiresolution format, our ability to search efficiently through our memory for images may be enhanced.

Threshold and Recognition

Image-compression methods link visual sensitivity measurements to an engineering application. This makes sense because threshold sensitivity plays a role in image compression; perceptually lossless compression methods, by definition, tolerate threshold-level differences between the reconstructed image and the original.

For the applications apart from compression, however, sensitivity is not the key psychological measure. Since low-resolution images do not look the same as the high-resolution images, sensitivity to differences is not the key behavioral measure. To understand when progressive image-transmission methods work well, or which low-resolution version is the best approximation to a high-resolution version of an image, we need to be informed about which multiresolution representations permit people to recognize quickly or search for an item in a large collection of low-resolution images quickly. Just as the design of multiresolution image-compression methods requires knowing visual sensitivity to different spatial-frequency bands, so too multiresolution methods for progressive image transmission require knowing how important different resolution bands will be for expressing the information in an image.

As we study these applications, we will learn about new properties of human vision. To emphasize some of the interesting properties that can arise, I will end this section by reviewing a perceptual study by Bruner and Potter (1964). This study illustrates some of the counterintuitive properties we may discover as we move from threshold to recognition studies.

Bruner and Potter studied subjects' ability to recognize common objects from low-resolution images. Their subjects were shown objects using slides projected onto a screen. In 1964 low-resolution images were created much more quickly and easily than today; rather than requiring expensive computers and digital framebuffers, low-resolution images were created by blurring the focus knob on the projector. Bruner and Potter compared subjects' ability to recognize images in a few ways. I want to abstract two key observations from their results.[10]

---

[10] There are a number of important methodological features of the study I will not repeat here, and I encourage the reader to return to the primary sources to understand more about the design of these experiments.

Figure 8.13 illustrates three different measurement conditions. Observers in one group saw the image develop from very blurry to only fairly blurry over a two-minute period. At the end of this period the subjects were asked to identify the object in the image. They were correct on about a quarter of the images. Observers in a second group only began viewing the image after 87 seconds. They first saw the image at a somewhat higher resolution, but then they could watch the image develop for only about a half minute. The difference between the second group and the first group, therefore, was whether they saw the image in a very blurry state during the first 87 seconds. The second group of observers performed substantially better, recognizing the object 44 percent of the time, rather than 25 percent. Surprisingly, the initial 87 seconds of viewing the image come into focus made the recognition task more difficult. A third group was also tested. This group only saw the image come into focus during the last 13 seconds. The third group did not see the first 107 seconds as the image came into focus. This group also recognized the images correctly about 43 percent of the time.

Seeing these images come into focus slowly made it harder for the observers to recognize the image contents. Observers who saw the images come into focus over a long period of time formulated hypotheses as to the image contents. These hypotheses were often wrong and ultimately interfered with their recognition judgments.

To illustrate the same phenomenon in a different way, Bruner and Potter showed one group of observers the image sequence coming into focus and a second group the same image sequence going out of focus. This was the same set of images, shown for the same amount of time; the difference between the stimuli was the time-reversal. Subjects who saw the images come into focus recognized the object correctly 44 percent of the time. Subjects who saw the image going out of focus recognized the object correctly 76 percent of the time. Seeing a low-resolution version of an image can interfere with our subsequent ability to recognize the contents of an image.

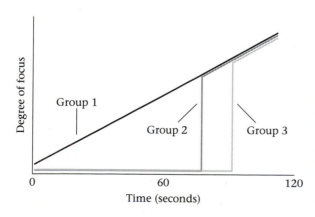

8.13 THE EXPERIMENTAL VIEWING CONDITIONS USED BY BRUNER AND POTTER IN THEIR RECOGNITION EXPERIMENT. One group saw the picture come into focus slowly and continuously over a period of 122 seconds. A second group saw nothing for 87 seconds and then watched the remainder of the image come into focus. The final group only saw the image after the first 107 seconds. Surprisingly, the group that watched the image come into focus for the full 122 seconds had the lowest recognition rate. Source: Bruner and Potter, 1964.

You should not draw too strong a conclusion from this study about the problems progressive image enhancement will create. There are a number of features of this particular experiment that make the data quite unlike applications we might plan for progressive image transmission. Most important, in this study subjects never saw very clear images. At the best focus, only half of the subjects recognized the pictures at all. Also, the durations over which the images developed were quite slow, lasting minutes. These conditions are sufficiently unlike most planned applications of progressive image transmission that we cannot be certain that the results will apply. I have presented the results here to emphasize that, even after the algorithms are in place, human testing will remain an important element of the system design.

Exercises

1. Answer these questions concerning the relations between image compression algorithms and visual perceptions.

    (a) What factors make it possible to achieve large compression ratios with natural images?

    (b) What properties of the human optics are important for compression? Do these have any implications for compression of color images?

    (c) The neuron doctrine states that a stimulus that generates a strong neural response defines what the neuron codes, usually called the neuron's *trigger feature*. In this chapter we have defined the image feature corresponding to a transform coefficient. How does the definition we have used in this chapter compare with the definition of a feature used in the neuron doctrine? Explain how the definition in this chapter could be stated in terms of a physiological hypothesis.

    (d) There are certain properties, such as shadows and surface curvature, that are common across many different images. How might one take advantage of the properties of the image-formation process to design more efficient image compression algorithms?

2. There are two ways in which compression can be useful. One is for representing the physical image efficiently. A second reason to compress image data is to obtain a form that is efficient for subsequent visual calculations of motion, color, and form. Answer the following questions relating these two aspects of image compression.

    (a) Make a hypothesis about where in the visual pathways you would make a master representation of the input data, and how other cortical areas might retrieve data from this site.

    (b) What properties would be computed by the separate cortical areas?

    (c) What properties would define an efficient central representation of visual information?

    (d) How would you test your hypotheses with physiological or behavioral experiments?

3. Answer these questions about the JPEG-DCT image compression algorithm and image pyramids.

    (a) Describe the JPEG-DCT computation in terms of convolution and sampling.

    (b) What is the main difference between the JPEG-DCT convolution/sampling process and the image pyramid convolution/sampling process?

    (c) At what stage is information lost in compression algorithms?

    (d) Why is it better to quantize the DCT coefficients rather than the individual pixels?

4. Here are some specific formulas concerning the DCT. Suppose that the data in an image block are given by $p(j,k)$. The DCT formula is

$$P(u,v) = \frac{4c(u)c(v)}{n^2} \sum_{j=0}^{n-1}\sum_{k=0}^{n-1} p(j,k)$$

$$\cdot \cos\left(\frac{(2j+1)u\pi}{2n}\right)\cos\left(\frac{(2k+1)v\pi}{2n}\right)$$

where $P(u,v)$ are the transform coefficients and c is a normalizing function defined as

$$c(w) = \begin{cases} 1/\sqrt{2} & \text{if } w = 0 \\ 1 & \text{otherwise} \end{cases}$$

Answer the following questions about the DCT.

    (a) Prove that the inverse of the DCT is

$$p(j,k) = \sum_{u=0}^{n-1}\sum_{v=0}^{n-1} c(u)c(v)P(u,v)$$

$$\cdot \cos\left(\frac{(2j+1)u\pi}{2n}\right)\cos\left(\frac{(2k+1)v\pi}{2n}\right)$$

   (Notice that, except for a scale factor, this formula is nearly the same as the forward DCT formula. Because of this, we say that the DCT is *self-inverting*.)

    (b) The DCT is separable with respect to the rows and columns of the input image block. This means that we can express the DCT calculation as a matrix product $D_r P D_c$ where the matrix P represents the image data, $p(j,k)$, and the matrices D_r and D_c represent the DCT transformation. Create the matrices D_r and D_c. How are they related?

5. Separability and circular symmetry are desirable properties. There is only one function that is both separable and circularly symmetric. What is it? Prove the result.

*H*ELMHOLTZ WROTE (quoted in Southall's *Physiological Optics*, Vol. III, p. 2): "The general rule determining the ideas of vision that are formed whenever an impression is made on the eye, is that *such objects are always imagined as being present in the field of vision as would have to be there in order to produce the same impression on the nervous mechanism* [italics in the original]."

Helmholtz's advice is at the center of much modern vision science. Helmholtz recommends that we think of our perceptions as mental representations of the object most likely to explain the sensory input. To understand the logic of perception, therefore, we should study how to use the retinal image to estimate the object properties. The interest in understanding perceptions as estimates of the physical properties of objects joins computational vision together with physiology and psychology. As we consider color appearance, motion and depth perception, and seeing in the next chapters we will find several ways in which Helmholtz's general advice has succeeded in specific cases.

Like many good ideas, Helmholtz's idea has often been rediscovered. Marr's (1982) influential book amplifies Helmholtz's point, and by using the word computational, rather than inferential, Marr also linked vision to the computer metaphor. Roger Shepard has championed this approach as well under the banner of "psychophysical complementarity."

PART THREE

Interpretation

When we pose vision-science questions as an estimation problem—what objects could give rise to the sensory input?—we place biology, psychology, and computation on common ground. Each discipline can formulate its experiments and theories in terms of a fundamental computational objective. The neural response, the behavior, and the computation all are seen as part of the goal of defining an object and estimating object properties.

In the next few chapters, then, we will engage in some free-wheeling abstract thinking about visual inferences. We will ask what sensory information is available in the retinal image that could be used to estimate object properties, first for color, and then for motion and depth. We will consider abstract algorithms to extract this information, and then we will consider how the neural substrate represents and analyzes this information.

Color Appearance

In the next chapter we will analyze the visual inferences that lead to color appearance. The color appearance of an object is predicted better by the object's surface-reflectance function than by the light scattered from the object. We will study how the visual system can, in principle, use the light scattered from a surface to infer an object's surface-reflectance function, and then we will compare people's color-appearance judgments with this standard.

As is common in biology and behavior, the performance does not match the absolute best limits. But there are some important similarities, so that we obtain an excellent framework for understanding behavior and the neural representation by beginning with the computational questions. For example, we will consider how computational analyses of color can help us understand some of the basic properties of the neural response to wavelength, such as opponent-colors signals.

We are at the beginning stages of discovering the neural mechanisms of color appearance. The clinical literature documents many cases of individuals who have lost their ability to organize color appearance as a consequence of strokes located in the visual area. We will consider the logic of these clinical case studies. Then, we will review some of the experimental evidence that seeks to connect color appearance and neural responses. The most important aspect of this review is that it will get us thinking about the general methods we have available to relate perception and brain activity.

Motion and Depth

Many of the same issues arise in Chapter 10, as I discuss motion and depth perception. I have grouped motion and depth perception because they are closely related computational tasks. Image changes arising from an observer's motion yield a rich source of information about depth.

It will also become clear that, just as color is not a direct representation of wavelength, perceived motion is not a direct representation of physical motion. Rather, motion perception is a mental inference that relies on computations implemented in the visual pathways.

For motion perception, more than any other percept, there is strong evidence to identify a particular visual stream as an important component of motion judgments. This visual stream can be traced from the retina to visual area MT (see Chapters 5 and 6). We will review the evidence that this stream plays a role in motion perception, and we will review new experiments that expand our repertoire of techniques for connecting brain activity and behavior.

Seeing

In the final chapter, I review how information about pattern, color, motion and depth is combined to create our visual experience; that is, how we see. Two types of observations are particularly informative about the principles of seeing. First, there are the experiences of individuals who were optically blinded at a young age and whose optics were restored later in life. These individuals quickly learn to detect patterns and colors and motion; but, they struggle to learn to recognize objects or to see the relationship between different views of an object.

Second, we can learn much about the principles of seeing from studying examples where vision fails us; that is, by studying visual illusions. Many illusions arise because the visual assumptions we use to interpret images are violated by the illusion. For example, we ordinarily interpret images as collections of surfaces; we see these surfaces in a three-dimensional space; we use information about occlusion to infer the depth relationship among these surfaces. Illusions can reveal the assumptions about physical processes we rely on when we interpret images, that is, when we see.

9

Color

Edwin Land was one of the great inventors and entrepreneurs in American history; among other achievements, he created instant developing film and founded the Polaroid Corporation. The first instant developing film made black and white reproductions, and after a few years Land decided to create a color version of the film. In order to learn about color appearance, Land returned to his laboratory to experiment with color. He was so surprised by his observations that he decided to write a paper summarizing them. The paper was published in the *Proceedings of the National Academy of Sciences*, and in it Land startled many people by arguing that there are only two, not three, types of cones. He further went on to dismiss the significance of the color-matching experiments. He wrote: "We have come to the conclusion that the classical laws of color mixing conceal great basic laws of color vision" (Land, 1959, p. 115). Land's sharp words, an arrow aimed at the heart of color science, provoked heated rejoinders from two leading scientists, Deane Judd (1960) and Gordon Walls (1960).

What was it that Land, a brilliant man, found so objectionable about color-matching? It seems that Land's reading of the literature led him to believe that the curves we measure in the color-matching experiment could be used to predict color appearance. When he set the textbooks down and began to experiment with color, he was sorely disappointed. He found that the color-matching measurements do not answer many important questions about color appearance.

Land's observation is consistent with our review of color-matching in Chapter 4. The results from the color-matching experiment can be

9.1 COLOR APPEARANCE IN A REGION DEPENDS ON THE SPATIAL PATTERN OF CONE ABSORPTIONS.
The two square regions are physically identical and thus create the same local rate of photopigment absorption. Yet, they appear to have different lightness because of the difference in their relative absorptions compared to nearby areas.

used to predict when two lights will look the same, but they cannot be used to tell us what the two lights look like. As Color Plate 2 illustrates, the experimental results in the color-matching experiment can be explained by the matches between the cone photopigment absorptions at a point, while color appearance forces us to think about the pattern of photopigment absorptions spread across the cone mosaics. Figure 9.1 illustrates this point again. The two squares in the image reflect the same amount of light to your eye. Yet, because the squares are embedded in different surroundings, we interpret the squares very differently, seeing one as light and the other as dark.

Land's paper contained a set of interesting qualitative demonstrations that illustrate these same points. While the limitations of the color-matching experiment were new to Land and the reviewers of his paper, they were not new to most color scientists. For example, Judd (1940) had worked for years trying to understand these effects. Later in this chapter I will review work at Kodak and in academic laboratories, contemporaneous with that of Land, that was designed to elucidate the mechanisms of color appearance. This episode in the history of color science remains important, however, because it reminds us that the phenomena of color appearance are very significant and very compelling, enough so to motivate Land to challenge whether the color establishment had answered the right questions. As to Land's additional and extraordinary claim in those papers, that there are two, not three, types of photoreceptors, well, we all have off days.[1]

Color Constancy: Theory

If the absolute rates of photopigment absorptions do not explain color appearance, what does? The illusions in Color Plate 2 and Figure 9.1 both suggest that color appearance is related to the *relative* cone absorption rates. Within an image, bright objects generate more cone absorp-

---

[1] Of course, even on his off days, Land was worth a billion dollars.

tions than dark objects; red objects create more L-cone absorptions, and blue objects create more S-cone absorptions. Hence, one square in Figure 9.1 appears light because it is associated with more cone absorptions than its neighboring region, while the other appears dark because it is associated with fewer cone absorptions. The relative absorption rate is very closely connected to the idea of the stimulus contrast that has been so important in this book. Color appearance depends more on the local contrast of the cone absorptions than on the absolute level of cone absorptions.

The dependence on relative, rather than absolute, absorption rates is a general phenomenon, not something that is restricted to a few textbook illusions. Consider a simple thought experiment that illustrates the generality of the phenomenon. Suppose you read this book indoors. The white part of the page reflects about 90 percent of the light toward your eye, while the black ink reflects only about 2 percent. Hence, if the ambient illumination inside a reading room is 100 units, the white paper reflects 90 units, and the black ink reflects 2 units. When you take the book outside, the illumination level can be 100 times greater, or 10,000 units. Outside, the black ink reflects 200 units toward your eye, which far exceeds the level of the white paper when you were indoors. Yet, the ink continues to look black. As we walk about the environment, then, we must constantly be inferring the lightness and color of objects by comparing the spatial pattern of cone absorptions.[2]

This thought experiment also illustrates that the color we perceive informs us mainly about objects. The neural computation of color is structured so that objects retain their color appearance whether we encounter them in shade or sun. When the color appearance of an object changes, we think that the object itself has changed. The defining property of an object is not the absolute amount of light it reflects, but rather how much light it reflects relative to other objects. From our thought experiment, it follows that the color of an object imaged at a point on the retina should be inferred from the relative level of cone absorptions caused by an object. To compute the relative level of cone absorptions, we must take into account the spatial pattern of cone absorptions, not just the cone absorptions at a single point.

On this view, color appearance is a mental explanation of why an object causes relatively more absorptions in one cone type than another object. The physical attribute of an object that describes how well the object reflects light at different wavelengths is called the object's **surface reflectance**. Objects that reflect mainly long-wavelength light usually appear red; objects that reflect mainly short-wavelength light usually appear blue. Yet, as we shall explore in the next few pages, interpreting the cone absorption rates in terms of the surface-reflectance functions is not trivial. How the nervous system makes this interpretation is an essential question in color appearance. A natural place

---

[2] This example was used by Hering (1964).

to begin our analysis of color appearance, then, is with the question, How can the central nervous system infer an object's surface-reflectance function from the mosaic of cone absorptions?

Spectral Image Formation

To understand the process of inferring surface reflectance from the light incident at our eyes, we must understand a little about how images are formed. The light incident at our corneas and absorbed by our cones depends in part on the properties of the objects that reflect the light and in part on the wavelength composition of the ambient illumination. We must understand each of these components, and how they fit together, to see what information we might extract from the retinal image about the surface-reflectance function. A very simple description of the imaging process is shown in Figure 9.2.

Ordinarily, image formation begins with a light source. We can describe the spectral properties of the light source in terms of the relative

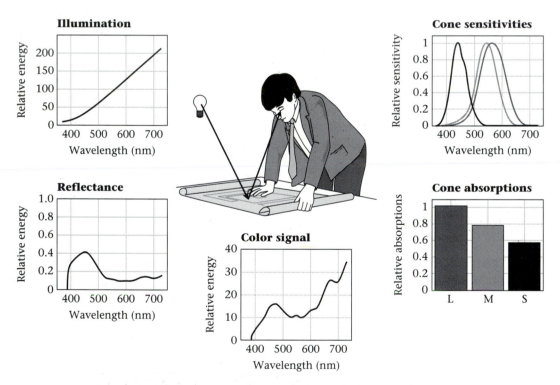

9.2   A DESCRIPTION OF SPECTRAL IMAGE FORMATION. Light from a source arrives at a surface and is reflected toward an observer. The light at the observer is absorbed by the cones and ultimately leads to a perception of color. The functions associated with the imaging process, represented by the graphs, include (counterclockwise from upper left) the spectral power distribution of the light source; the surface-reflectance function of the object; the result of multiplying these two functions to create the color signal incident at the eye; and the cone absorptions caused by the incident signal, which in turn are dependent on the cone sensitivities.

amount of energy emitted at each wavelength, namely the spectral power distribution of the light source (see Chapter 4). The light from the source is either absorbed by the surface or reflected. The fraction of the light reflected by the surface defines the surface-reflectance function. As a first approximation, we can calculate the light reflected toward the eye by multiplying the spectral power distribution and the surface-reflectance function together. We will call this light the **color signal** because it serves as the signal that ultimately leads to the experience of color. The color signal leads to different amounts of absorptions in the three cone classes, and it is the interpretation of these cone absorptions by the nervous system that is the basis of our color perception.

In Chapter 4, I reviewed some properties of illuminants and sensors; but this is the first time we have considered the surface-reflectance function. It is worth spending time thinking about some of the properties of how surfaces reflect light. Figure 9.3 shows the reflectance function of four matte papers, that is, papers with a smooth, even surface free from shine or highlights. Because these curves describe the fraction of light reflected, they range between 0 and 1. While it is common to refer to an object as having a surface-reflectance function (as I have just done), in a certain sense, the notion of a surface-reflectance function is a ruse. If you look about the room you are in, you will probably see some surfaces that are shiny or glossy. As you move around, changing the geometrical relationship between yourself, the lighting, and the surface, the light reflected to your eye changes considerably. Hence, the tendency of the surface to reflect light toward your eye does not depend

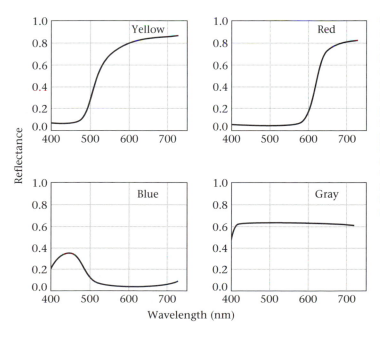

9.3 THE SURFACE-REFLECTANCE FUNCTION measures the proportion of light scattered from a surface at each wavelength. The panels show the surface-reflectance functions of various colored papers along with the color name associated with the paper. Surface reflectance is correlated with the color appearance; as Newton (1704) wrote "colours in the object are nothing but a disposition to reflect this or that sort of ray more copiously than the rest."

only on the surface; the light scattered to your eye also depends on the viewing geometry.[3]

The surface reflectance depends on viewing geometry because the reflected light arises from several different physical processes that occur when light is incident at the surface. Each of these processes contributes simultaneously to the light scattered from a surface, and each has its own unique properties. The full model describing reflectance appears to be be complex, but Shafer (1985) has created a simple approximation of the reflection process, called the **dichromatic reflection model**, that captures several important features of surface reflectance. Figure 9.4A sketches the model, which applies to a broad collection of materials called dielectric[4] surfaces (Shafer, 1985; Klinker et al., 1988; Nayar and Bolle, 1993, Wolff, 1994).

According to the dichromatic reflection model, dielectric material consists of a clear substrate with embedded colorant particles. One way light is scattered from the surface is by a mirror-like reflection at the interface of the surface. This process is called **interface reflection**. A second scattering process takes place when the rays enter the material. These rays are reflected randomly between the colorant particles. A fraction of the incident light is absorbed by the material, heating it up, and part of the light emerges. This process is called **body reflection**.

The spatial distributions of light scattered by these two mechanisms are quite different (Fig. 9.4B). Light scattered by interface reflection is quite restricted in angle, much as a mirror reflects incident rays. Conversely, the light scattered by body reflection emerges equally in all directions. When a surface has no interface reflections, but only body reflections, it is called a matte or Lambertian surface. Interface reflection is commonly called specular reflection and is the reason why some objects appear glossy.

The different geometrical distribution in how body and interface reflections are reflected is the reason why specular highlights on a surface appear much brighter than diffuse reflection. Nearly all of the specular scattering is confined to a small angle; the body reflection is divided among many directions. The interface reflections provide a strong signal, but because they can only be seen from certain angles they are not a reliable source of information. As the object and observer change their geometric relationship the specular highlight moves along the surface of the object, or it may disappear altogether.

For many types of materials, interface reflection is not selective for wavelength. The spectral power distribution of the light scattered at the interface is the same as the spectral power distribution of the incident

---

[3] Also, some types of materials fluoresce, which is to say they absorb light at one wavelength and emit light at another (longer) wavelength. This is also a linear process, but too complex to consider in this discussion.

[4] Dielectrics are nonconducting materials.

(A)

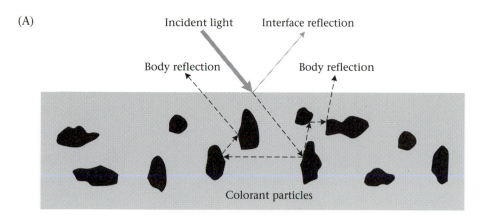

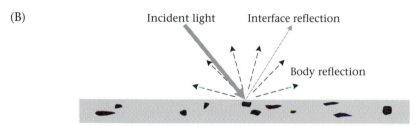

9.4 THE DICHROMATIC REFLECTION MODEL OF SURFACE REFLECTANCE IN INHOMOGENEOUS MATERIALS. (A) Light is scattered from a surface by two different mechanisms. Some incident light is reflected at the interface (interface reflection). Other light enters the material, interacts with the embedded particles, and then emerges as reflected light (body reflection). (B) Interface reflection is likely to be concentrated in one direction. Body reflection emerges with nearly equal likelihood in many different directions. Because interface reflections are concentrated in certain directions, light reflected by this process can be much more intense than light reflected by body reflection.

light. This is why specular highlights take on the color of the illumination source. Body reflection, on the other hand, does not return all wavelengths uniformly. The particles in the medium absorb light selectively, and it is this property that distinguishes objects in terms of their color appearance. Ordinarily, when people refer to the surface reflectance of an object, they mean to refer to the body reflection of the object.

We can describe the reflection of light by a matte surface with a simple mathematical formula. Suppose that the illuminant spectral power distribution is $e(\lambda)$. We suppose that the body reflectance is $s(\lambda)$. Then the color signal, that is, the light arriving at the eye, is

$$c(\lambda) = s(\lambda)e(\lambda) \tag{9.1}$$

Figure 9.5 shows several examples of the light reflected from matte surfaces. The shaded graph in Figure 9.5A is the spectral power distribution of an illuminant similar to a tungsten bulb. The other panels show the

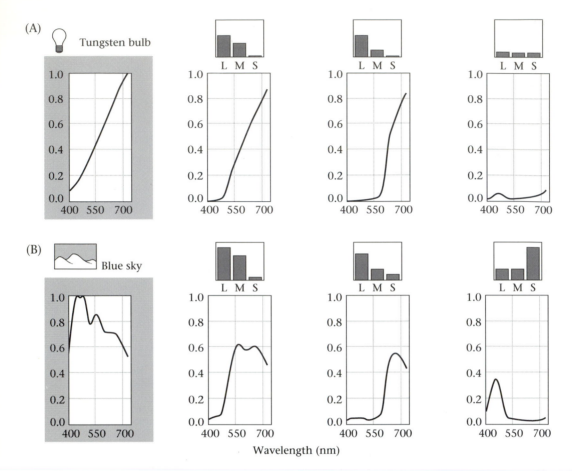

9.5 THE LIGHT REFLECTED FROM OBJECTS CHANGES AS THE ILLUMINANT CHANGES. (A) The shaded panel on the left shows the spectral power distributions of a light source similar to a tungsten bulb. The three graphs on the right show the light reflected from the yellow, red, and blue papers in Figure 9.3 when illuminated by this source. The bar plots above the graphs show the three cone absorption rates caused by the color signal. (B) When the light source is similar to blue sky, as in the shaded panel on the left, the light reflected from the same papers is quite different.

spectral power distribution of light that would be reflected from the yellow, red, and blue papers in Figure 9.3. The shaded graph in Figure 9.5B shows the spectral power distribution similar to blue sky illumination and the light reflected from the same three papers. Plainly, the spectral composition of the reflected light changes when the illuminant changes.

We can calculate the cone absorption rates caused by each of these color signals (see Chapter 4). These rates are shown in the bar plots above the individual graphs of reflected light in Figure 9.5. By comparing the bar graphs in parts A and B of the figure, you can see that the cone absorption rates from each surface change dramatically when the illumination changes. This observation defines a central problem in understanding color appearance. Color is a property of objects; but the reflected light and thus the cone absorptions vary with the illumination. If color must describe a property of an object, the nervous system must *interpret* the mosaic of photopigment absorptions and estimate something about the surface-reflectance function. This is an estimation problem. How can the nervous system use the information in the cone absorptions to infer the surface-reflectance function?

Surface-Reflectance Estimation

There are some very strong limitations on what we can achieve when we set out to estimate surface reflectance from cone absorptions. First, notice that the color signal depends on two spectral functions that are continuous functions of wavelength: the spectral power distribution of the ambient illumination and the surface-reflectance function. The light incident at the eye is the product of these two functions; so any illuminant and surface combination that produces this same light will be indistinguishable to the eye.

One easy mathematical way to see why this is so is to consider the color signal. Recall that the color signal is equal to the product of the illuminant spectral power distribution $e(\lambda)$ and the surface-reflectance function, $s(\lambda)$:

$$c(\lambda) = s(\lambda)e(\lambda) \qquad (9.2)$$

Suppose we replace the illuminant with a new illuminant, $f(\lambda)e(\lambda)$, and replace all of the surfaces with new functions, $s(\lambda)/f(\lambda)$. This change has no effect on the color signal,

$$c(\lambda) = [s(\lambda)/f(\lambda)][f(\lambda)e(\lambda)] = s(\lambda)e(\lambda) \qquad (9.3)$$

and thus no effect on the photopigment absorption rates. Hence, there is no way for the visual system to discriminate between these two illuminant and surface pairs.

Now, consider a second limitation to the estimation problem. The visual system does not measure the spectral power distribution directly. Rather, the visual system only encodes the absorption rates of the three different cone types, so the nervous system cannot be certain which of the many metameric spectral power distributions is responsible for causing the observed cone absorption rates (see Chapter 4). This creates even more uncertainty for the estimation problem.

In the introduction to this part of the book, I quoted Helmholtz's suggestion: the visual system imagines those objects being present that could give rise to the retinal image. We now find that the difficulty we have in following this advice is not that there are no solutions, but rather that there are too many. We encode so little about the color signal that many different objects could all have given rise to the retinal image.

Which of the many possible solutions should we select? The general strategy we should adopt is straightforward: pick the most likely one. Will this be a helpful estimate, or are there so many likely signals that encoding the most likely one is hardly better than guessing with no information?

Perhaps the most important point that we have learned from color-constancy calculations over the last ten years is this: the set of surface and illuminant functions we encounter is not so diverse as to make estimation from the cone catches useless. Some surface-reflectance functions and some illuminants are much more likely than others, and even with only three types of cones, it is possible to make educated guesses that do more good than harm.

The surface-reflectance estimation algorithms we will review are all based on this principle. They differ only in the set of assumptions they make concerning what the observer knows and what we mean by "most likely." I review them now because some of the tools are useful and interesting, and some of the summaries of the data are very helpful in making practical calculations and experiments.

Linear Models

To estimate which lights and surfaces are more probable, we need to do two things. First, we need to measure the spectral data from lights and surfaces. Second, we need a way to represent the likelihood of observing different surface and illuminant functions.

Since the early part of the 1980s, linear models of surface and illuminant functions have been used widely to represent our best guess about the most likely surface and illuminant functions. A linear model of a set of spectral functions, such as surface reflectances, is a method of efficiently approximating the measurements. There are several ways to build linear models, including **principal-components analysis**, **centroid analysis**, or **one-mode analysis**. These methods have much in common, but they differ slightly in their linear model formulation and error measures (Judd et al., 1964; Cohen, 1964; Maloney, 1986; Marimont and Wandell, 1993).

As an example of how to build a linear model, we will review a classic paper by Judd, Macadam, and Wyszecki (1964). These authors built a linear model of an important source of illumination, daylight spectral power distributions. They collected more than 600 measurements of the spectral power distribution of daylight at different times of day, under different weather conditions, and on different continents. To measure the spectral power distribution of daylight we place an object with a known reflectance outside. It is common to use blocks of pressed magnesium oxide as a standard object because such blocks reflect light of all wavelengths nearly equally. Moreover, the material is essentially a pure diffuser: a quantum of light incident on the surface from any angle is reflected back with equal probability in all other directions above the surface.

Since they were interested in the relative spectral composition, not the absolute level, Judd et al. normalized their measurements so that they were all equal to the value 100 at 560 nm. Their main interest was in the wavelength regime visible to the human eye, so they made measurements roughly from 400 nm to 700 nm. Their measurements were spaced every 10 nm. Hence, they could represent each daylight measurement by a set of 31 numbers. Three representative daylight spectral power distributions, normalized to coincide at 560 nm, are shown in Figure 9.6.

The data plotted in Figure 9.6 show that measured daylight relative spectral power distributions can differ depending on the time of day and the weather conditions. But, after examining many daylight functions, Judd et al. found that the curves do not vary wildly and unpredictably; the data are fairly regular. Judd et al. captured the regularities in the data by building a linear model of the observed spectral power distributions. They designed their linear model, a principal-components model, using the following logic.

First, they decided that they wanted to approximate their observations in the **squared-error** sense. That is, suppose $e(\lambda)$ is a measurement, and $\hat{e}(\lambda)$ is the linear-model estimate of the measurement. Then, they decided to select the approximation in order to minimize the squared error

$$\sum_{\lambda}[e(\lambda) - \hat{e}(\lambda)]^2$$

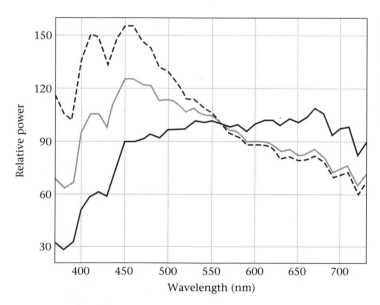

9.6 THE RELATIVE SPECTRAL POWER DISTRIBUTION OF DAYLIGHT UNDER THREE TYPICAL CONDITIONS. The curves drawn here are typical daylight measurements; the curves are normalized to coincide at 560 nm. Source: Judd et al., 1964.

When we consider the collection of observations as a whole, the function that approximates the entire data set with the smallest squared error is the mean. The mean observation from Judd et al.'s data set, $e_0(\lambda)$, is the solid curve in Figure 9.7.

Once we know the mean, we need only approximate the difference between the mean and each individual measurement. We build the linear model to explain these differences as follows. First, we select a fixed set of **basis functions**. Basis functions, like the mean, are descriptions of the measurements. We approximate a measurement's difference from the mean as the weighted sum of the basis functions. For example, suppose $\Delta e_j(\lambda)$ is the difference between the jth daylight measurement and the mean daylight. Further, suppose we select a set of N basis functions, $E_i(\lambda)$. Then, we approximate the differences from the mean as the weighted sum of these basis functions, namely,

$$\Delta e_j(\lambda) \approx \sum_{i=1}^{i=N} \omega_i E_i(\lambda) \tag{9.4}$$

The basis functions are chosen to make the sum of the squared errors between the *collection* of measurements and their approximations as small as possible. The number of basis functions, N, is called the **dimension** of the linear model. The values ω_i are called the linear-model **weights** or **coefficients**. They are chosen to make the squared error between an *individual* measurement and its approximation as small as possible. They serve to describe the properties of the specific measurement.

As the dimension of the linear model increases, the precision of the

9.7 A LINEAR MODEL FOR DAYLIGHT SPECTRAL POWER DISTRIBUTIONS. The curve labeled "Mean" is the mean spectral power distribution of a set of daylights whose spectral power distributions were normalized to a value of 100 at 560 nm. The curves labeled "1st" and "2nd" show the two basis curves used to define a linear model of daylights. By adding together the mean and weighted sums of the two basis functions, one can generate examples of typical relative spectral power distributions of daylight. Source: Judd et al., 1964.

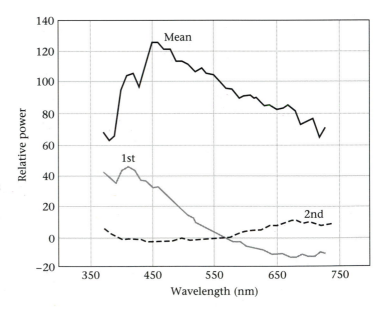

linear-model approximation improves. The dimension one chooses for an application depends on the required precision.[5]

Judd et al. found an excellent approximation of the daylight measurements using the mean and two basis functions. The linear-model representation expresses the measurements efficiently. The mean and two basis functions are fixed, side conditions of the model. Their linear-model approximation of each measurement uses only two weights. The empirical results have been confirmed by other investigators, and the results have been adopted by the international color standards organization to create a model of daylights (Sastri and Das, 1965; Dixon, 1978). The mean and two basis terms from the international standard are plotted in Figure 9.7.

Because daylight varies in absolute spectral power distributions, not just in the relative distribution, we should extend Judd et al.'s linear model to a three-dimensional linear model that includes absolute intensity. A three-dimensional linear model we might use consists of the mean and the two derived curves. In this case the three-dimensional linear model approximation becomes:[6]

$$e(\lambda) = \sum_{i=1}^{3} \omega_i E_i(\lambda) \tag{9.5}$$

We can express the linear model in Equation 9.5 as a matrix equation, $\mathbf{e} = \mathbf{B_e} \boldsymbol{\omega}$ in which $\mathbf{e}$ is a vector representing the illuminant spectral power distribution, the three columns of $\mathbf{B_e}$ contain the basis functions $E_i(\lambda)$, and $\boldsymbol{\omega}$ is a three-dimensional vector containing the linear-model coefficients ω_i.

We can see why linear models are efficient by writing Equation 9.4 in matrix form:

$$
\begin{pmatrix} \vdots \\ e(\lambda) \\ \vdots \end{pmatrix}
=
\begin{pmatrix} \vdots & \vdots & \vdots \\ E_1(\lambda) & E_2(\lambda) & E_3(\lambda) \\ \vdots & \vdots & \vdots \end{pmatrix}
\begin{pmatrix} \omega_1 \\ \omega_2 \\ \omega_3 \end{pmatrix}
$$

[5] The basis functions that minimize the squared error can be found in several ways, most of which are explained in widely available statistical packages. If the data are in the columns of a matrix, one can apply the singular-value decomposition to the data matrix and use the left singular vectors. Equivalently, one can find the eigenvectors of the covariance matrix of the data.

[6] It is possible to improve on this model slightly, but as a practical matter these three curves do quite well as basis functions.

The single spectral power distribution, the vector on the left, consists of measurements at many different wavelengths. The linear model summarizes each measurement as the weighted sum of the basis functions, which are the same for all measurements, and a few weights, $\boldsymbol{w}$, which are unique to each measurement. The linear model is efficient because we represent each additional measurement using only three weights, $\boldsymbol{w}$, rather than the full spectral power distribution.

Simple Illuminant Estimation

Efficiency is useful, but if efficiency were our only objective we could find more efficient algorithms. The linear models are also important because they lead to very simple estimation algorithms. As an example, consider how we might use a device with three color sensors, like the eye, to estimate the spectral power distribution of daylight. Such a device is vastly simpler than the spectroradiometer Judd et al. needed to make many measurements of the light.

Suppose we have a device with three color sensors, whose spectral responsivities are, say, $R_i(\lambda), i = 1, 2, 3$. The three sensor responses will be:

$$r_1 = \sum_\lambda R_1(\lambda)e(\lambda)$$

$$r_2 = \sum_\lambda R_2(\lambda)e(\lambda)$$

$$r_3 = \sum_\lambda R_3(\lambda)e(\lambda) \tag{9.6}$$

We can group these three linear equations into a single matrix equation

$$\mathbf{r} = \mathbf{S}\mathbf{e} \tag{9.7}$$

where the column vector $\mathbf{r}$ contains the sensor responses, the rows of the matrix $\mathbf{S}$ are the sensor spectral responsivities, and $\mathbf{e}$ is the illuminant spectral power distribution.

Before Judd et al.'s study, one might have thought that three sensor responses are insufficient to estimate the illumination. But from their data we have learned that we can approximate $\mathbf{e}$ with a three-dimensional linear model, $\mathbf{e} \approx \mathbf{B_e}\boldsymbol{w}$. This reduces the equation to

$$\mathbf{r} \approx (\mathbf{SB_e})\boldsymbol{w} \tag{9.8}$$

The matrix $\mathbf{SB_e}$ is 3×3, and its entries are all known. The sensor responses, $\mathbf{r}$, are also known. The only unknown is $\boldsymbol{w}$. Hence, we can estimate, $\boldsymbol{w}$, and use these weights to calculate the spectral power distribution, $\mathbf{B_e}\boldsymbol{w}$.

This calculation illustrates two aspects of the role of linear models. First, linear models represent a priori knowledge about the likely set of inputs. Using this information permits us to convert underdetermined linear equations (Equation 9.7) into equations we can solve (Equation 9.8). Linear models are a blunt but useful tool for representing probabilities. Using linear models, it becomes possible to use measurements from only three color sensors to estimate the full relative spectral power distribution of daylight illumination.

Second, linear models work smoothly with the imaging equations. Since the imaging equations are linear, the estimation methods remain linear and simple.

Surface Reflectance Models

Daylight represents an important class of signals for vision. For most of the history of the earth, daylight was the only important light source. There is no similar set of surface-reflectance functions. I was reminded of this once by the brilliant color scientist, G. Wyszecki. When I was just beginning my study of these issues, I asked him why he had not undertaken a study of surfaces similar to those in the daylight study. He shrugged at me and answered, "How do you sample the universe?"

Wyszecki was right, of course. The daylight measurement study could begin and end in a single paper. There is no specific set of surfaces that is of equal importance to daylight, so we have no way to perform a similar analysis on surfaces. But, there are two related questions we can investigate. First, we can ask what the properties are of certain collections of surfaces that are of specific interest to us, say, for practical applications. Second, we can ask what the visual system, with only three types of cones, can infer about surfaces.

Over the years linear models for special sets of materials have been used in many applications. Printer and scanner manufacturers may be interested in the reflectance functions of inks. Computer graphics programmers may be interested in the reflectance factors of geological materials, or tea pots. Color scientists have repeatedly measured the reflectance functions of standard color samples used in industry.[7] These cases can be of practical value and interest in printing and scanning applications (e.g., Drew and Funt, 1992; Marimont and Wandell, 1992; Farrell and Wandell, 1993; Vrhel and Trussell, 1994). To discover the regularities in surface functions, then, we should measure the body reflection terms. From the studies that have taken place over the last several years, it has become increasingly clear that in the visible wavelength region the surface-reflectance functions tend to be quite smooth and thus exhibit a great deal of regularity. Hence, linear models serve to describe the reflectance functions quite well.

[7] Such as the Munsell chips, which are described later in this chapter.

For example, Cohen (1964), Maloney (1986), and Parkkinen et al. (1989) studied the reflectance properties of a variety of surfaces including special samples and some natural objects. For each of the sets studied by these authors, the data can be modeled nearly perfectly using a linear model with fewer than six dimensions. Excellent approximations, though not quite perfect, can be obtained by three-dimensional approximations.

As an example, I have built a linear model to approximate a small collection of surface-reflectance functions for a color target, the **Macbeth ColorChecker**, which is used widely in industrial applications. The target consists of 24 square patches laid out in a 4 × 6 array. The surfaces in this target were selected to have reflectance functions similar to a range of naturally occurring surfaces. They include reflectances similar to human skin, flora, and other materials (McCamy et al., 1976). To create the linear model, I measured the surface-reflectance functions of these patches with a spectral radiometer in my laboratory. The original data set, then, consisted of measurements from 370 nm to 730 nm in 1-nm steps for each of the 24 patches. Then, using conventional statistical packages, I calculated a three-dimensional linear model to fit all of these surface-reflectance functions. The linear model basis functions, $S_i(\lambda)$, were selected to minimize the squared error:[8]

$$\left[s(\lambda) - \sum_{i=1}^{N} \sigma_i S_i(\lambda) \right]^2 \tag{9.9}$$

The values σ_i are called the **surface coefficients**, and we will represent them as a vector, $\boldsymbol{\sigma} = (\sigma_1, \ldots, \sigma_N)$. There are fewer surface coefficients than data measurements. If we create a matrix whose columns are the basis functions, $\mathbf{B_s}$, then we can express the linear model approximation as $\mathbf{B_s}\boldsymbol{\sigma}$.

The shaded lines in Figure 9.8 show the reflectance functions of six of the 24 surfaces. The solid curves within each row of the figure contain the approximations using linear models with different dimensionality. The bottom row shows a one-dimensional linear model; in this case the approximations are scaled copies of one another. As we increase the dimensionality of the linear model the approximations become very similar to the originals. In the three-dimensional model, the approximations are quite close to the true functions.

The low-dimensional linear model approximates these surface-reflectance functions because the functions vary smoothly as a function of wavelength. The linear model consists of a few, slowly varying basis functions, as shown in Figure 9.9. The first basis function captures the light–dark variation of the surfaces. The second basis function captures a red–green variation, and the third captures a blue–yellow variation.

---

[8] I calculated the singular value decomposition of the matrix whose columns consist of the surface reflectance vectors. I used the left singular vectors as the basis functions.

(A)

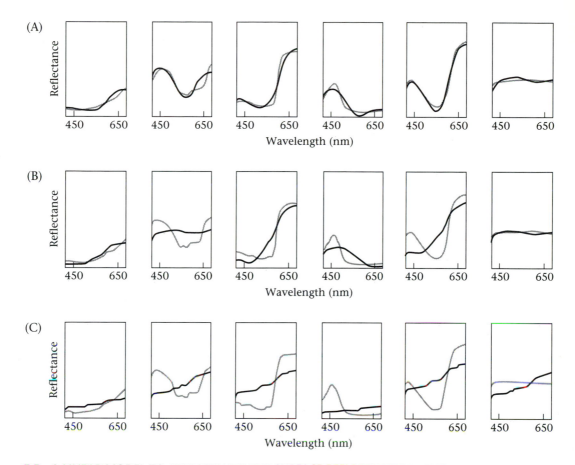

9.8 A LINEAR MODEL TO APPROXIMATE THE SURFACE REFLECTANCES IN THE MACBETH COLORCHECKER. The panels in each row of this figure show the surface-reflectance functions of six colored surfaces (shaded lines) and the approximation to these functions using a linear model (solid lines). The approximations using linear models with (A) three, (B) two, and (C) one dimension are shown.

Although the approximations are quite good, there are differences between the surface-reflectance functions and the three-dimensional linear model. We might ask whether these differences are visually salient. This question is answered by the renderings of these surface approximations in Color Plate 4. The one-dimensional model looks like a collection of surfaces in various shades of gray. For the blue-sky illumination used in the rendering, linear models with three or more dimensions appear very similar to a rendering using the complete set of data.

Sensor-Based Error Measures

I have described linear models that minimize the squared error between the approximation and the original spectral function. As the last analysis showed, however, when we choose linear models to minimize the

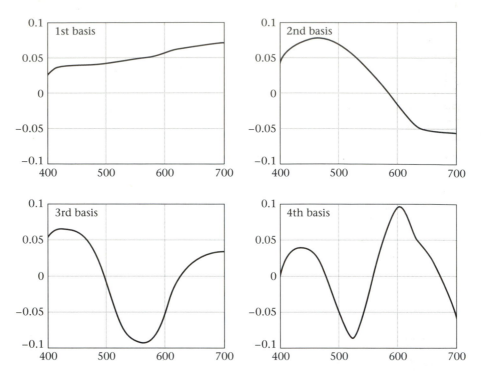

9.9 BASIS FUNCTIONS OF THE LINEAR MODEL FOR THE MACBETH COLORCHECKER. The surface-reflectance functions in the collection vary smoothly with wavelength, as do the basis functions. The first basis function is all positive and explains the most variance in the surface-reflectance functions. The basis functions are ordered in terms of their relative significance for reducing the error in the linear-model approximation to the surfaces.

spectral error we are not always certain whether we have done a good job in minimizing the visual error. In some applications, the spectral error may not be the objective function that we care most about minimizing. When the final consumer of the image is a human, we may only need to capture that part of the reflectance function that is seen by the sensors.

If we are modeling reflectance functions for a computer graphics application, for example, there is no point in modeling the reflectance function at 300 nm, since the human visual system cannot sense light in that part of the spectrum anyway. For these applications, we should be careful to model accurately those parts of the function that are most significant for vision. In these cases, one should select a linear model of the surface reflectance by minimizing a different error measure, one that takes into account the selectivity of the eye.

The procedure for creating linear models that are appropriate for the eye is described in Marimont and Wandell (1992). That study considers how to define linear models that minimize the root-mean-squared

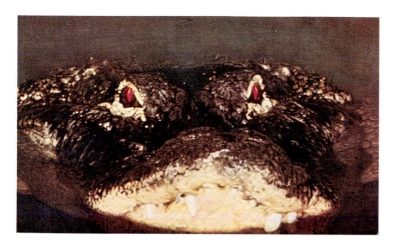

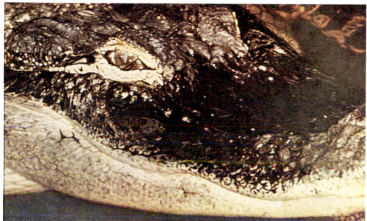

1   In its regenerated form, the rod photopigment rhodopsin appears purple. (Top) The pigment can be seen easily in light reflected from the eyes of an alligator that had been kept in the dark for several hours. (Bottom) After exposure to light, rhodopsin bleaches and becomes transparent; only the alligator's reflective white tapetum is visible after light exposure. From Rushton, 1962.

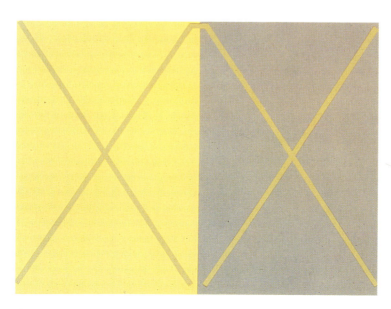

2   This collage by Josef Albers shows that the results of the color-matching experiment cannot explain color appearance. Although the light reflected from the two "X" shapes have the same spectral power distribution (as can be seen at the top of the figure where the X's join), and thus have the same effect on the photopigments, their appearance differs. This illustration demonstrates that the photopigment responses in a small region do not determine color appearance in that region; rather, color appearance depends on the spatial structure of the image as a whole. From Albers, 1975.

3   Our visual experience of color depends on the spatiotemporal frequency range of the stimulus. The graph divides the spatiotemporal plane into three regions corresponding to three basic color appearance regimes. At low spatiotemporal frequencies, color perception is trichromatic: we perceive blue–yellow, red–green, and light–dark variations in contrast. At moderate spatiotemporal frequencies, color perception is dichromatic: we fail to perceive blue–yellow contrast variations. At high spatiotemporal frequencies, color perception is monochromatic: we perceive all image contrast as light–dark modulations of the mean color.

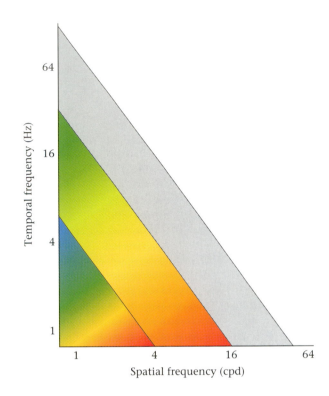

4   Linear-model approximations to the Macbeth ColorChecker are shown rendered under a blue-sky illumination; the linear model dimension of each approximation is listed above the images. In the one-dimensional approximation, the surfaces appear monochromatic, varying only in lightness. As the dimension of the linear-model increases, the approximations appear more similar to the original. For these surfaces, this illuminant, and this method of creating a linear model, the original is visually indistinguishable from the approximations when we use four or more linear-model dimensions.

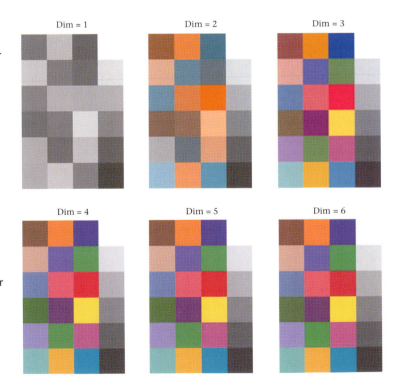

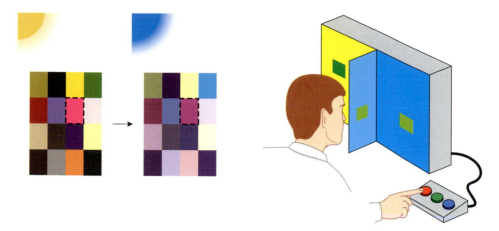

5 The memory-matching (left) and haploscopic (right) methods for measuring asymmetric color matches. In the memory-matching method, the subject sees a target under one illumination, remembers its appearance, and then identifies a matching target after adapting to a second illumination. In the haploscopic method, the observer adapts each eye separately and makes a simultaneous appearance match. An important feature of the haploscopic apparatus depicted is that the bipartite test field is divided by a perpendicular, two-sided mirror that enlarges the size of the background presented to each eye. If a black dividing screen is used instead of a mirror, shifting the gaze between right and left visual fields causes significant changes in the mean illumination.

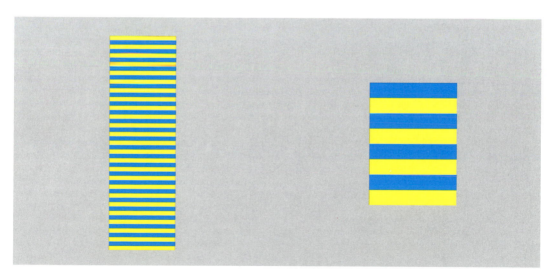

6 These two square-wave patterns were printed using the same ink, and hence the colored bars reflect the same light toward your eyes. The color appearance differs, however, because they are printed at different spatial frequencies. At many viewing distances, the thin bars on the left appear relatively green while the thick bars on the right appear relatively blue. You can also influence the color appearance of the bars by modifying the temporal frequencies of the two patterns: move the book up and down rapidly while viewing the patterns. From Wandell, 1993.

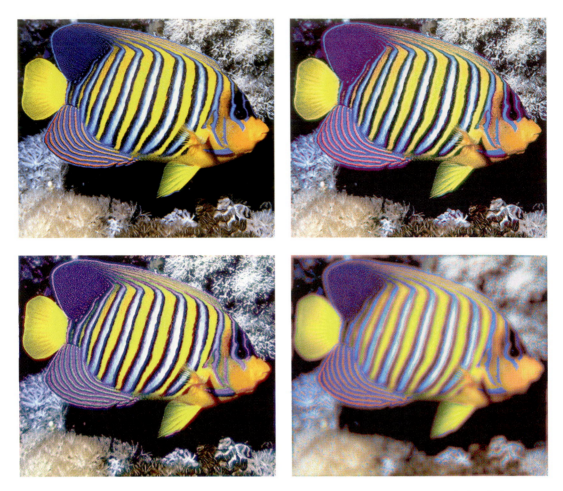

7 The apparent spatial sharpness, or focus, of a color image depends mainly on the light–dark components of the image rather than the opponent-colors components. Using a digital representation, the image at top left was decomposed into three separate red–green, blue–yellow, and light–dark contrast images. Three new versions of the original were made by blurring each of the three contrast images in turn and then combining the contrast images. The results of blurring the red–green (top right), blue–yellow (bottom left), or light–dark (bottom right) contrast image are shown. Although the physical defocus of each contrast image prior to recombination was the same, only the reproduction with a blurred light–dark contrast image appears defocused. Courtesy of Hagit Hel-Or.

error in the photopigment absorption rates, rather than the root-mean-squared error of the spectral curves. The method is called one-mode analysis. For many applications, the error measure minimized by one-mode analysis is superior to root-mean-squared error of the spectral curves.

Surface and Illuminant Estimation Algorithms

There is much regularity in daylight and surface functions, so it makes sense to evaluate how well we estimate spectral functions from sensor responses. Estimation algorithms rely on two essential components.

First, we need a method of representing our knowledge about the likely surface and illuminant functions. For example, linear models can be used to encode our a priori knowledge.[9] Second, all modern estimation methods assume that the illumination varies either slowly or not at all across the image. This assumption is important because it means that the illumination adds very few new parameters to estimate.

Consider an example of an image with p points. We expect to obtain three cone absorption rates at each image point, so there are $3p$ measurements. If we can use a surface three-dimensional model for the surfaces, then there are $3p$ unknown surface coefficients; and there is a linear relationship between the measurements and the unknown quantities. If the illuminant is known, then the problem is straightforward to solve.

Additional unknown illuminant parameters make the problem a challenge. If the illuminant can vary from point to point, there will be $6p$ unknown parameters and the mismatch between known and unknown parameters will be very great. However, if the illuminant is constant across the image, we only have three additional parameters. In this case, by making some modest assumptions about the image, we can find ways to infer these three parameters and then proceed to estimate the surface parameters.

Modern estimation algorithms work by finding a method to overcome the mismatch between the measurements and the unknowns. We can divide existing estimation algorithms into two groups. The majority of estimation algorithms infer the illumination parameters by making one additional assumption about the image contents. For example, suppose we know the reflectance function of one surface. Then, we can use the sensor responses from that surface to measure the illuminant parameters. Knowing the reflectance function of one surface in the image compensates for the three unknown illuminant parameters. There are several implementations of this principle. The most important is the assumption that the average of all the surfaces in the image is gray, which

---

[9] More sophisticated methods are based on using Bayesian estimation as part of the calculation. For example, see D'Zmura and Iverson (1993) and Freeman and Brainard (1994).

is called the **gray-world assumption** (Buchsbaum, 1980; Land, 1986). Other algorithms are based on the assumption that the brightest surface in the image is a **uniform perfect reflector** (McCann et al., 1977). An interesting variant on both of these assumptions is the idea that we can identify **specularities** or glossy surfaces in the image. Since specularities reflect the illumination directly, often without altering the illuminant's spectral power distribution, the sensor responses to glossy surfaces provide information about the illuminant (D'Zmura and Lennie, 1986; Lee, 1986; Tominaga and Wandell, 1989, 1990).

A second group of estimation algorithms compensates for the mismatch in measurements and parameters by suggesting ways to acquire more data. For example, Maloney and Wandell (1986; Wandell, 1987) showed that by adding a fourth sensor (at three spatial locations), one can also estimate the surface and illuminants. D'Zmura and Iverson (1993a, b) explored an interesting variant of this idea. They asked what information is available if we observe the same surface under several illuminants. Pooling information about the same object seen under different illuminants is much like acquiring additional information from extra sensors (e.g., see Wandell, 1987).

Illuminant Correction: An Example Calculation

Before returning to experimental measurements of color appearance, we will perform a calculation that is of some practical interest as well as of some interest in understanding how the visual system might compensate for illumination changes. By working this example, we will start to consider what neural operations might permit the visual pathways to compensate for changes in the ambient illumination.

First, we will consider the general expression that shows how the surface and illuminant functions combine to yield the cone absorption rates. The three equations for the three cone types (L, M, and S), are:

$$r_1 = \sum_\lambda R_1(\lambda)E(\lambda)S(\lambda)$$

$$r_2 = \sum_\lambda R_2(\lambda)E(\lambda)S(\lambda)$$

$$r_3 = \sum_\lambda R_3(\lambda)E(\lambda)S(\lambda) \tag{9.10}$$

Next, we replace the illuminant and surface functions in Equation 9.10 with their linear-model approximations. This yields a new relationship between the coefficients of the surface-reflectance linear model, $\boldsymbol{\sigma}$, and the three-dimensional vector of cone absorptions, $\mathbf{r}$,

$$\mathbf{r} \approx \Lambda_e \boldsymbol{\sigma} \tag{9.11}$$

We call the matrix Λ_e that relates these two vectors the **lighting matrix**. The entries of this matrix depend upon the illumination, **e**. The ijth entry of the lighting matrix is

$$\sum_{\lambda} \left(\sum_k \omega_k E_k(\lambda) \right) R_i(\lambda) S_j(\lambda) \tag{9.12}$$

We can compute two lighting matrices (Equation 9.11) from the spectral curves we have been using as examples. For one lighting matrix, I used the mean daylight spectral power distribution, and for the other I used the spectral power distribution of a tungsten bulb. I used the linear model of the Macbeth ColorChecker for the surface basis functions and the Stockman and MacLeod cone absorption functions (see Fig. 3.3). The lighting matrix for the blue-sky illumination is

$$\begin{pmatrix} 591.48 & 223.05 & -643.05 \\ 477.62 & 376.93 & -564.48 \\ 267.61 & 487.46 & 350.39 \end{pmatrix}$$

and the lighting matrix for the tungsten bulb is

$$\begin{pmatrix} 593.45 & 168.37 & -646.71 \\ 445.79 & 312.79 & -564.33 \\ 152.46 & 278.51 & 185.47 \end{pmatrix}$$

Notice that the largest differences between the matrices are in the third row. This is the row that describes the effect of each surface coefficient on the S-cone absorptions. The blue-sky lighting matrix contains much larger values than the matrix for the tungsten bulb. This makes sense because that is the region of the spectrum where these two illuminant spectral power distributions differ the most (see Fig. 9.5).

Imagine the following way in which the visual system might compensate for illumination changes. Suppose that the cortical analysis of color is based upon the assumption that the illumination is always that of a blue sky. When the illumination is different from the blue sky, the retina must try to provide a neural signal that is similar to the one that would have been observed under a blue sky. What computation does the retina need to perform in order to transform the cone absorptions obtained under the tungsten-bulb illuminant into the cone absorptions that would have occurred under the blue sky?

The cone absorptions from a single surface under the two illuminants can be written as:

$$\mathbf{r} \approx \Lambda_e \boldsymbol{\sigma}$$

$$\mathbf{r}' \approx \Lambda_e' \boldsymbol{\sigma}$$

By inverting the lighting matrices and recombining terms, we find that the cone absorptions under the two illuminants should be related linearly as,

$$\mathbf{r} \approx \Lambda_e \Lambda_e'^{-1} \mathbf{r}' \tag{9.13}$$

Hence, we can transform the cone absorptions from a surface illuminated by the tungsten bulb into the cone absorptions of the same surface illuminated by the blue sky by the following:

$$\mathbf{r} = \begin{pmatrix} 0.8119 & 0.2271 & 0.0550 \\ -0.0803 & 1.1344 & 0.1282 \\ 0.0429 & -0.0755 & 1.8091 \end{pmatrix} \mathbf{r}' \tag{9.14}$$

The retina can compensate for the illumination change by linearly transforming the observed cone absorptions, $\mathbf{r}'$, into a new signal, $\mathbf{r}$.

Now, what does it mean for the retina to compute a linear transformation? The linear transformation consists of a simple series of multiplications and additions. For example, consider the third row of the matrix in Equation 9.14. This row defines how the new S-cone absorptions should be computed from the observed absorptions. When we write this transformation as a single linear equation we see that the observed and transformed signals are related as

$$S = 0.0429 \, L' + -0.0755 \, M' + 1.8091 \, S' \tag{9.15}$$

The transformed S-cone absorption is mainly a scaled version of the observed absorptions. Because the tungsten bulb emits much less energy in the short-wavelength part of the spectrum, the scale factor is larger than 1. In addition, to be absolutely precise, we should add in a small amount of the observed L-cone signal and subtract out a small amount of the observed M-cone signal. But, these contributions are relatively small compared to the contribution from the S-cones. In general, for each of the cone types, the largest contributions to the transformed signal are scaled copies of the same signal type.

In this matrix, and in many practical examples, the only additive term that is not negligible is the contribution of the M-cone response to the transformed L signal. As a rough rule, because the diagonal terms are much larger than the off-diagonal terms, we can obtain good first-order approximation to the proper transformation by simply scaling the observed cone absorptions (see Foster and Nascimento, 1994).

Compensating for the illumination change by a purely diagonal scaling of the cone absorptions is called the **von Kries coefficient law**. The correction is not as precise as the best linear correction, but it frequently provides a good approximation. As we shall see in the next section, the von Kries coefficient law describes certain aspects of human color-appearance measurements as well.

Color Constancy: Experiments

> In woven and embroidered stuffs the appearance of colors is pro-
> foundly affected by their juxtaposition with one another (purple, for
> instance, appears different on white than on black wool), and also
> by differences of illumination. Thus embroiderers say that they often
> make mistakes in their colors when they work by lamplight, and use
> the wrong ones.
>
> Aristotle, *Meteorologica*

Asymmetric Color-Matching Experiments

To formulate some ideas about how the visual pathways compute color
appearance, we adopted the view that color appearance is a psychological estimate of the surface-reflectance function (body reflectance). By
thinking about computational methods of estimating body reflectance,
we have discovered how the cone absorptions from an object vary with
illuminant changes. Finally, we have seen that it is possible to compensate approximately for these changes by applying a linear transformation to the cone absorptions.

From the computational analysis, we have discovered a good question to examine in experimental studies of color appearance: What is
the relationship between the cone absorptions of objects that appear
the same under different illuminants? The computational analysis suggests that the cone absorptions of lights with the same color appearance, but seen under different illuminants, are related by a linear transformation.

It is up to the experimentalist, then, to find a method to use for
measuring the cone absorptions that correspond to the same color
appearance when seen in different viewing contexts. Color Plate 5 illustrates two methods of making such measurements. Panel A shows
a **memory-matching** method. In this method, the subject studies the
color of a target that is presented under one illumination source and
then must select a target that looks the same under a second illumination source. These measurements identify the stimuli, and thus the
cone absorptions, of targets that appear the same under the two illuminants. The drawback of the method is that making such matches is
very time-consuming because the subject must adapt to the two illumination sources completely, a process which can take two minutes or
more.

Color Plate 5B shows a second method called **dichoptic matching**.
In this experiment the observer views the two scenes simultaneously in
different eyes. One eye is exposed to a large neutral surface illuminated
by, say, a daylight lamp. The other eye is exposed to an equivalent large
neutral surface illuminated by, say, a tungsten lamp. These surfaces define a background stimulus that is different for each eye. The two backgrounds fuse in appearance and appear as a single large background. To

establish the asymmetric color matches, the experimenter places a test object on top of the standard background seen by one eye. The observer selects a matching object from an array of choices seen by the second eye. The color-appearance mapping is defined by measuring the cone absorptions of the test and matching objects, usually small colored papers, seen under their respective illuminants.

The dichoptic method has the advantage that the matches may be set quickly, avoiding the tedious delays required for visual adaptation in memory matches. The method has the disadvantage of making the assumption that adaptation occurs independently, prior to binocular combination.[10]

The experimental methods shown in Color Plate 5 generalize the conventional color-matching experiment. These methods are called **asymmetric color-matching** because, unlike standard color-matching, in these experiments the matches are set between stimuli presented in different contexts. As we have already seen, because color appearance discounts estimated changes of the illumination, matches set in the asymmetric color-matching experiment are *not* cone-absorption matches. Rather, the observer is establishing a match at a more central site following the correction for the properties of the scene.

The asymmetric color-matching experiment is directly relevant to the questions raised by our computational analysis of color appearance. Moreover, the experiment has a central place in the study of color appearance simply for practical experimental reasons. There are many general questions we might ask about color appearance. For example, we would like to be able to measure which colors are similar to one another; which colors have a common hue, saturation, or brightness; and so forth. If we had to study these questions separately under each illuminant, the task would be overwhelming. By beginning with the asymmetric color-matching experiment, we can divide color appearance measurements into two parts and reduce our experimental burden. The asymmetric matches define a mapping between the cone absorptions of objects with the same color appearance seen under different illuminants. From these experiments, we learn how to convert a target seen under one illuminant into an equivalent target under a standard illuminant. This transformation saves a great deal of experimental effort since we can focus most of our questions about color appearance on studies using just one standard illuminant.

---

[10] This binocular method makes sense if one accepts the view that the adjustment for the illumination is mediated primarily before the signals from the two eyes are combined, in the superficial layers of area V1. The coherence of the experimental method can be tested psychophysically by examining transitivity. The observer matches a test on backgrounds L and R_1, and then on backgrounds L and R_2. The experimenter then places R_1 in the left eye and R_2 in the right eye and verifies that the matching lights match one another. There is no guarantee, of course, that these measurements are governed by precisely the same visual mechanisms that govern adaptation under normal viewing conditions.

The Linearity of Asymmetric Color Matches

We have seen measurements of superposition to test linearity through-out this volume. Tests of linearity in asymmetric color-matching appear very early in the color-appearance literature. When von Kries (1902, 1905) introduced the coefficient law, he listed several testable empirical results. Among the predictions, he listed the basic test of linearity, namely,

> . . . there exist several very simple laws, which also appear to be specially adapted for experimental test. Namely, it must be that if L_1 on one retinal region causes the same result as L_2 on another, and similarly M_1, working on the first, causes the same effect as M_2 on the other, in every case also $L_1 + M_1$ must have here the same effect as $L_2 + M_2$ there.
> . . . The extended studies of Wirth (1900–1903) show that the law can be considered as nearly valid for reacting lights that are not too weak.

Evidently, von Kries not only raised the question of linearity of asymmetric color-matching, but by 1905 he considered it answered affirmatively.

While von Kries considered the question settled, not everyone was persuaded. Over the years, there have been many separate experimental tests of linearity in the asymmetric color-matching experiment. I am particularly impressed by a series of papers by Elaine Wassef, working first in London and then at the University College for Girls in Cairo. Wassef wrote at roughly the same time E. H. Land was working at Polaroid. In her papers, she reports on new studies and provides a review of the experimental tests of asymmetric color-matching linearity (Wassef, 1952, 1958, 1959).[11] Like von Kries, Wassef asked whether one could predict asymmetric color matches using the principle of superposition. Like von Kries, she concluded that the weight of the experimental evidence supported the linearity hypothesis: when the illumination changes, the cone absorptions of the test and matching lights are related by a linear transformation.

I have replotted some of Wassef's data to illustrate the nature of the measurements and the size of the effect (Figure 9.10). The illuminant spectral power distributions she used in her dichoptic matching experiment are plotted in Figure 9.10A. To plot her results, I have converted Wassef's reported measurements into cone absorptions. I have plotted the cone absorptions of the surfaces that matched in color appearance when seen under the two illuminants. Figure 9.10B shows the L- and M-cone absorptions of the surfaces under the two illuminants, and Figure 9.10C shows the L- and S-cone absorptions. The cone absorptions for objects seen under a tungsten illuminant are plotted as open circles;

---

[11] Interestingly, one of the largest sets of data she reviewed was a series of experiments performed at the Kodak research laboratories, Polaroid's competitor.

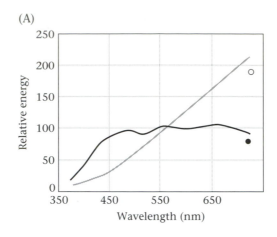

(A)

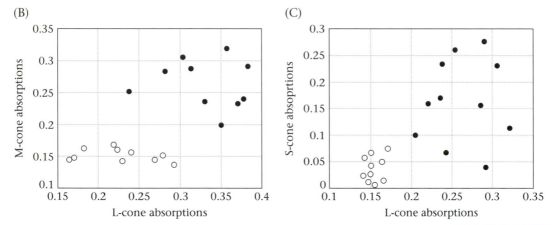

9.10 DATA FROM AN ASYMMETRIC COLOR-MATCHING EXPERIMENT USING THE DICHOPTIC METHOD. The test and matching lights are viewed in different contexts and appear identical; but the two lights have very different cone absorption rates. Hence, appearance matches made across an illuminant change are not cone absorption matches. (A) The spectral power distributions of two illuminants, one approximating mean daylight and the other a tungsten illuminant are shown. (B) Cone absorptions for targets that appear identical to one another in these two contexts are shown as scatterplots for the L- and M-cones, and (C) for the L- and S-cones. The points plotted as open circles are cone absorptions for tests seen under the first illuminant; matches seen under the second illuminant are plotted as filled circles. The stimuli represented by the absorptions have the same color appearance, but they correspond to very different cone absorptions. Source: Wassef, 1959.

the cone absorptions for objects seen under a blue-sky illumination are plotted as filled circles. The size of the effect is quite substantial. Two sets of points show the cone absorptions of targets that look identical in their respective contexts, yet the cone absorption values from the surfaces under these illuminants do not even overlap in their values.

Taken together, the color matching and asymmetric color matching results show the following. When the objects are in the same context, equating the cone absorptions equates appearance, but when the two objects are seen under different illuminants, equating cone absorptions does not equate appearance. Within each context the observer uses the pattern of cone absorptions to infer color appearance, probably by comparing the relative cone absorption rates. Color appearance is an interpretation of the physical properties of the objects in the image.

The von Kries Coefficient Law: Experiments

Through his coefficient law, von Kries sought to explain these asymmetric color matches by a simple physiological mechanism. He suggested that the visual pathways adjust to the illumination by scaling the signals from the individual cone classes. This hypothesis has a simple experimental prediction: if we plot, say, the S-cone absorptions of the test and match surfaces on a single graph, the data should fall along a straight line through the origin. The slope of the predicted line is the scale factor for the illuminant change.

Neither von Kries nor Wassef knew the cone spectral curves; hence, they could not create the graph they needed to test the von Kries coefficient law directly. However, using an indirect measurement based on estimation of the eigenvectors of the measured linear transformations, Burnham et al. (1957) and Wassef (1959) rejected von Kries scaling. Despite this rejection, von Kries's hypothesis continued to be used widely to explain how color appearance varies with illumination. Among theorists, for example, E. H. Land relied entirely on von Kries scaling as the foundation of his retinex theory (Brewer, 1954; Brainard and Wandell, 1986; Land, 1986).

Today, we have good estimates of the spectral sensitivities of the cone photopigments, and it is possible to convert Wassef's data into cone absorptions and to analyze the von Kries coefficient law directly. Figure 9.11 shows a graphical evaluation of von Kries's hypothesis for the data in Figure 9.10. Each panel plots the cone absorptions of corresponding test and match targets for one of the three cone types. As

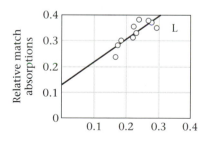 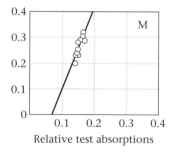 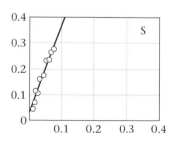

Relative test absorptions

9.11 GRAPHICAL EVALUATION OF VON KRIES'S HYPOTHESIS for the data in Figure 9.10. These appearance matches were made by presenting the test and match objects to different eyes. The illuminant for one eye was similar to a tungsten bulb, and the other eye was blue skylight. As predicted by von Kries, the cone absorptions of the test and match surfaces approximate a straight line. However, the von Kries coefficient law predicts that the line should pass through the origin of the graph; while not precisely correct, the rule is a helpful starting point. Source: Wassef, 1959.

predicted by von Kries, the cone absorptions of the test and match targets fall along a line. Moreover, the slopes of the lines relating the cone absorptions also make sense. The slope is largest for the S-cones, where illuminant change has its largest effect. The data are not perfectly consistent with von Kries scaling, however, because the lines through the data do not pass through the origin, as required by the theory.[12]

There is an emerging consensus in many branches of color science that the von Kries coefficient law explains much about how color appearance depends on the illumination. Von Kries's simple hypothesis is important partly because of its practical utility and partly because of its implications for the representation of color appearance within the brain. The hypothesis explains the major adjustments for color constancy in terms of the photoreceptor signal and how the photoreceptor signals combine within the retina (Chapter 4). Hence, von Kries's hypothesis implies that either (a) the main adjustment takes place very early, or (b) the photoreceptor signals can be separated in the central representation. This topic will come up again later, when we review some of the phenomena concerning color appearance in the central nervous system.

How Color-Constant Are We?

Finally, we will consider how well the visual pathways correct for illumination change. On this point there is some consensus: the asymmetric color matches do not compensate completely for the illumination change (Helson, 1938; Judd, 1940).

Brainard and Wandell (1991b, 1992) described this phenomenon using an apparatus consisting of simulated surfaces and illuminants and an asymmetric color-matching experiment based on memory-matches. Subjects were presented with images of simulated colored papers, rendered under a diffuse daylight illuminant, on a CRT display. The subjects memorized the color appearance of one of the surfaces. Next, the simulated illuminant was changed, slowly over a period of two minutes, giving subjects a chance to adapt to the new illuminant. Then, the subject adjusted the appearance of a simulated surface to match the color appearance of the surface he or she had memorized.

We can represent the difference between the two simulated illuminants by plotting the illuminant change. The filled symbols in Figure 9.12 show the illuminant changes in two experimental conditions. The top panel shows an illuminant change that increased the short-wavelength light and decreased the long-wavelength light. The bottom panel shows an illuminant change that increased the energy at all wavelengths.

---

[12] Indeed, this is equally a failure of the simple linearity that Wassef uses to summarize the data, and more in line with some of the conclusions that Burnham et al. (1957) drew about their data.

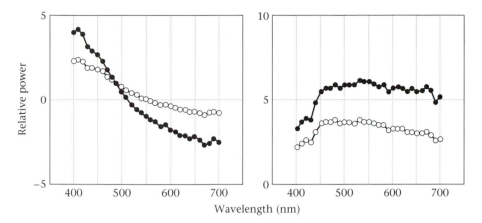

9.12 A COMPARISON OF THE ILLUMINANT CHANGE AND THE SUBJECTIVE ILLUMINANT CHANGE, as inferred from an asymmetric matching experiment. The simulated illuminant change and subjective illuminant changes are shown by the filled and open circles, respectively. Subjects behave as if the illuminant change is about half of the true illuminant change. Source: Brainard and Wandell, 1991b.

Suppose that subjects equated the perceived surface reflectance, but that the illuminant change they estimated was different from the true illuminant change. In that case, we can use the observed matches to infer the the subjects' illuminant estimates, which are plotted as the open symbols in two panels of Figure 9.12. Subjects are acting as if the illuminant change they are correcting for is similar to the simulated illuminant change, but smaller. Subjects' performance is conservative, correcting for about half the true illuminant change.

The experiments in Brainard and Wandell (1991b, 1992) were conducted on display monitors, and the images were far less complex than full natural scenes. It is possible that, given additional clues, subjects may come closer to true illuminant estimation. But in most laboratory experiments to date, subjects do not compensate fully for changes in the illumination. When the illumination changes, color appearance changes less than it might if color were defined by the cone absorptions, but it changes more than it would if the nervous system used the best possible computational algorithms.

The Perceptual Organization of Color

In this section, I will review some of the methods for describing the perceptual organization of color appearance. Specifically, we will consider the relationship between different colors and some of the systems for describing color appearance. In addition to the implications this organization has for understanding the neural representation of color appearance, there are also many practical needs for descriptive systems of color appearance. Artists and designers need ways to identify and specify the color appearance of a design. Further, they need ways of organizing colors and finding interesting color harmonies. Engineers need to assess the appearance and discriminability of colors used for highway signs, for labeling parts and packaging, and for designing software icons.

Language provides us with a useful start for organizing color appearance. Spoken English in the United States consists of 11 color terms that are widely and consistently used.[13] While the number of terms used differs across cultures, there is a remarkable hierarchical organization to the order in which color names appear. Cultures with a small number of basic color names always include white, black and red. Color terms such as purple and pink enter later (Berlin and Kay, 1969; Boynton and Olsen, 1987).

Color names are a coarse description of color experience. Moreover, names list but do not organize color experience. Thus, they are not helpful when we consider issues such as color similarity or color harmony. A more complete organization of color experience is based on the three perceptual attributes called **hue, saturation**, and **brightness**. Hue is the attribute that permits a color to be classified as red, yellow, green, and so forth. Saturation describes a color's similarity to a neutral gray or white. A gray object with a small reddish tint has little saturation, while a red object, with little white or gray, is very saturated. An object's brightness tells us about the relative ordering of the object on the dark-to-light scale.

Based on psychological studies of the similarity of colored patches with many different hues, saturations, and brightnesses, the artist Albert Munsell created a book of colored samples. The samples are organized with respect to hue, saturation, and brightness. Furthermore, the colored samples are spaced in equal perceptual steps. Munsell organized the samples within his book using a cylindrical organization as shown in Figure 9.13. The *Munsell Book of Colors* is sold by the Munsell Color Company, and is used as a reference in many design and engineering applications.

Perceptually, both saturation and brightness can be arranged using a linear ordering from small to large; hue, however, does not follow a linear ordering. Therefore, Munsell organized lightness along the main axis of the cylinder, and saturation as the distance from the center of the cylinder to the edge. The circular hue dimension was mapped around the circumference of the cylinder.

Munsell developed a special notation to refer to each of the samples in his book. To distinguish his notation from the colloquial usage, Munsell substituted the word **value** for lightness and the word **chroma** for saturation. He retained the word hue, apparently finding no adequate substitute. In the Munsell notation, the words hue, chroma, and value have specific and technical meanings. Each colored paper is described

[13] White, black, red, green, yellow, blue, brown, purple, pink, orange, and gray.

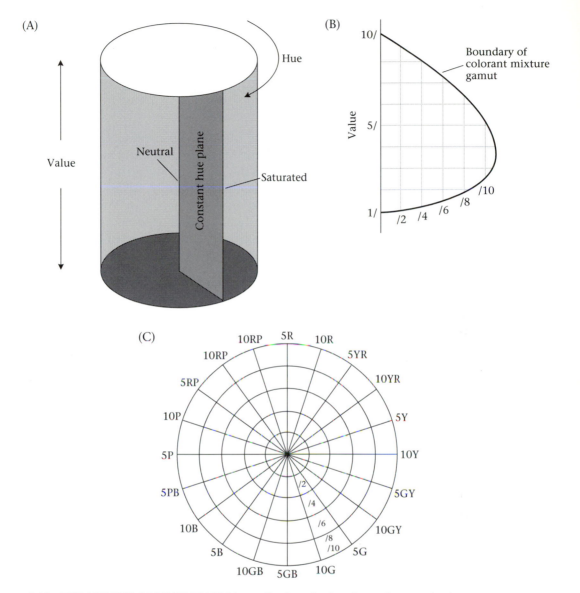

9.13 THE *MUNSELL BOOK OF COLORS* is a collection of colored samples organized in terms of three perceptual attributes of color. (A) The samples are arranged using a cylindrical geometry. The main axis of the cylinder codes lightness; the distance from the center of the cylinder to the edge codes the Munsell property called value (saturation); the position around the circumference of the cylinder codes the Munsell property called chroma (hue). (B) A cross-section of the cylinder through the main axis represents a single hue, but different values and chroma. Not all combinations of hue, chroma and value can be reproduced; the general shape of the reproduction boundary is shown. (C) A cross-section perpendicular to the main axis includes samples at a single value but with different hues and chroma. Regions around the circle are lableled with basic color names (e.g., R = red, Y = yellow, GB = green-blue). These regions are divided into ten steps, though usually only the positions corresponding to steps 5 and 10 are shown. The hues are arranged so that similar hues are near to one another and complementary hues are on opposite sides of the circle.

using a three-part syntax of hue chroma/value. For example, 3YR 5/3 refers to a colored paper with the hue called 3YR, the chroma level 5, and the value level 3.

The *Munsell Book of Colors* was created before the CIE color standards described in Chapter 4. With the advent of the CIE measurement standard, based on the color-matching functions, there was a need for a method to convert the Munsell representation into the CIE standard representation. A committee of the Optical Society (Newhall et al., 1943) measured the CIE values of the Munsell samples in the published book, and the Munsell Corporation agreed to produce the colored samples to measurement standards defined by the Optical Society of America. The new standard for the *Munsell Book of Colors*, based on CIE values rather than pigment formulas, is called the **Munsell Renotation System**. Calibration tables that describe the color measurements of the Munsell samples are available, for example, in Wyszecki and Stiles (1982).

Opponent Colors

One of the most remarkable and important insights about color appearance is the concept of **opponent colors**, first described by Hering (1878). Hering pointed out that there is a powerful psychological relationship between the different hues. While some pairs of hues can coexist in a single color sensation, others cannot. For example, orange is composed of red and yellow while cyan is composed of blue and green. But we never experience a hue that is simultaneously red and green. Nor do we experience a color sensation that is simultaneously blue and yellow. These two hue pairs, red–green and blue–yellow, are called **opponent colors**.

There is no physical reason why these two opponent-color pairs must exist. That we never perceive red and green, while we easily perceive red and yellow, must be due to the neural representation of colors. Hering argued that opponent colors exist because the sensations of red and green are encoded in a single visual pathway. The excitation of the pathway causes us to perceive one of the opponent colors; inhibition of the pathway causes us to perceive the other.

Hering made his point forcefully and extended his theory to explain various other aspects of color appearance, as well. But his insights were not followed by a set of quantitative studies. Perhaps for this reason, his ideas languished while the colorimetrists used color-matching to set standards for all of modern technology. This is not to say that Hering's work was forgotten. Colorimetrists who thought about color appearance invariably turned to Hering's insights. In a well-known review article (Judd, 1951), the eminent scientist D. B. Judd wrote (p. 836):

> The Hering (1905) theory of opponent colors has come to be fairly well accepted as the most likely description of color processes in the optic nerve and cortex. Thus this theory reappears in the final stage in the stage theories of von Kries-Schrodinger (von Kries, 1905; Schrodinger,

1925), Adams (1923, 1942) and Muller (1924, 1930). By far the most completely worked out of these stage theories is that of Muller. . . . There is slight chance that all of the conjectures are correct, but, even if some of the solutions proposed by Muller prove to be unacceptable, he has nevertheless made a start toward the solution of important problems that will eventually have to be faced by other theorists.

Hue Cancellation

Several experimental observations, beginning in the mid-1950s, catapulted opponent-colors theory from a special-purpose model, known only to color specialists, to a central idea in vision science. The first was a behavioral experiment that defined a procedure for measuring opponent colors, the **hue-cancellation experiment**. The hue cancellation experiment was developed in a series of papers by Jameson and Hurvich (1955, 1957). By providing a method of quantifying the opponent-colors insight, Hurvich and Jameson made the idea accessible to other scientists, opening a major line of inquiry.

In the hue-cancellation experiment, the observer is asked to judge whether a test light appears to be, say, reddish or greenish. If the test light appears reddish, the subject adds green light in order to cancel precisely the red appearance of the test. If the light appears greenish, then the subject adds red light to cancel the green appearance. The added light is called the **canceling light**. Once the red or green hue of the test light is canceled, the test plus canceling light appears yellow, blue, or gray. The same experiment can be performed to measure the blue–yellow opponent-colors pairing. In this case the subject is asked whether the test light appears blue or yellow, and the canceling lights also appear blue or yellow.

Figure 9.14 shows a set of hue-cancellation measurements obtained by Jameson and Hurvich (1955, 1957). Subjects canceled the red–green or blue–yellow color appearance of a series of spectral lights. The vertical axis shows the relative intensity of the canceling lights, scaled so that when equal amounts of these lights are superimposed the result did not appear, say, red or green. The canceling lights always have positive intensity, but the intensity of the green and blue canceling lights are plotted as negative to permit you to distinguish which canceling light was used.

To what extent can we generalize from red–green measurements using monochromatic lights to other lights? To answer this question we must evaluate the linearity of the hue-cancellation experiment. If the experiment is linear, we can use the data in Figure 9.14 to predict whether any test light will appear red or green (or blue or yellow) since all lights are the sum of monochromatic lights. If the experiment is not linear, then the data represent only an interesting collection of observations.

To evaluate the linearity of the hue-cancellation experiment, one can perform the following experiment. Suppose the test light t_1 ap-

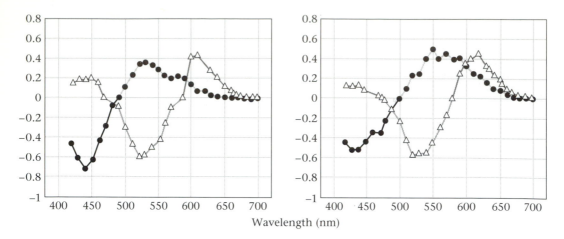

Wavelength (nm)

9.14 MEASUREMENTS FROM THE HUE-CANCELLATION EXPERIMENT. An observer is presented with a monochromatic test light. If the light appears red then some amount of a green canceling light is added to cancel the redness. If the light appears green, then a red canceling light is added to cancel the greenness. The horizontal axis of the graph measures the wavelength of the monochromatic test light, and the vertical axis measures the relative intensity of the canceling light. The entire curve (open triangles) represents the red–green appearance of all monochromatic lights. A similar procedure is used to measure blue–yellow hue cancellation (filled circles). The two graphs show results from two observers. Source: Hurvich and Jameson, 1957.

pears neither red nor green, and the test light t_2 appears neither red nor green. Does the superposition of these two test lights, $t_1 + t_2$, also appear neither red nor green? In general, the hue-cancellation experiment fails this test of linearity. If we superimpose two lights, neither of which appears red or green, the result can appear red; if we add two lights neither of which appears blue or yellow, the result can appear yellow. Hence, although the hue-cancellation studies provide a useful benchmark, we need a more complete (nonlinear) model before we can apply the hue-cancellation data in Figure 9.14 to predict the opponent-colors appearance of polychromatic test lights (Larimer et al. 1975; Burns et al., 1984; Ayama and Ikeda, 1989; Chichilnisky, 1995).

Opponent-Colors Measurements at Threshold

In addition to color-appearance judgments, one can also demonstrate the presence of essential opponent-colors signals behaviorally by **color test-mixture experiments**. These color experiments are direct analogues of the pattern-mixture experiments reviewed in Chapter 7 (see Figs. 7.7 and 7.9). A set of threshold measurements from a color test-mixture experiment are shown in Figure 9.15. The axes represent the absorption rates of the L- and M-cones. Each point represents a combination of absorption rates at detection threshold. The smooth curve fit through the data points is an ellipse.

The intersection of the ellipse with the horizontal axis, shows the relative L-cone absorption rate at detection threshold. The intersection

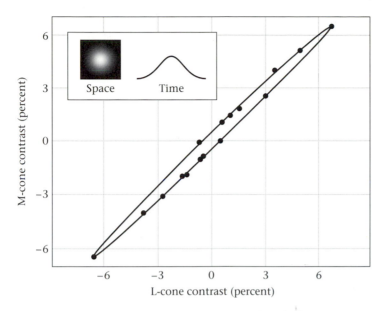

9.15 COLOR TEST-MIXTURE EXPERIMENTS demonstrate opponent-colors processes. The axes measure percentage change in cone absorption rates for the L- and M-cones. The points show the cone absorption rates at the detection threshold measured using different colored test lights. The smooth curve is an ellipse fit through the data points. The mixture experiment shows that the L- and M-cone signals cancel one another, so that lights that excite a mixture of L- and M-cones are harder to see than lights that stimulate just one of these two cone classes. The insets show the spatially blurred appearance of the test stimulus and the gradual timecourse as the stimulus contrast increases and then decreases. Source: Wandell, 1985.

of the ellipse with the vertical axis shows the relative M-cone absorption rate at detection threshold. The shape of the ellipse shows that signals that stimulate the L- and M-cones simultaneously are less visible than signals that stimulate only one or the other. At the most extreme points on the ellipse, the cone absorptions of the L- and M-cones are more than five times the rate required to detect a signal when each cone class is stimulated alone. The poor sensitivity to mixtures of signals from these two cone types shows that the signals must oppose one another. The cancellation of threshold-level signals from the L- and M-cones, as well as between the S-cones and the other two classes (not shown), has been observed in many different laboratories and under many different experimental conditions (e.g., Boynton et al., 1964; Pugh, 1976; Pugh and Mollon, 1979; Mollon and Polden, 1977; Sternheim, 1979; Wandell and Pugh, 1980a, b; Stromeyer et al., 1985).

In addition to demonstrating opponent colors, these threshold data reveal a second interesting and surprising feature of visual encoding. Two neural signals that are visible when they are seen singly become invisible when they are superimposed. It seems odd that the visual system should be organized so that plainly visible signals can be made invisible. From the figure we can see that this is a powerful effect, suppressing a signal that is more than five times threshold. This observation tells us that in many operating conditions absolute sensitivity is not the dominant criterion. The visual pathways can sacrifice target visibility in order to achieve the goals of the opponent-colors encoding.

Opponent Signals in the Visual Pathways

In addition to these two types of behavioral evidence, there is also considerable physiological evidence that demonstrates the existence of opponent-colors signals in the visual pathway. In a report that gained widespread attention, Svaetichin (1956) measured the responses of three types of retinal neurons in a fish. He reported that the electrical responses were roughly consistent with Hering's notion of the opponent-colors representation. In two types of neurons, the electrical response increased to certain wavelengths of light and decreased in response to other wavelengths, paralleling the red–green and blue–yellow opponency in color perception.[14] The electrical response of a third set of neurons increased to all wavelengths of light, as in a black–white representation. Shortly after Svaetichin's report, DeValois and his colleagues established the existence of opponent-colors neurons in the LGN of nonhuman primates. There is now a substantial literature documenting the presence of opponent-color signals in the visual pathways (e.g., DeValois et al., 1958a,b, DeValois, 1965a,b; DeValois et al., 1966; Wiesel and Hubel, 1966; Gouras, 1968; Derrington et al., 1984; Lennie et al., 1991).

The resemblance between the psychological organization of opponent colors measured in the hue-cancellation experiment and the neural opponent signals suggests a link from the neural responses to the perceptual organization. To make a convincing argument for the specific connection between opponent colors and a specific set of neural opponent signals, we must identify a linking hypothesis. The hypothesis should tell us how we can predict appearance from the activity of cells, and conversely how we can predict the activity of these cells from appearance.

A natural starting place is to suppose that there is a population of neurons whose members are excited when we perceive red and inhibited when we perceive green. From the linking hypothesis, we predict that neurons in this population will be unresponsive to lights that appear neither red nor green. There are two spectral regions that appear neither red nor green to human observers: one near 570 nm and a second near 470 nm. The question of whether there exists a population of neurons with the hypothetical response patterns was studied by DeValois and his collaborators in the LGN of the monkey. In their studies, DeValois and his colleagues studied the response of neurons to

---

[14] At first, it was thought that these responses reflected the activity of the the the cones. Subsequent investigations showed that the responses were from horizontal cells (Svaetichin and MacNichol, 1958).

monochromatic stimuli presented on a zero background. They found a weak correspondence between the neutral points of individual neurons and the perceptual neutral points (DeValois et al., 1966). More recently, Derrington et al. (1984) measured the responses of LGN neurons using contrast stimulus presented on a moderate neutral background. They estimated the input to these neurons from the different cone classes and confirmed the basic observations made by DeValois and his colleagues.

Derrington et al. (1984) reported that parvocellular neurons can be classified into two groups. One population of neurons receives opposing input from the L- and M-cones; the left panel of Figure 9.16 shows my estimate of the spectral sensitivity of this group of parvocellular neurons. While stimulus wavelengths near 570 nm are ineffective at exciting these cells, the precise wavelength of the zero-crossing varies widely across the neural population. Moreover, neurons in this population do not show a second zero-crossing near 470 nm that would parallel the human opponent-colors judgments in the hue-cancellation experiment. Hence, there is no strong evidence that this population of neurons represents red–green color appearance.

A second population of LGN neurons receives input from the S-cones and an opposing signal from a combination of the L- and M-cones. For these neurons, wavelengths near 500 nm are quite ineffective. The panel on the right of Figure 9.16 shows my estimate of the spectral sensitivity of this group of parvocellular neurons.

There was less order in the opponent-color signals of the magnocellular neurons. Many magnocellular units seemed to be driven by a difference between the L- and M-cones. A few parvocellular units and a few magnocellular units were driven by a positive sum of the signals from these two cone types.

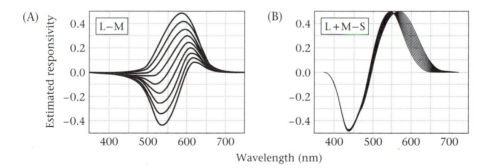

9.16 OPPONENT SIGNALS MEASURED IN LGN NEURONS. These spectral response curves are inferred from the measured responses of LGN neurons to many different colored stimuli presented on a monitor. The vast majority of LGN neurons in the parvocellular layers can be divided into two groups based on their response to modulations of colored lights. (A) One group of neurons receives an opponent contribution from the L- and M-cones alone. (B) The second group of neurons receives a signal of like sign from the L- and M-cones, and an opposing signal from the S-cones. Source: Derrington et al., 1984.

The spectral responses of these neural populations suggest that there is only a loose connection between the signals coded by the neurons and the perceptual coding into opponent hues; it is unlikely that excitation and inhibition causes our perception of red–green and blue–yellow as opponent colors. One difficulty is the imperfect correspondence between the neural responses and the hue-cancellation measurements. The second difficulty is that there is no substantial population of neurons representing a white–black signal. This is a very important perceptual dimension which must be carried in the signals of the LGN. Yet, no clearly identified group of neurons can be assigned this role.[15]

Decorrelation of the Cone Absorptions

The opponent signals measured in the LGN probably represent a code used by the visual pathways in communicating information from the retina to the brain. The psychological opponent-colors coding may be a consequence of the coding strategy used to communicate information from the retina to the cortex. What reason might there be for using an opponent-signals coding?

One reason to use an opponent-signal representation has to do with the efficiency of the visual encoding. Because of the overlap of the L- and M-cone spectral sensitivities, the absorption rates of these two cone types are highly correlated. This correlation represents an inefficiency in the visual coding of spectral information. As I described in Chapter 8, decorrelating the signals can improve the efficiency of the neural representation.

We can illustrate this principle by working an example, parallel to the one in Chapter 8. Consider the cone absorptions for a set of surfaces. Because of the overlap in spectral sensitivities, the cone absorptions between, say, the L- and M-cones will be correlated. To remove the correlation, we create a new representation of the signals consisting of the L- cone absorptions alone and a weighted combination of the L-, M-, and S-cone absorptions. We will choose the weighted combination of signals so that the new signal is independent of the L-cone absorptions. As we reviewed in the earlier chapter, by decorrelating the cone absorptions before they travel to the brain, we make effective use of the dynamic range of the neurons transmitting the information (Buchsbaum and Gottschalk, 1984).

The graphs in Figure 9.17 show examples of the correlation of the cone absorptions for a particular set of surfaces and illuminant. These

[15] Some authors have suggested that a single group of LGN neurons codes a white–black sensation for high-spatial-frequency patterns and a red–green sensation for low-spatial-frequency patterns. This is an interesting hypothesis that abandons the idea that there is a specific color sensation associated with the response of LGN neurons. Instead, the perceived hue depends on the pattern of neural activation (Derrington, et al., 1984; Ingling and Martinez, 1984).

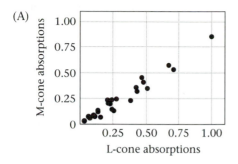 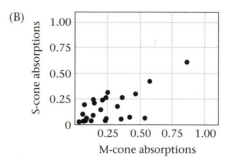

9.17 ABSORPTIONS IN THE THREE CONE CLASSES ARE HIGHLY CORRELATED.
The correlation between cone absorptions can be measured using correlograms. In
this figure, correlograms are shown for the cone absorptions from the surfaces in the
Macbeth ColorChecker illuminated by average daylight. (A) A correlogram of the L- and
M-cone absorptions. (B) A correlogram of the M- and S-cone absorptions.

plots represent the cone absorptions from light reflected by a Macbeth
ColorChecker viewed under mean daylight illumination. The correlations shown in these two plots are typical of natural images: the L- and
M-cone absorptions are highly correlated (panel A); the M- and S-cone
absorptions are also correlated (panel B).

As described in Chapter 8, we decorrelate the signals derived from
the cone absorptions by forming new signals that are weighted combinations of the cone absorptions. There are many linear transforms of
the cone absorptions that could serve to decorrelate these absorptions.
One such transformation is represented by the three linear equations,[16]

$$O_1(\lambda) = 1.0L(\lambda) + 0.0M(\lambda) + 0.0S(\lambda)$$

$$O_2(\lambda) = -0.59L(\lambda) + 0.80M(\lambda) + -0.12S(\lambda)$$

$$O_3(\lambda) = -0.34L(\lambda) + -0.11M(\lambda) + 0.93S(\lambda) \tag{9.16}$$

or, written in matrix form,

$$\begin{pmatrix} O_1(\lambda) \\ O_2(\lambda) \\ O_3(\lambda) \end{pmatrix} = \begin{pmatrix} 1.00 & 0.00 & 0.00 \\ -0.59 & 0.80 & -0.12 \\ -0.34 & -0.11 & 0.93 \end{pmatrix} \begin{pmatrix} L(\lambda) \\ M(\lambda) \\ S(\lambda) \end{pmatrix}$$

The new signals, $O_i(\lambda)$, are related to the cone absorptions by a linear
transformation. These three signals are decorrelated with respect to this
particular collection of surfaces and illuminant.

The spectral sensitivity of the three decorrelated signals are shown
in Figure 9.18. The two opponent spectral sensitivities are reminiscent of the hue-cancellation measurements and the opponent signals
measured in the LGN. One of the sensors has two zero-crossings, near

[16] The decorrelation is based on the singular value decomposition of the cone absorptions.

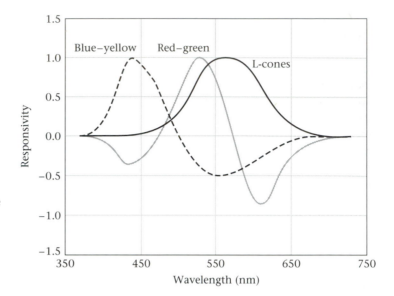

9.18   THE SPECTRAL RESPONSIVITY OF A SET OF COLOR SENSORS whose responses to the Macbeth ColorChecker under mean daylight are decorrelated. The spectral sensitivities of these sensors resemble the spectral sensitivities of LGN neurons and the color-appearance judgments measured in the hue-cancellation experiment.

570 nm and 470 nm. A second sensor has one zero-crossing at about 490 nm. The third sensor has no zero-crossings, as required for a white–black pathway. The similarity among the decorrelated signals, the opponent signals in the lateral geniculate nucleus, and the hue-cancellation experiment suggests a purpose for opponent-colors organization. Opponent colors may exist to decorrelate the cone absorptions and provide an efficient neural representation of color (Buchsbaum and Gottschalk, 1984; Derrico and Buchsbaum, 1991).

The opponent-colors representation is a universal property of color appearance for humans, just as the need for efficient coding is a simple and universal idea. We should expect to find a precise connection between opponent-colors appearance and neural organization in the central visual pathways. The hue-cancellation experiment provides us with a behavioral method of quantifying opponent-colors organization. Hue-cancellation measurements establish a standard for neurophysiologists to use when evaluating opponent signals in the visual pathways as candidates for the opponent-colors representation. Opponent-colors organization is a simple and important idea; pursuing its neural basis will lead us to new ideas about the encoding of visual information.

Spatial Pattern and Color

Color Plate 2 and Figure 9.1 show that the color appearance at a location depends on the local image contrast, that is, the relationship between the local cone absorptions and the mean image absorptions. The targets we used to demonstrate this dependence are very simple spatial patterns, squares or lines, with no internal spatial structure of their own. In this section, we will review how color appearance can also depend on the spatial structure, such as the texture or spatial frequency, of the target itself.

Color Plate 6 shows two square waves composed of alternating blue and yellow bars. One square wave is at a higher spatial frequency than the other. The average signal reflected from the regions containing the square waves is the same; that is, these are pure contrast modulations about a common mean field. If you examine the square waves from a close distance, you will see that bars in the square-wave patterns are drawn with the same ink. If you place this book a few meters away from you, say, across the room, the color of the bars in the high-spatial-frequency pattern will appear different from the color of the bars in the low-spatial-frequency pattern. The bars in the high-spatial-frequency patterns will appear to be light and dark modulations about the green average. The bars in the low-spatial-frequency pattern will continue to look like distinct blue and yellow bars.[17]

Poirson and Wandell (1993) used an asymmetric color-matching task to study how color appearance changes with spatial frequency of the square-wave pattern. Subjects viewed square-wave patterns whose bars were colored modulations about a neutral gray background; that is, the average of the two bars comprising the pattern was equal to the mean background level. Subjects adjusted the appearance of a 2-degree square patch to have the same color appearance as each of the bars in the pattern.

Two qualitative observations stood out in this study. First, spatial patterns of moderate- and high-spatial-frequency patterns (above 8 cpd) appear mainly light–dark, with little saturation. Thus, no matter what the relative cone absorptions of a high-spatial-frequency target, the target appeared to be a light–dark variation about the mean level. Second, the spatially asymmetric color appearance matches are not photopigment matches. This can be deduced from the first observation: because of axial chromatic aberration, moderate-frequency square-wave contrast patterns (4 and 8 cpd) cannot stimulate the S-cones significantly. Yet, subjects match the bars in these high-frequency patterns using a 2-degree patch with considerable S-cone contrast. The asymmetric color matches are established at neural sites central to the photoreceptors.

Poirson and I explained the asymmetric spatial color matches using a pattern–color separable model. In this model, we supposed that the color appearance of the target was determined by the response of three color mechanisms, and that the response of each mechanism was separable with respect to pattern and color. We derived the spatial and spectral responsivities of these pathways from the observers' color matches; the estimated sensitivities are shown in Figure 9.19.

Interestingly, the three color pathways that we derived from the asymmetric matching experiment correspond well to the opponent-color mechanisms derived from the hue-cancellation experiment. One pathway is sensitive mainly to light–dark variation; this pathway has

[17] You can also alter the relative color appearance of the patterns by moving the book rapidly up and down. You will see that the low-frequency square wave retains its appearance, while the high-frequency square wave becomes a green blur.

(A)

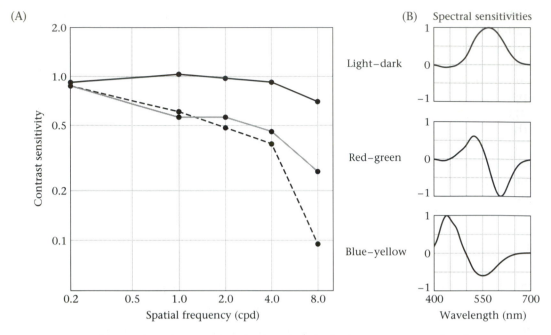

(B) Spectral sensitivities

Light–dark

Red–green

Blue–yellow

Contrast sensitivity

Spatial frequency (cpd)

Wavelength (nm)

9.19 ESTIMATES OF PATTERN–COLOR SEPARABLE SENSITIVITY of pathways mediating color appearance. By measuring spatially asymmetric color matches, it is possible to deduce the pattern and color sensitivity of three visual mechanisms that mediate color appearance judgments. (A) The pattern sensitivities and (B) the wavelength sensitivities derived from experimental measurements are shown for light–dark, red–green, and blue–yellow mechanisms. Source: Poirson and Wandell, 1993.

the best spatial resolution. The other two pathways are sensitive to red–green and blue–yellow variation. The blue–yellow pathway has the worst spatial resolution. Granger and Heurtley (1973), Mullen (1985), and Sekiguchi et al. (1993a, b) made measurements that presupposed the existence of opponent-color pathways and estimated similar pattern sensitivities of the three mechanisms. Notice that the derivation of the opponent-colors representation in this experiment did not involve asking the observers any questions about the hue or saturation of the targets. The observers simply set color-appearance matches; the opponent-colors mechanisms were needed to predict the color matches.

One of the more striking aspects of opponent-colors representations is that the apparent spatial sharpness, or focus, of a color image depends mainly on the sharpness of the light–dark component of the image; apparent sharpness depends very little on the spatial structure of the opponent-color image components. This is illustrated in the three images shown in Color Plate 7.

We can take advantage of the low spatial acuity of the opponent-colors representations when we code color images for image storage and transmission. We can allocate much less information about the opponent-colors components of color images without changing the apparent spatial sharpness of the image. This property of human perception was important in shaping broadcast television standards and digital image-compression algorithms. As a quantitative prediction, we should expect to find that neurons in the central visual pathways that represent light–dark information should be able to represent spatial information at a much higher resolution than neurons that code opponent-colors information. Consequently, we should expect that the largest fraction of central neurons encode light–dark, rather than the other two opponent-colors signals.

The differences between the light–dark encoding and the opponent-colors encoding are of great perceptual significance. Consequently, several authors have studied hypotheses based on the idea that opponent-colors signals and light–dark signals are found in separate areas of the brain. In the final section of this chapter, we will consider some of the evidence concerning the representation of color information in the visual cortex.

The Cortical Basis of Color Appearance

Clinical Studies

In 1974, Meadows reviewed case studies of 14 patients who had lost their ability to see colors due to brain injuries. For some patients, the colors of objects appeared wrong. Other patients saw the world entirely in shades of gray. However, these patients still had good visual acuity.

The syndrome Meadows reviewed, which I will call **cerebral dyschromatopsia**,[18] had been described in reports spanning a century (Zeki, 1990a,b). But the cases were rare, poor methods were used to study the patients, and the color loss was not well dissociated from other visual deficits. Consequently, at the time Meadows wrote his review, several well-known investigators had expressed doubt about even the existence of cerebral dyschromatopsia (e.g., Teuber et al., 1960).[19] By bringing together a number of new cases and studying them with much better methods, Critchley (1965), Meadows (1974), Zeki (1990b), and others (e.g., Green and Lesell, 1977; Domasio et al., 1980; Mollon, 1980;

[18] Some of the terms used to describe color loss vary between authors. The terms trichromacy, dichromacy, and monochromacy are precise, referring to the number of primary lights necessary to complete the color-matching experiment. Some authors use the phrase *cerebral achromatopsia*, meaning "without color vision," to describe a loss of color vision while others use *cerebral dyschromatopsia*. I prefer the second term because in these cases insensitivity to hue is often not complete and because these patients still distinguish the colors white and black. When the behavioral evidence warrants it, one might append a modifier, such as *monochromatic* dyschromatopsia, to describe the the color loss more precisely.

[19] In his book and in a long article, Zeki (1990b, 1993) argued that the skepticism concerning cerebral dyschromatopsia was due to the acceptance of a profoundly misguided theory concerning the significance of visual area V1. I agree with Meadows's gentler assessment; the early evidence in support of cerebral dyschromatopsia was spotty and poorly argued. There was room for some skepticism.

Heywood et al., 1987, 1992; Victor et al., 1987) have removed any doubt about the existence and significance of the syndrome.

Congenital Monochromacy

Usually, observers are dichromats or monochromats because they are missing one of the cone photopigments (see e.g., Alpern, 1974; Smith and Pokorny, 1972). There are also reports of congenital cone monochromacy of central origin. In a thorough and fascinating study, Weale (1953) searched England for individuals who (a) could not tell color photographs from black and white, (b) were not photophobic, and (c) had good visual acuity. [Requirements (b) and (c) eliminated rod monochromats]. Weale found three cone monochromats, that is, individuals who could adjust the intensity of a single primary light to match the appearance of any other test light. Yet, based on direct measurements of the photopigment in the eye of one of the observers, as well as behavioral measurements, some of these cone monochromats were shown to have more than one cone photopigment (Weale, 1959; Gibson, 1962; see also Alpern, 1974). Hence, Weale's subjects had a congenital dyschromatopsia caused by deficiencies central to the photopigments. At present, we know little more about them.

Regularities of the Cerebral Dyschromatopsia Syndrome

When color loss arises from damage to the brain, the distortion of color appearance can take several forms. In some cases, patients report that colors have completely lost their saturation and hue and the world becomes gray. In other cases, color appearance may become desaturated. Some observers can perform some simple color-discrimination tasks, but they report that the colors of familiar objects do not appear right. In many cases the loss is permanent, but there are also reports of transient dyschromatopsia. For example, Lawden and Cleland (1993) recently reported on the case of a woman who suffers from migraines. During the migraine attacks, her world becomes transiently colorless.

The variability in the case studies suggest that a variety of mechanisms may disturb color appearance. Across this variability, however, there are also some regularities. First, Meadows (1974) observed that every patient with dyschromatopsia was blind in some portion of the upper visual field.

Meadows also examined the reverse correlation: do patients with purely upper visual field losses tend to have cerebral dyschromatopsia? In the literature, he found 12 patients with a purely upper visual field loss, seven of whom had dyschromatopsia; of 16 patients with a purely lower visual field loss, none had dyschromatopsia. In humans, the upper visual field is represented along the lower part of the calcarine sulcus (Chapter 6). The correlation between field loss and dyschromatopsia suggests a second regularity: damage that leads to dyschromatopsia is either near the lower portion of the calcarine or somewhere along the path traced out by the nerve fibers whose signal enters the lower portion of the calcarine cortex.

Third, many of the patients suffer from a syndrome called **prosopagnosia**, the inability to recognize familiar faces. Twelve of the 14 patients described by Meadows had this syndrome. The patient with migraines also has transient prosopagnosia (Lawden and Cleland, 1993). The co-occurrence of dyschromatopsia and prosopagnosia suggests that the neural mechanisms necessary for recall of familiar faces and color are located close to one another or that they rely on the same visual signal. Based on his review of the literature, Meadows (1974, p. 622) concluded that, "The evidence on localization in cases of cerebral achromatopsia points to the importance of bilateral, inferiorly placed, posterior lesions of both cerebral hemispheres."[20]

Behavioral Studies of Patients with Cerebral Dyschromatopsia

Patients with cerebral dyschromatopsia often fail to identify any of the test patterns on the Ishihara plates (see Chapter 4).[21] Mollon et al. (1980) reported on a patient who failed to identify the targets on the Ishihara plates at reading distance, but who could distinguish the targets when the plates were viewed from a distance of 2 meters. At the 2-meter viewing distance, the neutral areas separating the target and background are barely visible, and the target and background appear contiguous. Twelve years after the original study, Heywood et al. (1992) replicated the finding on the same patient. They also showed that the patient could discriminate contiguous colors, but not colors separated by a gray stripe. Hence, in this patient, cerebral dyschromatopsia involves color and pattern together (see also Victor et al., 1987).

Cerebral dyschromatopsics score quite poorly on the Farnsworth–Munsell hue test (see Chapter 4). The pattern of errors does not correspond to the errors made by any class of dichromat. The results of the test of one such patient is shown in Figure 9.20. The errors are large in all directions, though there is some hint that the errors may be somewhat larger in the blue and yellow portions of the hue circle.

How Many Cone Types Are Functional?

The patients' errors on the Ishihara color plates and the Farnsworth–Munsell hue test are not consistent with visual-pigment loss. Nonetheless, we cannot tell from their performance on these tests whether the

---

[20] As Zeki (1990b) points out, Meadows's conclusion echoes a disputed suggestion made a century earlier. While studying a patient who reported a loss of color vision, the French physician, Verrey (1888) concluded, "Le centre du sense chromatique se trouverait dans la partie la plus inferieure du lobe occipital, probablement dans la partie posterieure des plis lingual et fusiforme." [Translation: The center of the chromatic sense will be found in the inferior part of the occipital lobe, probably in the posterior part of the lingual and fusiform gyrus.]

[21] Meadows (1974) and Victor et al. (1987) describe patients with cerebral dyschromatopsia who nonetheless could read all of the plates.

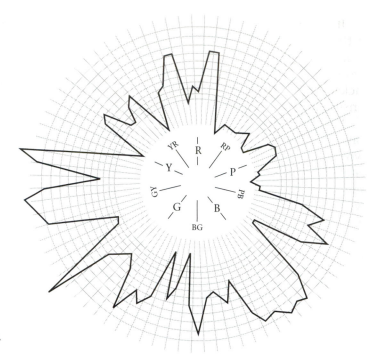

9.20 RESULTS OF THE FARNSWORTH–MUNSELL HUE TEST FROM A PATIENT SUFFERING CEREBRAL DYSCHROMATOPSIA. The patient's error scores are high in all hue directions. This pattern of scores is not consistent with any of the usual pattern of errors observed by cone dichromats who are missing one of their cone photopigments (see Figure 4.21). Source: Meadows, 1974.

separate cone classes are functioning or whether the loss of color perception is due, in part, to cone dysfunction.

Gibson (1962; see also Alpern, 1974; Mollon et al., 1980) developed a behavioral test to infer whether patients with cerebral dyschromatopsia had more than a single class of functioning cones. The logic of this behavioral test is based on the fact the cone signals are scaled to correct for changes in the ambient lighting conditions. For example, in the presence of a long-wavelength background, the sensitivity of the L-cones is suppressed, while the sensitivity of the S-cones remains unchanged.

Suppose a subject has only a single type of cone. For this observer, wavelength sensitivity is determined by the spectral sensitivity of a single cone photopigment. Changes of the background illumination will not change the observer's relative wavelength sensitivity. This is the situation for normal observers under scotopic viewing conditions, when we see only through the rods. Under scotopic conditions, wavelength sensitivity is determined by the rhodopsin photopigment; changing the background does not change in the relative sensitivity to different test wavelengths.[22]

---

[22] In a beautiful series of experiments, Stiles (1939, 1959, 1978) studied how sensitivity varies as one changes the wavelength and intensity of a test and background lights. He developed a penetrating analysis of this experimental paradigm and identified candidate processes which he believed might describe photoreceptor adaptation. He referred to these processes as π-mechanisms.

If an individual has two functional cone classes, however, changes in the sensitivity of one cone class relative to the other will change the behavioral wavelength sensitivity. Hence, we can detect the presence of two cone classes by measuring wavelength sensitivity on two different backgrounds and noting a change in the observer's relative wavelength sensitivity.

Mollon et al. (1980) measured a cerebral dyschromatopsic's relative wavelength sensitivity to test wavelengths (510 nm and 640 nm) on two different backgrounds (510 nm and 650 nm). I have replotted their data in Figure 9.21. When the background changes, the relative test-wavelength sensitivity changes, showing that the subject has at least two functional cone classes, as in the case of congenital monochromats.

Clinical studies of cerebral dyschromatopsia show that central lesions can disturb color vision severely, while sparing many other aspects

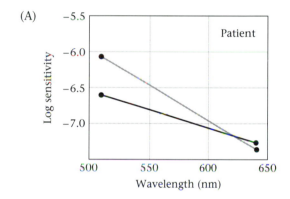

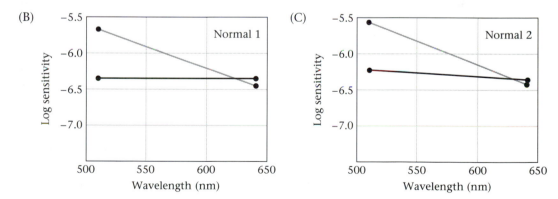

9.21 EXPERIMENTAL DEMONSTRATION THAT A PATIENT WITH CEREBRAL DYSCHROMATOPSIA HAS MORE THAN A SINGLE FUNCTIONING CONE CLASS.
(A) The patient's threshold sensitivity was measured to two monochromatic test lights on two different backgrounds. The change in background illumination changed the patient's relative wavelength sensitivity. (B, C) The results of performing the same experiment on normal observers. The results from the normal observers and the patient are quite similar. Source: Mollon et al., 1980.

of visual performance. This clinical syndrome suggests that some of the neural mechanisms essential to the sensation of color appearance may be anatomically separate from the mechanisms required for other visual tasks, such as acuity, motion perception, and depth perception. Clinical lesions are not neat and orderly, however, and the syndrome of cerebral dyschromatopsia is quite varied. Alternative hypotheses, for example, that neurons carrying color information are more susceptible to stroke damage than other neurons, are also consistent with the clinical observations (Mollon et al., 1980). To pursue the question of the neural representation of color information, we need to consider other forms of evidence concerning the localization of color appearance.

Physiological Studies of Color Appearance

Much of the agenda for modern research on the cortical representation of color appearance has been set by Zeki via a hypothesis he calls **functional segregation** (Zeki, 1974, 1993; see Chapter 6). Zeki argues that there is a direct correlation between the neural responses in cortical areas beyond V1 and various perceptual features, such as color, motion, and form. This is not the only hypothesis we might entertain for the relationship between brain structures and perceptual function. An alternative view has been expressed by Livingstone and Hubel (1984, 1987) who argue that perceptual function can be localized to groups of neurons residing within single visual areas. Specifically, they have argued that differences in the density of the enzyme cytochrome oxidase within cell bodies serves as a clue to the localization of perceptual processing (see Chapter 6). This criterion for identifying neural segregation of function seems relevant in areas V1 and V2, since the the anatomical interconnections between these areas appear to respect the differences in cytochrome oxidase density (Burkhalter et al., 1989).

Livingstone and Hubel's hypothesis need not conflict with Zeki's, since information may be interwined within peripheral visual areas only to be segregated later. But the presence of subdivisions within areas V1 and V2 raises the question of whether more detailed study might not reveal functional subdivisions within the other cortical areas as well (see e.g., Born and Tootell, 1992; Deyoe et al., 1994).

The principal line of evidence used to support Zeki's hypothesis of functional segregation is Barlow's neuron doctrine, namely, that the receptive field of a neuron corresponds to the perceptual experience the animal will have when the neuron is excited (Chapter 6). Based on this doctrine, neurophysiologists frequently assume that neurons with spatially oriented receptive fields are responsible for the perception of form; neurons that are inhibited by some wavelengths and excited by others are responsible for opponent-color percepts; neurons with motion-selective receptive fields are responsible for motion perception.

Zeki's suggestion that monkey area V4 is a color center and area MT is a motion center is based on differences in the receptive-field properties of neurons in these two areas. The overwhelming majority of neurons in area MT show motion direction selectivity. Zeki reported that many neurons in area V4 exhibited an unusual wavelength selectivity (Zeki, 1973, 1980, 1990a,b).

As we have already seen, qualitative observations concerning receptive neural wavelength selectivity is not a firm basis to establish these neurons as being devoted mainly to color. For example, the vast majority of neurons in the LGN respond with opponent signals, and these neurons have no orientation selectivity. Yet, we know that these neurons surely represent color, form, and motion information.

Moreover, the quality of the receptive-field measurements in area V4 has not achieved the same level of precision as measurements in the retina or area V1. Because these cells appear to be highly nonlinear, there are no widely agreed upon methods for fully characterizing their responses. Also, there have been disputes concerning even the qualitative properties of area-V4 receptive fields. For example, Desimone et al. (1985) report that many cells are selective for orientation, direction of motion, and spatial frequency. Like Zeki, these authors accept the basic logic of the neuron doctrine. They conclude from the variation of receptive field properties that "like V1, area V4 is not specialized to analyze one particular stimulus quality, but rather processes several in parallel" (p. 447). They then develop an alternative notion of the role of area V4 and later visual areas (Desimone and Schein, 1987).

Reasoning about the Cortex and Perception

While hypotheses about the roles of different cortical areas in perception are being debated, and although experiments to test these hypotheses have begun, we are at quite an early stage in our understanding of cortical function. This should not be too surprising; after all, the scientific investigation of the relationship between cortical responses and perception is a relatively new scientific endeavor, less than 100 years old. At this point in time we should expect some controversy and uncertainty regarding the status of early hypotheses. Much of the controversy stems from uncertainty concerning which experimental measurements will prove to be reliable sources of information and which will not.

In thinking about what we have learned about cortical function, I find it helpful to consider these two questions:

1. What do we want to know about cortical function?

2. What are the logical underpinnings of the experimental methods we have available to determine the relationship between cortical responses and perception?

When one discovers a new structure in the brain, it is almost impossible to refrain from asking: what does this part of the brain do? Once one poses this question, the answer is naturally formulated in terms of the *localization* of perceptual function. Our mindset becomes one of asking what happens where, rather than simply asking what happens. Hypotheses concerning the localization of function are the usual way to begin a research program on brain function. Moreover, I think any fair reading of the historical literature will show that hypotheses about what functions are localized within the brain region serve the useful purpose of organizing early experiments and theory.

On the other hand, in those portions of the visual pathways where our understanding is relatively mature, localization is rarely the central issue. We know that the retina is involved in visual function, and we know that some features of the retinal encoding are important for acuity, adaptation, wavelength encoding, and so forth. Our grasp of retinal function is sufficiently powerful so that we no longer frame questions about retinal function as a problem of localization. Instead, we pose problems in terms of the flow of information; we try to understand how information is represented and transformed within the retina.

For example, we know that information about the stimulus wavelength is represented by the relative absorption rates of the three cone photopigments. The information is not localized in any simple anatomical sense: no single neuron contains all the necessary information, nor are the neurons that represent wavelength information grouped together. Perhaps one might argue that acuity is localized, since acuity is greatest in the fovea. Even so, acuity depends on image formation, proper spacing of the photoreceptors, and appropriate representation of the photoreceptors in the optic tract. Without all of these other components in place, the observer will not have good visual acuity. The important questions about visual acuity are questions about the nature of the information and how the information is encoded and transmitted. That the fovea is the region of highest acuity is important, but not a solution to the question of how we resolve fine detail.

The most important questions about vision are those that Helmholtz posed: What are the principles that govern how the visual pathways make inferences from the visual image? How do we use image information to compute these perceptual inferences? We seek to understand these principles of behavior and neural representations with the same precision as we understand color-matching and the cone photopigments. We begin with spatial localization of brain function so that we can decide where to begin our work, not how to end it.

Thus, as our understanding becomes more refined we no longer formulate hypotheses based on localization of function alone. Instead, we use quantitative methods to compare neural responses and behavioral measurements. Mature areas of vision science relate perception and neural response by demonstrating correlations between the information in the neural signals and the computations applied to those signals. The information contained in the neural response and the transformations applied to that information are the essence of perception.

Summary and Conclusions

Color appearance, like so much of vision, is an inference. Mainly, color is a perceptual representation of the surface reflectance of an object. There are two powerful obstacles that make it difficult to infer surface reflectance from the light incident at the eye. First, the reflected light confounds information about the surface and the illuminant. Second, the human eye has only three types of cones to encode a spectral signal consisting of many different wavelengths.

We began this chapter by asking what aspects of color imaging might make it feasible to perform this visual inference. Specifically, we studied how surface reflectance might be estimated from the light incident at the eye. We concluded that it is possible to draw accurate inferences about surface-reflectance functions when the surface and illuminant spectral curves are regular functions that can be well approximated by low-dimensional linear models. When the input signals are constrained, it is possible to design simple algorithms that use the cone absorptions to estimate surface reflectance accurately.

Next, we considered whether human judgments of color appearance share some of the properties used by algorithms that estimate surface reflectance. As a test of the correspondence between these abstract algorithms and human behavior, we reviewed how judgments of color appearance vary with changes in the illumination. Experimental results using the asymmetric color-matching method show that color-appearance judgments of targets seen under different illuminants can be predicted by matches between scaled responses of the human cones. The scale factor depends on the difference in illumination. To a large degree, these results are consistent with the general principle we have observed many times: judgments of color appearance are described mainly by the local contrast of the cone signals, not their absolute level. By basing color-appearance judgments on the scaled signal, which approximates the local cone contrast, color appearance is more closely correlated with surface reflectance than with the light incident at the eye.

Then we turned to a more general review of the organizational principles of color appearance. There are two important means of organizing color experience. Many color representations, like the Munsell representation, emphasize the properties of hue, saturation, and lightness. A second organizational theme is based on Hering's observation that red–green and blue–yellow are opponent-colors pairs and that we never experience these hues together in a single color. The opponent-colors organization has drawn considerable attention with the discovery that many neurons carry opponent signals, increasing their response to some wavelengths of light and decreasing in response to others.

In recent years, there have been many creative and interesting attempts to study the representation of color information in the visual cortex. Most prominent among the hypotheses generated by this work is the notion that opponent-colors signals are spatially localized in the cortex. The evidence in support of this view comes from two types of experiments. First, clinical observations show that certain individuals lose their ability to perceive color although they retain high visual acuity. Second, studies of the receptive fields of individual neurons suggest that opponent-colors signals are represented in spatially localized brain areas. These hypotheses are new and unproven. But whether they are ultimately right or wrong, these hypotheses are the important opening steps in the modern scientific quest to understand the neural basis of conscious experience.

Exercises

1. Apart from surface reflectance, what other aspects of the material world might be represented by color vision?

2. Color vision has evolved separately in birds, fish, and primates. What does this imply about the significance of wavelength information in the environment?

3. We have used finite-dimensional linear models of surfaces and illuminants to understand how the visual system might infer surface reflectance from the responses of only three cone types.

   (a) Offer a definition of a linear model that relates them to the discrete Fourier series.
   (b) Describe the relationship between linear models used in this chapter and linear models used in spatial pattern sensitivity and multiresolution image representations.
   (c) List some reasons why light-bulb manufacturers would be interested in linear models for illuminants.
   (d) Using a linear model for daylight, we can design a device with two color sensors to estimate the relative spectral power distribution of daylight.
      i. Suppose a device has sensor sensitivities **S**. Write an equation showing how the sensor responses depend on the illuminant model basis functions and the illuminant coefficients.
      ii. Describe why you can solve this equation for the linear-model weights.
      iii. Once you have calculated the linear-model weights, how do you calculate the estimated spectral power distribution?

4. (a) What was von Kries's hypothesis concerning the biological mechanisms of color constancy?
   (b) How did Wassef test this theory experimentally?

(c) What was Land's view of color science and its role in understanding color appearance?

(d) In his recent book, Zeki (1993, p. 12) writes:

> Why did colour constancy play such a subsidiary role in enquiries on colour vision? Almost certainly because, until only very recently it has been treated as a departure from a general rule, although it is in fact the central problem of colour vision. That general rule supposes that there is a precise and simple relationship between the wavelength composition of the light reaching the eye from every point on a surface and the colour of that point.

Zeki also quotes Newton's famous passage in support of his view:

> Every Body reflects the rays of its own colour more copiously than the rest, and from their excess and predominance in the reflected light has its colour.

Does Newton's passage support Zeki's assertion that most authors thought it was the light at the eye that governs color appearance? Or, does Newton's passage support Helmholtz's view that surface reflectance determines appearance? What do *you* think, based on your reading of this chapter? Go to the historical literature and see what others have written on the topic.

5. (a) Design a neural wiring diagram such that the system will see yellow and blue at the same time, but not yellow and red.

    (b) Given the strong chromatic aberration of the eye, what spatial sensitivity properties would you assign to the blue–yellow neural pathway?

6. Stiles developed a sophisticated quantitative behavioral analysis of light adaptation to uniform fields. His papers were collected in a 1979 volume entitled *Mechanisms of Colour Vision*. Stiles's work makes substantial use of linear methods coupled with static nonlinearities. Read the experimental literature in this area and consider your answers to the following questions.

    (a) What role did homogeneity play in Stiles's analysis of the color mechanisms?

    (b) Which aspect of his measurements led him to believe that the data might be revealing the action of independent cone pathways?

    (c) As you read about Stiles's experiments, consider how you would perform experimental tests of superposition. Then, read the papers on the Stiles mechanisms by Pugh and Mollon (1979) and Wandell and Pugh (1980). How did they test superposition?

7. Speculate about why prosopagnosia (the inability to recognize familiar faces) and cerebral dyschromatopsia are frequently associated in patients. Make sure that you list some reasons that have to do with functional issues concerning visual computation and some that have to do with the organization of the neural and vascular structures related to vision. Design experimental tests of your hypotheses.

10

Motion and Depth

The perception of motion, like the perception of color, is a visual inference. The images encoded by the photoreceptors are merely changing two-dimensional patterns of light intensity. Our visual pathways *interpret* these two-dimensional images to create our perception of objects moving in a three-dimensional world. How it is possible, even in principle, to infer three-dimensional motion from the two-dimensional retinal image is one important puzzle of motion; how our visual pathways actually make this inference is a second.

In this chapter we will try first to understand abstractly the retinal image information that is relevant to the computation of motion estimation. Then, we will review experimental measurements of motion perception and try to make sense of these measurements in the context of the computational framework. Many of the experiments involving judgment of motion suggest that visual inferences concerning motion use information about objects and their relationships, such as occlusion and texture boundaries, to detect and interpret motion. Finally, we will review a variety of experimental measurements that seek to understand how motion is computed within the visual pathways. Physiologists have identified a visual stream whose neurons are particularly responsive to motion; in animals, lesions of this pathway lead to specific visual deficits of motion. The specific loss of motion perception, without an associated loss of color or pattern sensitivity, suggests that a portion of the visual pathways is specialized for motion perception.

It is useful to begin our review of motion with a few of the many behavioral observations that show motion to be a complex visual inference, and not a simple representation of the physical motion. One demonstration of this, called **apparent motion**, can be seen in many downtown districts. There you will find displays consisting of a sequence of flashing marquee lights that appear to be moving, drawing your attention to a theater or shop. Yet, none of the individual lights in the display is moving; the lights are fixed in place, flashing in sequence. Even though there is no physical motion, the stimulus evokes a sense of motion in us. Even a single pair of lights, flashing in alternation, can provide a distinct visual impression of motion.

A second example of a fixed stimulus that appears to move can be found in **motion aftereffects**. Perhaps the best known motion aftereffect is the **waterfall illusion**, described in the following passage from Addams (1834):

> Whilst on a recent tours of the highlands of Scotland, I visited the celebrated Falls of Foyers near Loch Ness, and there noticed the following phaenomenon.
> Having steadfastly looked for a few seconds at a particular part of the cascade, admiring the confluence and decussation of the currents forming the liquid drapery of waters, and then suddenly directed my eyes to the left, to observe the vertical face of the sombre age-worn rocks immediately contiguous to the waterfall, I saw the rocky surface as if in motion upwards, and with an apparent velocity equal to that of the descending water, which the moment before had prepared my eyes to behold this singular deception.

The waterfall Addams described is shown in Figure 10.1. Notice that in the waterfall illusion, the object that appears to move (in this case, the rock) does not have the same shape or texture as the object that causes the motion aftereffect (the waterfall).

A third way to convince yourself that motion is an inference is to consider the fact that many behavioral experiments show that perceived velocity, unlike physical velocity, depends on the color and contrast of an object. We know that the color of an object and its contrast relative to the background are not good cues about motion. Indeed, the physical definition of motion does not depend on color or contrast at all. Yet, some of the effects are quite large. For example, by proper selection of the color and pattern, a peripheral target moving at 1 degree per second can be made to appear as though it were still. These effects show that the visual inference of motion is imperfect because it is influenced by image features that are irrelevant to physical motion (Cavanagh and Anstis, 1991).

Motion computations and stereo depth perception are closely related. For example, as an observer moves, the local motion of image points contain useful visual information about the distance from the observer to various points in the scene. Points in the image change in a predictable way that depends on the direction of the observer's motion and the distance of the point from the observer. Points that are farther away generally move smaller amounts than points that are closer; and points along the direction of the observer's motion move less than

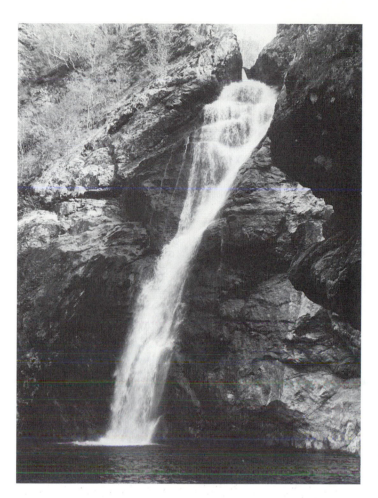

10.1 THE FALLS OF FOYERS
where Addams (1834)
observed the motion aftereffect
called the waterfall illusion.
The illusion demonstrates that
perceived motion is different
from physical motion; we
see motion in the aftereffect,
although there is no motion
in the image. Courtesy of
Nicholas Wade.

points lying in other directions. Information from the image motion informs us about the position of objects in space relative to the viewer (Gibson, 1950).

The collective motion of points in an image from one moment to the next is called the **motion flow field**. By drawing our attention to this source of depth information, Gibson (1950) established an important research paradigm that relates motion and depth perception: define an algorithm for measuring the motion flow field, and then devise algorithms to extract information about observer motion and object depth from the motion flow field. In recent years, this problem has been substantially solved. It is now possible to use motion flow fields to estimate both an observer's motion through a static scene and a depth map from the observer to different points within the scene (Koenderink, 1990; Heeger and Jepson, 1992; Tomasi and Kanade, 1992).

These computational examples show that motion and stereo depth algorithms are related by their objectives: both inform us about the positions of objects in space and the viewer's relationship to those objects.

Because motion and stereo depth estimation have similar goals, they use similar types of stimulus information. Stereo algorithms use the information in our two eyes to recover depth information, relying on the fact that the two images are taken from slightly different points of view. Motion algorithms use a broader range of information that may include multiple views obtained as the observer moves or as objects change their position with respect to the viewer. Most of this chapter is devoted to a review of the principles in the general class of motion-estimation algorithms. In a few places, because the goals of motion and stereo depth are so similar, I have inserted some related material concerning stereo depth perception.

Computing Motion

Figure 10.2 shows an overview of the key elements used in motion-estimation algorithms. The left panel of the figure shows the input data, a series of images acquired over time. Because the observer and objects move over time, each image in the sequence is a little different from the previous one. The image differences are due to the new geometric relationship among the camera, objects, and light source. The goal of most motion- and depth-estimation algorithms is to use these changes to infer motion of the observer, the motion of the objects in the image, or the depth map relating the observer to the objects.

The arrows drawn in the center panel of Figure 10.2 show the motion flow field. These arrows represent the changes in the position of points over small periods of space and time. The direction and length of the arrows correspond to the local motions that occur when the observer travels forward, down the road.

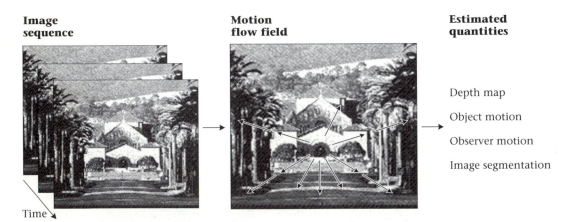

Image sequence

Time

Motion flow field

Estimated quantities

Depth map

Object motion

Observer motion

Image segmentation

10.2 THE OVERALL LOGIC OF MOTION-ESTIMATION ALGORITHMS. The input stimulus consists of an image sequence. The motion flow field at each moment in time is computed from the image sequence. Various quantities relating to motion and depth can be calculated from the motion flow fields.

In the right panel of Figure 10.2 is a list of several quantities that can be estimated from the motion flow fields. As I have already reviewed, the motion flow field contains information relevant to the depth map and observer motion. In addition, the motion flow field can be used to perform **image segmentation**, that is, to identify points in the image that are part of a common object. In fact, we shall see that the motion flow field defined by a set of moving points, but devoid of boundaries and shading, is sufficient to give rise to an impresson of a moving three-dimensional object.

Finally, the motion flow field contains information about object motion. This information is important for two separate reasons. First, as we have already reviewed, an important part of motion algorithms is establishing the spatial relationship between objects and the viewer. Second, object motion information is very important for guiding **smooth pursuit** eye movements. The structure of our retina, in which only the fovea is capable of high spatial resolution, makes it essential that we maintain good fixation on targets as we move or as the object moves in our visual field. Information derived from motion estimation is essential to guide the eye movement system as we track moving objects in a dynamic environment (Komatsu and Wurtz, 1989; Movshon et al., 1990; Schiller and Lee, 1993).

Stimulus Representation: Motion Sampling

I begin this review of motion algorithms by asking a simple question about the input data. In any practical system, the input stimulus is a sampled approximation of the continuous motion. The sampling rate should be rapid enough so that the input images provide a close approximation to the true continuous motion. How finely do we need to sample temporally the original scene in order to create a convincing visual display?

Beyond its significance for the science of motion perception, this question is also of great practical interest to people who design visual displays. A wide variety of visual display technologies represent motion by presenting a temporal sequence of still images. For example, movies and television displays both present the observer with a set of still images, each differing slightly from the previous one. In designing these display systems, engineers must select a temporal sampling rate for the display so that the observer has the illusion of smooth motion.[1]

---

[1] Different display technologies solve this problem using various special-purpose methods. For example, television in the United States displays a sequence of 30 static images per second. Each image is displayed in two frames; even-numbered lines in the image are presented in one frame, and odd-numbered lines in the second frame. Hence, the display shows 60 frames (30 images) per second. Movie projectors display only 24 images per second, but each image is flashed three times so that the temporal flicker rate is 72 frames per second. Modern computer displays present complete images at 72 frames per second or higher. This rate is fast enough that they rarely need special tricks to avoid temporal flicker artifacts for typical image sequences.

To answer the question of how finely we should sample an image sequence, we must include specifications about the image sequence and the human observer. First, consider why the answer must depend on the image sequence. Suppose that we are trying to represent a scene in which both objects and observer are still. In that case, we only need to acquire a single image. Next, suppose the image sequence contains a rapidly moving object. In that case, we need to acquire many images in order to capture all of the relevant scene information. If the image sequence contains rapidly moving objects, or if the observer moves rapidly, we must use high temporal sampling rates.

We will analyze the information in an image sequence using several simple representations shown in Figure 10.3. When we analyze the image sequence in order to estimate motion, we can call the image sequence the *motion signal* or **motion sequence.** Figure 10.3A represents the motion sequence as a three-dimensional data set: the volume of data includes two spatial dimensions (x, y) and time (t). Each point in this volume sends an amount of light to the eye, $I(x, y, t)$. The data in Figure 10.3A illustrate an image sequence consisting of a dark bar on a light background moving to the right.

Next, consider two simplified versions of this three-dimensional data. Figure 10.3B shows a cross-section of the data in the (x, y) plane. This image represents the dark bar at a single moment in time. Figure 10.3C shows a cross-section of the motion volume in the (t, x)

(A)

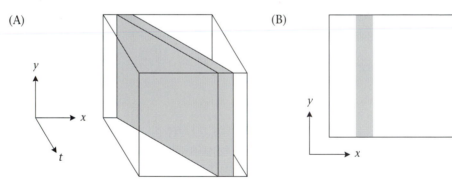

(B)

(C)

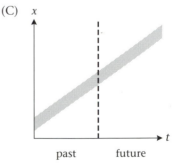

10.3 A MOTION SEQUENCE is a series of images measured over time. (A) The motion sequence of images can be grouped into a three-dimensional volume of data. (B) Cross sections of the volume show the spatial pattern at a moment in time. (C) Time (t) may be plotted against one dimension (x) of space. When the spatial pattern is one-dimensional, the (t, x) cross-section provides a complete representation of the stimulus sequence.

plane at a fixed value of y. In this plot, time runs from the left (past) to the right (future) of the graph. The present is indicated by the dashed vertical line. The image intensity along the x direction is shown as the gray bar across the vertical axis.

When the spatial stimulus is one-dimensional, (i.e., constant in one direction) we can measure only the motion component perpendicular to the constant spatial dimension. For example, when the stimulus is an infinite vertical line, we can estimate only the motion in the horizontal direction. In this case, the (t, x) cross section is the same at all levels of y so that the (t, x) cross section contains all of the information needed to describe the object's motion. In the motion literature, the inability to measure the motion along the constant spatial dimension is called the **aperture problem.**[2]

We can use the (t, x) plot to represent the effect of temporal sampling. First, consider the (t, x) representation of a smoothly moving stimulus shown in Figure 10.4A. Now, suppose we sample the image intensities regularly over time. The sampled motion can be represented as a series of dashes in the (t, x) plot, as shown in Figure 10.4B. Each dash represents the bar at a single moment in time, and the separation between the dashes depends on the temporal sampling rate and target velocity. If the sampling rate is high, the separation between the dashes is small, and the sequence will appear similar to the original continuous image. If the sampling rate is low, the separation between the dashes is large, and the sequence will appear quite different from the continuous motion.

The separation between the dashes in the sampled representation also depends on the object's velocity. As the bar pattern moves faster, the dashes fall along a line of increasing slope. Thus, for increasing velocities the separation between the dashes will increase. Hence, the difference between continuous motion and sampled motion is larger for faster-moving targets.

The Window of Visibility

Next, we will use measurements of visual spatial and temporal sensitivity to predict the temporal sampling rate at which a motion sequence appears indistinguishable from continuous motion. The basic procedure reviewed here has been described by several independent sources; Watson et al. (1983) call the method the **window of visibility** (see also Pearson, 1975; Fahle and Poggio, 1981)

---

[2] "Aperture problem" is something of a misnomer. It was selected because it is impossible to create infinite one-dimensional stimuli experimentally. Instead, subjects are presented finite one-dimensional patterns, such as a line segment, through an aperture that masks the endpoints of the line segment, making the stimulus effectively one-dimensional. The source of the uncertainty concerning the direction of motion, however, is not the aperture itself, but rather the fact that the information available to the observer is one-dimensional.

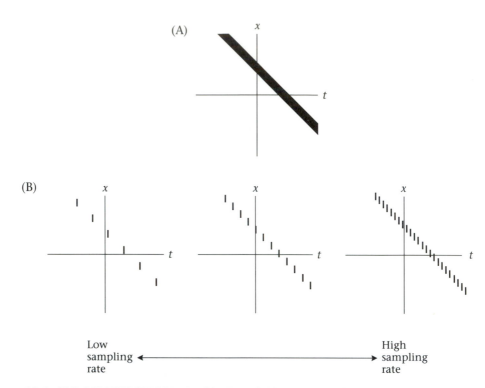

10.4 THE REPRESENTATION OF CONTINUOUS AND TEMPORALLY SAMPLED MOTION. (A) The continuous space–time plot of a moving line. (B) Temporal sampling of the continuous stimulus is represented by a series of dashes. As the temporal sampling rate increases (from left to right), the sampled stimulus becomes more similar to the continuous stimulus.

The window-of-visibility method begins by transforming the images from the (t, x) representation into a new representation based on spatial and temporal harmonic functions. We can convert from the (t, x) representation to the new representation by using the Fourier transform (see Chapter 2 and Appendix A). In the new representation, the stimulus is represented by its intensity with respect to the spatial and temporal frequency dimensions, (f_t, f_x). We convert the motion signal from the (t, x) form to the (f_t, f_x) form because, as we shall see, it is easy to represent the effect of sampling in the latter representation.

In the (t, x) graph, a moving line is represented by a straight line whose slope depends on the line's velocity. In the (f_t, f_x) graph, a moving line is also represented by a straight line whose slope depends on the line's velocity. You can see how this comes about by considering the units of spatial frequency, temporal frequency, and velocity. The units of f_t and f_x are cycles/sec and cycles/deg, respectively. The units of velocity, v, are deg/sec. It follows that spatial frequency, temporal frequency, and velocity are related by the linear equation $f_t = v f_x$.

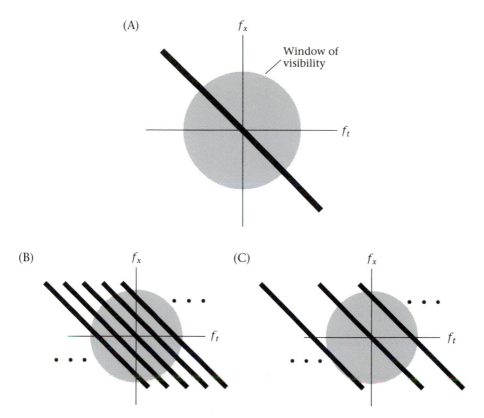

10.5 A GRAPHICAL METHOD TO DECIDE WHEN SAMPLED MOTION CAN BE DISCRIMINATED FROM CONTINUOUS MOTION. The axes of the graphs represent the spatial and temporal frequency values of the stimulus. (A) The solid line represents the spatial and temporal frequency content of a vertical line moving continuously. The shaded area represents the range of visible spatial and temporal frequencies, that is, the window of visibility. (B) Temporally sampling the image introduces replicas. The spacing of the replicas depends on the temporal sampling rate. When the rate is low, the replicas are closely spaced and there is significant energy inside the window of visibility. (C) When the sampling rate is high, the replicas are widely spaced and there is little energy inside the window of visibility. If the replicas fall outside the window, then the sampled and continuous motion will be indistinguishable.

Now, a still image has zero energy at all nonzero temporal frequencies. Suppose an object begins to move at velocity v. Then, each spatial-frequency component associated with the object moves at this same velocity and creates a temporal modulation at the frequency $v f_x$. Consequently, an object moving at v will be represented by its spatial frequencies, f_x, and the corresponding temporal frequencies, $f_t = v f_x$. In the (f_t, f_x) graph, this collection of points defines a line whose slope depends on the velocity, as shown in Figure 10.5A.[3]

---

[3] Speaking more precisely, the Fourier transform maps the intensities in the (t, x) plot into a set of complex numbers. The plot shown in Figure 10.5A represents the locations of the nonzero components of the data after applying the Fourier transform.

We use the (f_t, f_x) representation because it is easy to express the sampling distortion in that coordinate frame. A basic result of Fourier theory is that temporally sampling a continuous signal creates a set of replicas of the original continuous signal in the (f_t, f_x) representation.[4] The temporal sampling replicas are displaced from the original along the f_t axis; the size of the displacement depends on the sampling rate. When the sampling is very fine, the replicas are spaced far from the original. When the sampling is very coarse, the replicas are spaced close to the original.

Panels B and C of Figure 10.5 contain graphs representing temporally sampled motion. In panel B, the temporal sampling rate is low, and the replicas are spaced close to the original signal. At this sampling rate, the sampled motion is plainly discriminable from the continuous motion. In panel C, the temporal sampling rate is high, and the replicas are far from the original signal. To make the sampled image appear like continuous motion, we must set the temporal sampling rate high enough so that the sampling distortion is invisible. The problem that remains is to find the sampling rate at which the replicas will be invisible.

The shaded area in each panel of Figure 10.5 shows the window of visibility. The window describes the spatiotemporal frequency range that is detectable to human observers. The boundary of the window is a coarse summary of the limits of space–time sensitivity that we reviewed in Chapter 7. Spatial signals beyond roughly 50 cpd, or temporal signals beyond roughly 60 Hz, are beyond our perceptual limits. If the sampling replicas fall outside the window of visibility, they will not be visible, and the difference between the continuous and sampled motion will not be perceptible. Hence, to select a temporal sampling rate at which sampled motion will be indiscriminable from continuous motion, we should select a temporal sampling rate such that the replicas fall outside of the window of visibility.

The window-of-visibility method is a very useful approximation to use when we evaluate the temporal sampling requirements for different image sequences and display technologies. But, the method has two limitations. First, the method is very conservative. There will be sampled motion signals that fail to contain energy within the window for which the sampled motion will still appear to be continuous motion. This will occur because the unwanted energy that falls within the window of visibility may be masked by the energy from the continuous motion (see Chapter 7 for a discussion of masking).

Second, the method is a limited description of motion. By examining the replicas, we can decide that the stimulus looks the same as

---

[4] I do not have a simple intuitive explanation for why the distortions are arranged in this way. Ordinarily, this effect of sampling is proved by appeal to properties of the Fourier transform that are slightly beyond the scope of this book. But, the interested reader can find a proof of the consequences of sampling, and many other useful properties of the Fourier transform, in Bracewell (1978) and Oppenheim et al. (1983).

the original continuous motion; the method does not help us to decide what the motion looks like (i.e., the velocity and direction). We next will analyze how to estimate motion from image sequences.

Image Motion Information

What properties of the data in an image sequence suggest that motion is present? We can answer this question by considering the representation of a one-dimensional object, say, a vertical line, in the (t, x) plot. When the observer and object are still, the intensity pattern does not change across time. In this case the (t, x) plot of the object's intensity is the same for all values of t and is simply a horizontal line. When the object moves, its spatial position, x, changes across time so that in the (t, x) plot the path of the moving line includes segments that deviate from the horizontal. The value of the orientation of the trajectory in the (t, x) plot depends on the object's velocity. Large velocities are near the vertical; small velocities are near the horizontal orientation of a still object. Hence, orientation in the (t, x) representation informs us about velocity (Adelson and Bergen, 1985; Watson and Ahumada, 1985).

The connection between orientation in the (t, x) plot and velocity suggests a procedure for estimating motion. Suppose we wish to create a neuron that responds well to motion at a particular velocity but responds little to motion at other velocities. Then, we should create a neuron whose space–time receptive field is sensitive to signals with the proper orientation in the (t, x) plot.

Figure 10.6 shows the idea of a space–time-oriented receptive field. In Figure 10.6A, I have represented the space–time receptive field of the neuron using the same conventions that we used to represent the space–time receptive field of neurons in Chapters 5 and 6: the excitatory region of the receptive field is shown as the light area, and the inhibitory regions are shown as the shaded area. The horizontal axis represents time, and the dashed line represents the present moment in time. This graph has much in common with the ordinary notation showing an oriented two-dimensional spatial receptive field. The graph is somewhat different from the conventional spatial receptive field because the space–time receptive field always responds to recent events in the past, and so it travels in time just behind the line denoting the present.

Neurons with oriented space–time receptive fields respond differently to stimuli moving in different directions and velocities. Figure 10.6B shows the response to a line moving in a direction that is aligned with the space–time receptive field. The upper portion of the graph shows the relationship between the stimulus and the neuron's receptive field at several points in time. Because the stimulus and the receptive field share a common orientation, the stimulus fills inhibitory, excitatory, and then inhibitory portions of the receptive field in turn.

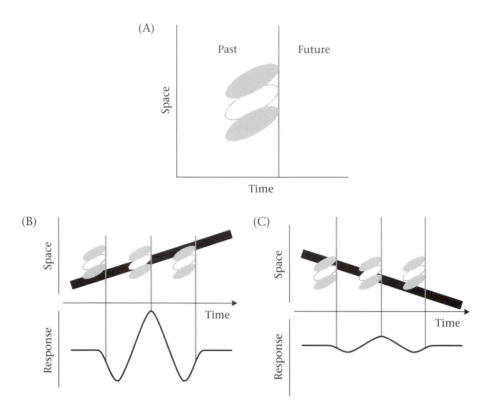

10.6 SPACE–TIME-ORIENTED RECEPTIVE FIELD. (A) The space–time receptive field of a neuron is represented on a (t, x) plot. The neuron always responds to events in the recent past, so the receptive field moves along the time axis with the present. The dark areas show an inhibitory region, and the light area shows an excitatory region. (B) The upper portion of the graph shows a (t, x) plot of a moving line and the space–time receptive field of a linear neuron. The neuron's receptive field is shown at several different moments in time, indicated by the vertical dashed lines. The common orientation of the space–time receptive field and the stimulus motion produce a large amplitude response, shown in the bottom half of the graph. (C) When the same neuron is stimulated by a line moving in a different direction, the stimulus motion aligns poorly with the space–time receptive field. Consequently, the response amplitude is much smaller.

Consequently, the neuron will have a large amplitude response to the stimulus, as shown in the lower portion of Figure 10.6B.

Figure 10.6C shows the response of the same neuron to a stimulus moving in a different direction. The space–time orientation of this stimulus is not well aligned with the receptive field, so the stimulus falls across the inhibitory and excitatory receptive-field regions simultaneously. Consequently, the response amplitude to this moving stimulus is much smaller. Just as neurons with oriented receptive fields in (x, y) space respond best to bars with the same orientation, so too neurons with oriented receptive fields in a (t, x) plot respond best to signals with a certain velocity.

It is possible, in principle, to create cells with space–time-oriented receptive fields by combining the responses of the simple cells in area

V1 of the cortex. One of many possible methods is shown in Figure 10.7. Consider an array of neurons with adjacent spatial receptive fields. The spatial receptive fields are shown at the top of Figure 10.7A. The responses of these neurons are added together after a temporal delay, Δt. The sum of these responses drives the output neuron as indicated at the bottom of Figure 10.7A.

Figure 10.7B shows the (t, x) receptive field of the output neuron. The receptive fields plotted along the x dimension are the one-dimensional receptive fields of the neurons in Figure 10.7A, that is, the receptive fields measured using a one-dimensional stimulus that is constant along the y axis. The spatial receptive fields of the input neurons are adjacent to one another, so they are shifted along the x dimension of the graph. The temporal response of the neurons, measured at each point in the receptive field, is also shown in Figure 10.7B. Since the responses of the input neurons are delayed prior to being summed, the temporal receptive fields are shifted along the t dimension. The shift in both the x and t dimensions yields an output receptive field that is oriented in the space–time plot.

When a neuron has a space–time-oriented receptive field, its response amplitude varies with the image velocity (see Figure 10.6). Thus, to measure stimulus velocity we need to compare the response amplitudes of an array of neurons, each with its own preferred motion. There are various methods of computing the amplitude of the time-varying response of a neuron and comparing the results among different neurons. Generally, these methods involve simple squaring and summing

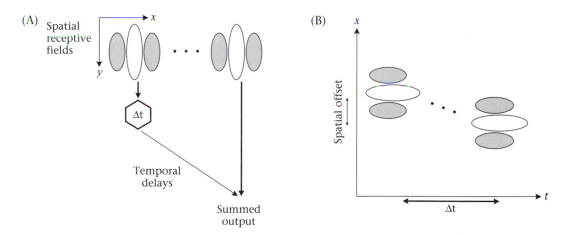

10.7   A METHOD FOR CREATING A SPACE–TIME-ORIENTED RECEPTIVE FIELD.
(A) A pair of spatial receptive fields, displaced in the x direction, is shown at the top. The response of the neuron on the left is delayed and then added to the response of the neuron on the right. (B) The (t, x) receptive field of the output neuron in panel (A). The temporal response of the neuron on the left is delayed compared to the temporal response of the neuron on the right. The combination of spatial displacement and temporal delay yields an output neuron whose receptive field is oriented in space–time.

operations applied to the responses. In recent years, several specific computational methods for extracting the amplitude of the neural responses have been proposed (Adelson and Bergen, 1985; van Santen and Sperling, 1985; Watson and Ahumada, 1985). We will return to this topic again after considering a second way to formulate the problem of motion estimation.

The Motion Gradient Constraint

The (t, x) representation of motion clarifies the requirements for a linear receptive field that is capable of discriminating motion in different directions and with different velocities. There is a second way to describe the requirements for motion estimation which provides some additional insights. In this section, we will derive a motion-estimation computation based on the assumption that in small regions of the image motion causes a displacement of the point intensities without changing the intensity values. This assumption is called the **motion gradient constraint**.

The motion gradient constraint is an approximation, and sometimes not a very good one. As the relative positions of the observer, objects, and light sources change, the spatial intensity pattern of the reflected light changes as well. For example, when one object moves behind another the local intensity pattern changes considerably. Or, as we saw in Chapter 9, in viewing a specular surface, the spatial distribution of the light reflected to the eye varies as the observer changes position. As a practical matter, however, there are often parts of an image sequence for which the motion gradient constraint is a good approximation. In some applications the approximation is good enough so that we can derive useful information.

To estimate local velocity using the motion gradient, we first describe the image intensities in the sequence as $I(a, b, t)$, the intensity at location (a, b) and time t. Suppose the velocities in the x and y directions at a point (a, b, t) are described by the **motion vector**, (v_x, v_y). Further, suppose that images in the motion signal are separated by a single unit of time. In that case, the intensity at point (a, b) will have shifted to a new position in the next frame,

$$I(a, b, t) = I(a + v_x, b + v_y, t + 1) \tag{10.1}$$

[Remember that v_x and v_y depend on the spatial position and the moment in time, (a, b, t).]

Our goal is to use the changing image intensities to estimate the motion vector, (v_x, v_y), at each position. We expand the right-hand side of Equation 10.1 in terms of the partial derivatives of the intensity pattern with respect to space and time,

$$I(a + v_x, b + v_y, t + 1) \approx I(a, b, t) + v_x \frac{\partial I}{\partial x} + v_y \frac{\partial I}{\partial y} + \frac{\partial I}{\partial t} \tag{10.2}$$

The terms $\frac{\partial I}{\partial x}$, $\frac{\partial I}{\partial y}$, and $\frac{\partial I}{\partial t}$ are the partial derivatives of $I(a, b, t)$ in the spatial and temporal dimensions. Grouping Equations 10.1 and 10.2, we obtain the **gradient constraint equation**:

$$v_x \frac{\partial I}{\partial x} + v_y \frac{\partial I}{\partial y} + \frac{\partial I}{\partial t} \approx 0 \qquad (10.3)$$

Equation 10.3 is a linear relationship between the space–time derivatives of the image intensities and the local velocity. Since there is only one linear equation and there are two unknown velocity components, the equation has multiple solutions. All the solutions fall on a **velocity-constraint line**, as shown in the graph in Figure 10.8.

Because the data at a single point do not define a unique solution, to derive an estimate we must combine the velocity-constraint lines from a number of nearby points. There will be a unique solution, that is, all of the lines will intersect in a single point, if (a) the motion gradient constraint is true, (b) nearby points share a common velocity, and (c) there is no noise in the measurements. If the lines do not come close to a single intersection point, then the motion gradient constraint is a poor local description of the image motion or the nearby points do not share a common motion. In the Appendix, I discuss some of the issues related to finding the best solution to the motion-gradient-constraint equations of multiple points in the presence of measurement noise.

Space–Time Filters and the Motion Gradient Constraint

We have seen that we can use the response amplitudes of space–time-oriented linear filters to measure local image velocity. Now, studying the motion gradient constraint, we find that we can combine the spatiotemporal derivatives of the image intensities to measure the local ve-

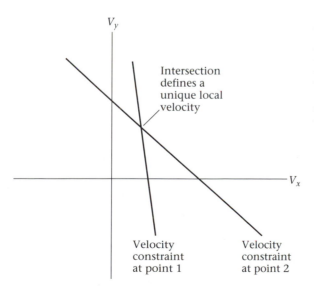

10.8 A GRAPHICAL REPRESENTATION OF THE MOTION GRADIENT CONSTRAINT. According to the motion gradient constraint, the spatial and temporal derivatives at each image point constrain the local velocities to fall somewhere along a line. The intersection of the constraint lines derived from nearby points yields a local velocity estimate that is consistent with the motion of all the local points.

locity. These two methods of measuring local motion are closely linked, as the following argument shows (Simoncelli, 1993).

To explain the relationship using pictures, we will consider only one-dimensional spatial stimuli and use the (t, x) graph. With this simplification, the motion gradient constraint has the reduced form

$$v_x \frac{\partial I}{\partial x} + \frac{\partial I}{\partial t} = 0 \tag{10.4}$$

Since the stimuli are one-dimensional, we can only estimate a single directional velocity, v_x.

How can we express the computation in Equation 10.4 in terms of the responses of space–time receptive fields? It is possible to compute spatial and temporal image derivatives by creating neurons with the appropriate space–time receptive fields. First, the receptive field must compute a weighted average of the local image intensities over a small space–time region.[5] We can describe this space–time averaging as a convolution with a Gaussian weighting function $g(x, t)$. Second, we compute the spatial and temporal derivatives by applying the appropriate partial derivative operator to the averaged data. We can group the spatial averaging and derivative operations to create a spatial receptive field, $\frac{\partial g}{\partial x}$, and a temporal receptive field, $\frac{\partial g}{\partial t}$. Images of the space–time receptive fields that compute these two derivative operations are shown in the (t, x) graphs at the top of Figure 10.9A.

One way to compute the velocity, according to Equation 10.4, is to multiply these spatial and temporal receptive fields with the image. The ratio of the spatial and temporal derivative responses is equal to the velocity, v_x. An equivalent way to perform the same calculation is to create an array of neurons whose receptive fields are various weighted sums of the two derivative operators for different values, v_x. The receptive fields of such an array of neurons are shown in Figure 10.9A. Each receptive field is oriented in space–time, and the orientation depends on the velocity used as a weight, v_x. The pattern of response amplitudes of these neurons can be used to estimate the stimulus motion. For example, the receptive field of the neuron shown in Figure 10.9B is aligned with the stimulus motion and has a large response amplitude. The receptive field of the neuron shown in panel C of Figure 10.9 has a small response amplitude. We can deduce the local image velocity from the pattern of response amplitudes.

This set of pictures shows that the motion gradient constraint can be understood in terms of the responses of space–time-oriented receptive fields; hence, space–time-oriented receptive fields and the motion gradient constraint are complementary ways of thinking about local motion.

---

[5] Some space–time averaging of the image intensities is inevitable because of physiological factors, such as optical blurring and temporal sluggishness of the neural response.

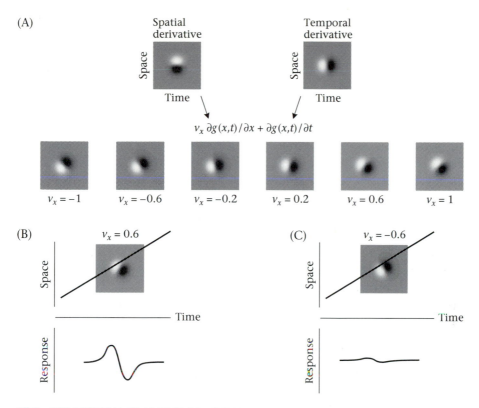

10.9 THE MOTION GRADIENT CONSTRAINT REPRESENTED IN TERMS OF SPACE–TIME RECEPTIVE FIELDS. (A) The spatial and temporal derivatives can be computed using neurons whose (t, x) receptive fields are shown at the top. We can form weighted sums of these neural responses to create new receptive fields that are oriented in space–time. The response amplitudes of these neurons can be used to identify the motion of a stimulus. The receptive field of the neuron represented in (B) responds strongly to the stimulus motion while the receptive field of the neuron in (C) responds weakly. By comparing the response amplitudes of the array of neurons, one can infer the stimulus motion.

Depth Information in the Motion Flow Field

We now have several ways of thinking about motion-flow-field estimation. But, remember that estimation of the motion flow field itself is not our main goal. Rather, we would like to be able to use the information in the motion-flow-field estimate to make inferences about the positions of objects in the scene. Much of the computational theory of motion and depth is concerned with how to calculate these quantities from the motion flow field. I do not provide a general review of such algorithms here. However, I do explain one principle concerning the computation of a depth map from observer motion, illustrated in Figure 10.10, that is important to understanding many of these algorithms (Koenderink and van Doorn, 1975; Longuet-Higgins and Prazdny, 1980).

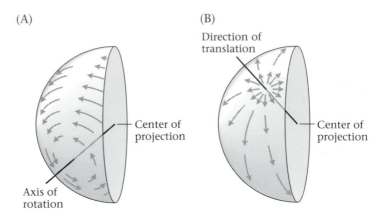

(A)

(B)

Direction of
translation

Center of
projection

Center of
projection

Axis of
rotation

**10.10   THE MOTION-FLOW-FIELD COMPONENTS ASSOCIATED WITH OBSERVER
MOTION.** A change in the observer's viewpoint causes two separate changes in the
motion flow field. The total flow-field vector is a sum of the rotation and translation
components. (A) When the viewpoint rotates, the rotation component of the motion
flow field is the same for all points, regardless of their distance. (B) When the viewpoint
translates, the motion flow field varies as a function of the image point distance from the
observer and the observer's direction of heading. After Longuet-Higgins and Prazdny,
1980.

We can partition each motion-flow-field vector into two components that are associated with different changes in the observer's viewpoint. The first component is due to a pure rotation of the viewpoint,
and the second component is due to a pure translation of the viewpoint. Each motion-flow-field vector is the sum of a change due to the
rotational and translational viewpoint changes.

These two flow-field components contain different information
about the distance of the point from the viewer. The change caused
by a viewpoint *rotation* does not depend on the distance to the point.
When the viewpoint rotates, the local flow field of all points, no matter what their distance from the observer, rotates by same amount.
Hence, the rotational component of the motion flow field contains no
information about the distance to different points in the image (Figure 10.10A).

The flow-field component caused by a *translation* of the viewpoint
depends on the distance to the image point in two ways. First, along
each line of sight the points closer to the viewpoint are displaced more
than distant points. Second the direction of the local flow field depends
on the direction of the translation (Figure 10.10B). You can demonstrate
these effects for yourself by closing one eye and looking at a pair of objects, one near and one distant. As you move your head from side to
side, the image of the nearby point shifts more than the image of the
distant point (i.e., motion parallax). Hence, the translational component of the motion-flow-field vectors contains information about the
distance between the viewer and the point.

Experimental Observations of Motion

Each of the main theoretical ideas we have reviewed concerning motion and depth has an experimental counterpart. For example, there are behavioral studies that analyze the role of the motion gradient constraint in visual perception (Adelson and Movshon, 1982). And, the cat visual cortex contains neurons with space–time-oriented receptive fields (DeAngelis et al., 1993a,b; McLean et al., 1994).

In addition to confirmations of the importance of the computational ideas, the experimental literature on motion perception has provided new challenges for computational theories of motion perception. Most computational theories are based on measurements of image intensities and their derivatives. Experimental evidence suggests that motion perception depends on more abstract image features, such as surfaces or objects, as well. In Chapter 9 we saw that surfaces and illuminants are important components of our analysis of color vision. Similarly, the experimental literature on motion perception shows us that we need to incorporate knowledge about surfaces and objects to frame more mature theories of motion perception (Ramachandran et al., 1988; Stoner et al., 1990; Anderson and Nakayama, 1994; Hildreth et al., 1995; Treue et al., 1995).

The experimental work defines new challenges and guidelines for those working on the next generation of computational theories. As we review these results, we shall see that motion perception is far from perfect; we make many incorrect judgments of velocity and direction. Moreover, perception of surfaces and occlusion are integral parts of how we interpret motion and depth. A complete computational theory of motion perception will need to include representations of surfaces and objects, as well as explanations of why image features such as contrast and color influence motion perception.

Motion Gradients: The Intersection of Constraints

Adelson and Movshon (1982) studied how the some of the ideas of the motion gradient constraint apply to human perception. They utilized a motion-superposition experiment that measures how people integrate motion information from separate image features when observers infer motion. The principle behind Adelson and Movshon's measurements is shown in Figure 10.11.

The motion of a one-dimensional pattern is ambiguous. We cannot measure whether a one-dimensional pattern, say, a bar, has moved along its length. Figure 10.11A shows three images from an image sequence of a moving bar and the set of possible velocities that are consistent with the image sequence. The graph is called a **velocity diagram**, and the set of possible motions defines what is called the **constraint**

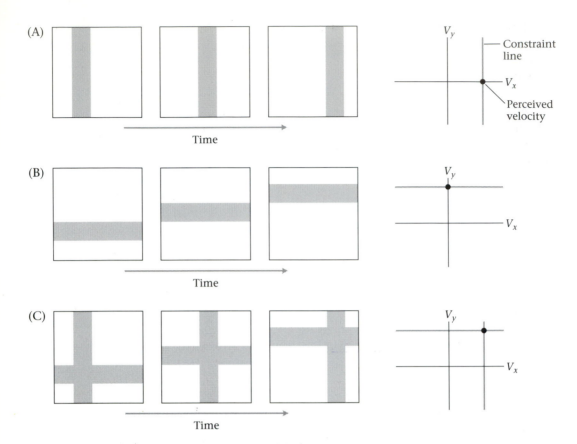

10.11   THE INTERSECTION OF CONSTRAINTS. The physical motion of a one-dimensional stimulus is inherently ambiguous. The physical motion in the display is consistent with a collection of possible velocities that may be plotted as a line in velocity space. (A) A set of images of a vertical line moving to the right; the set of physical motions consistent with the stimulus information corresponds to points along the velocity-constraint line. The dot shows the perceived physical motion. (B) A similar set of graphs for a horizontal line. (C) When the two lines are superimposed, there is only a single physical motion that is consistent with the stimulus information. That motion corresponds to the intersection of the two velocity-constraint lines shown in the graph at right.

line. The image sequence constrains the bar's horizontal velocity, but the data tell us nothing about the bar's vertical velocity. Although the information in the image sequence is ambiguous, subjects' perception of the motion is not ambiguous: the bar appears to move to the right. This perceived velocity is indicated on the velocity diagram by the black dot.

Panel B of Figure 10.11 shows the image sequence and constraint line of a horizontal bar. In this case, the stimulus information is only informative about the the vertical motion. This stimulus defines a different constraint line in the velocity diagram, and in this case, subjects see the line moving upward.

Panel C of Figure 10.11 shows the superposition of the two lines. In this stimulus, each bar separately determines a single constraint line;

the **intersection of constraints** is the only point in the velocity diagram that is consistent with the image sequence information. The only consistent interpretation that groups the two lines into a single stimulus is that the pair of lines moves up and to the right. This is what subjects see.

Adelson and Movshon (1982) described a set of measurements in which they evaluated whether observers generally saw the motion of the superimposed stimuli moving in the direction predicted by the intersection of constraints. In that study, they used one-dimensional sinusoidal gratings as stimuli, rather than bars.[6] They altered the contrast, orientation, and spatial frequency of the two gratings. As parameters varied, observers generally saw motion near the direction of the intersection of constraints. Often, however, observers saw the two gratings as two different objects, sliding over one another, an effect called **motion transparency**. Transparency is a case in which the observer perceives two motions at each point in the image. This fact alone has caused theorists to scurry back to their chalkboards and reconsider their computational motion algorithms.

The behavioral experiments show that representations like the intersection of constraints are helpful in some cases. But even in these simple mixture experiments, observers see objects and surfaces, concepts that are not represented in the motion computations. This finding indicates that perceptions of surfaces are important elements of human motion perception. A second way to see the close relationship between motion and surfaces is through a visual demonstration, described in Figure 10.12, called a **random-dot kinematogram**.

The demonstration described in Figure 10.12 consists of an image sequence in which each individual frame is an array of dots. From frame to frame, the dots change position as if they were painted on the surface of a moving object. In a single frame the observer sees nothing but a random dot pattern; the only information about the object is contained in the dot motions. The motions of the dots painted on the surface of a transparent cylinder are shown in Figure 10.12. The cylinder is also shown, though in the actual display the cylinder outline is not shown.

Random-dot kinematograms reveal several surprising aspects of how the visual system uses motion information. First, the visual system seems to integrate local motions into globally coherent structures. The ability to integrate a set of seemingly independent local motions into a single coherent percept is called **structure from motion**. The demonstration described in Figure 10.12 is particularly impressive on this point. The image sequence contains a representation of dots on a transparent object. Because some of the dots are painted onto the front and some onto the back of the transparent object, each region of the image contains dots moving in opposite directions. Despite the apparent

---

[6] The superposition of two gratings at different orientations looks like a plaid, so this design is often called a *motion-plaid* experiment.

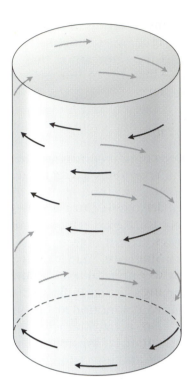

10.12 DESCRIPTION OF A RANDOM-DOT KINEMATOGRAM.
Suppose that an observer views a random collection of dots and
that each dot is moving as if it is attached to the surface of a
transparent cylinder. Observers perceive the surface of an implicit
rotating cylinder, even though there is no shading or edge
information in the image. Because the cylinder is transparent, dots
move in both directions in each local region of the image. The
dots are perceived as being attached to the near or far surface
consistent with their direction of motion.

jumble of local motions, observers automatically segregate the local dot
motions and interpret the different directions and speeds, yielding the
appearance of the front and back of a rotating and transparent object.

Second, the ability to integrate these dot motions into an object
seems to be carried out by a visual mechanism that infers the presence
of a surface without regard to the stability of the surface texture. We
can draw this conclusion from the fact that the stability and temporal
properties of the individual dots have very little effect on the overall
perception of the moving object. Single dots can be deleted after only
a fraction of a second; new dots can be introduced at new surface locations on the implicit surface without disrupting the overall percept.
Even as dots come and go, the observer sees a stable moving surface.
The local space–time motions of the dots are important for revealing
the object, but the object has a perceptual existence that is independent
of any of the individual dots (Treue, 1991).

The shapes we perceive using random-dot kinematograms are very
compelling, but they do not look like real moving surfaces. The motion
cue is sufficient to evoke the shape, but many visual cues are missing,
and the observer is plainly aware of their absence. Random-dot kinematograms are significant because they seem to isolate certain pathways
within the visual system. Random-dot kinematograms may permit us
to isolate the flow of information between specialized motion mecha-

nisms and shape recognition. By studying motion and depth perception using these stimuli, we learn about special interconnections in the visual pathway. Studies with these types of stimuli have played a large role in the physiological analysis of the visual pathways, which we turn to next.

Contrast and Color

The contrast or color of an object is not a cue about the object's velocity. Yet while velocity judgments should be independent of contrast and color, perceived velocity in fact depends on these stimulus variables. Models of human performance must be able to predict this dependence and to explain why judged velocity depends on these extraneous variables.

Stone and Thompson (1992) measured how perceived speed depends on stimulus contrast. Subjects compared the speed of a standard grating drifting at 2 deg/sec with the speed of a test grating. The data points measure the chance that the test appeared faster than the standard as a function of the speed of the test grating. The data points near the curve in the middle of Figure 10.13 are from a control condition in

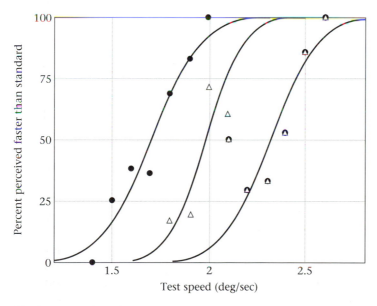

10.13 PERCEIVED SPEED DEPENDS ON STIMULUS CONTRAST. The horizontal axis measures the velocity of a test grating. The vertical axis measures the probability that the test grating appears to be moving faster than a standard grating whose speed is always 2 deg/sec. The three separate curves show measurements for test gratings at three different contrasts. The curve on the left is for a test at seven times the contrast of the standard; the curve in the middle is for a test at the same contrast as the standard; the curve on the right is for a test at one-seventh the contrast of the standard. The spatial frequency of the test and standard were always 1.5 cpd. Source: Stone and Thompson, 1992.

which the test and standard had the same contrast. In the control condition, the test and standard had the same apparent speed when they had the same physical speed. The curve on the left shows the results when the test grating had seven times more contrast than the standard. In this case the test and standard had equal perceived speed when the test speed was 1.6 deg/sec, significantly slower than the standard. The data points near the curve on the right show the results when the test grating had one-seventh the contrast of the standard grating. In this condition the test had equal perceived speed to the standard speed at 2.4 deg/sec, considerably faster than the standard. High-contrast targets appear to move faster than low-contrast targets.

Our velocity judgments also depend on other irrelevant image properties, such as the pattern of the stimulus (e.g., Smith and Edgars, 1991) and the color of the stimulus (e.g., Moreland, 1982; Cavanagh et al., 1984). Taken together these experiments suggest that some properties of the peripheral representation, while helpful in representing color and form information, have unwanted side-effects on motion perception. The initial encoding of the signal by the visual system must be appropriate for many different kinds of visual information. Given these practical requirements, interactions between irrelevant image properties and motion estimation may be unavoidable.

Long- and Short-Range Motion Processes

Creative science often includes a clash between two opposing tendencies. The search to unify phenomena in a grand theory is opposed by the need to distinguish phenomena with separate root explanations. The tension is summarized in Einstein's famous remark: "Everything should be made as simple as possible, but not simpler." Perhaps the best-known effort to classify motion into different processes is Braddick's (1974) classification into **long- and short-range motion processes**.

In 1888, Exner first demonstrated that even very coarsely sampled motion generates a visual impression of motion. Such motion is easily distinguished from continuous motion, but there is no doubt that, to viewers, something appears to be moving. The motion impression created by viewing coarsely sampled stimuli is called **apparent motion**.[7] The properties of apparent motion were studied by many of the Gestalt psychologists, such as Wertheimer (1912) and Korte (1915), who describe the conditions under which the motion illusion is most compelling.

Braddick (1974) found two differences in how people perceive classical apparent motion and random-dot kinematograms. First, he found that the spatial and temporal sampling necessary to perceive motion

---

[7] This term is peculiar since all perceived motion is apparent.

with classical apparent-motion stimuli, such as large spots, is quite different from the sampling limits necessary to perceive motion using random-dot kinematograms. Specifically, he found that subjects perceive motion in a random-dot kinematogram only when the spatial separations between frames are less than about 15 minutes of arc. When the spatial displacements are larger than this, observers see flickering dots but no coherent motion. This is a much smaller spatial limit than the sampling differences at which subjects report seeing apparent motion. The upper limit on the spatial displacement at which motion is perceived is called D_{max} in the motion literature.

Second, Braddick found a difference in how binocular information is integrated when viewing classical apparent motion versus random-dot kinematograms. He found that subjects perceive motion when the two spots in classical apparent motion are presented either to the same eye or when they are presented alternately to two eyes. Alternating frames of a random-dot kinematogram between the two eyes, however, is less effective at evoking a sense of motion.

Based on the different responses to classical apparent motion stimuli and random-dot kinematograms, Braddick suggested that there are two different motion systems that he called the long- and short-range motion systems. He argued that these pathways were separately responsible for the perception of classical apparent motion and random-dot kinematogram motion. A wide range of experimental findings have been interpreted within this classification of motion (see e.g., Braddick, 1980; Anstis, 1980; Nakayama, 1985).

In the discussion of temporal sampling of motion (see Figure 10.5), I described how the ability to discriminate continuous from sampled motion depends on the spatial and temporal properties of the image display. It is not too surprising that the conditions necessary to perceive motion also vary with the spatiotemporal properties of the stimulus. When Cavanagh and Mather (1989) reviewed measurements relating the spatiotemporal stimulus properties to motion perception, they found that the differences between classical apparent motion and random-dot kinematograms that Braddick observed, as well as many other differences, can be explained by the general spatiotemporal organization of the visual system. For example, the value of D_{max} is proportional to the size of the elements in the random-dot field for dot sizes larger than 15 min; it does not appear to be a fixed constant that divides the sensitivity of the two motion systems (Cavanagh et al., 1985).

Based on their review, Cavanagh and Mather concluded that Braddick's division of motion perception into long- and short-range motion systems is explained more simply as a consequence of spatiotemporal sensitivity of motion mechanisms. The long- and short-range motion classification is still widely used, so understanding the classification is important. But I suspect the classification will not last (see also Chang and Julesz, 1983; Shadlen and Carney, 1986).

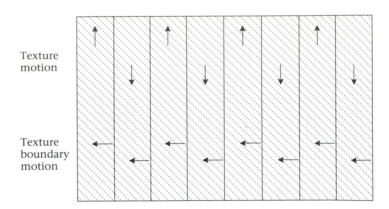

Texture motion

Texture boundary motion

10.14 A SECOND-ORDER MOTION STIMULUS. The stimulus consists of a set of texture patterns which are set into motion in two different ways. First, the texture in the separate bands moves up or down, alternately. The up/down motion of the texture bands defines a set of boundaries that are easily perceived even though there is no line separating the bands. (In the actual stimulus, there is no real edge to separate the texture bands. The lines are only drawn here to clarify the stimulus.) The boundaries separating the texture bands move continuously from right to left. This motion is also easily perceived. The leftward motion of the stimulus is very ineffective at creating a response from linear space–time-oriented filters. Source: Cavanagh and Mather, 1989.

First- and Second-Order Motion

Some authors have classified motion perception based on whether or not a stimulus activates neurons with space–time-oriented receptive fields followed by simple squaring operations (Anstis, 1980; Chubb and Sperling, 1988). According to this classification, whenever a stimulus evokes a powerful response from these sensors, the motion can be perceived by the **first-order motion system**. Chubb and Sperling (1988) show precisely how to create stimuli that are ineffective at stimulating the first-order system but still appear to move. They propose that these moving stimuli are seen by a **second-order motion system**.[8]

Figure 10.14 presents an example of a stimulus that is ineffective at stimulating space–time-oriented filters and yet appears to move. At each moment in time, the stimulus consists of a single uniform texture pattern. The stimulus appears to contain a set of vertical boundaries because the local elements in different bands move in opposite (up/down) directions. In addition to this up/down motion, the positions of the bands drift from right to left. This stimulus does not evoke a powerful leftward response from space–time-oriented filters. Yet, the pattern plainly appears to drift from right to left (Cavanagh and Mather, 1989).

These second-order motion stimuli can also be interpreted as evidence that surfaces and objects play a role in human motion percep-

---

[8] In their original paper, Chubb and Sperling (1988) called the two putative neural pathways *Fourier* and *non-Fourier* motion systems. Cavanagh and Mather (1989) used the terms *first-* and *second-order* motion systems to refer to a broad class of similar motion phenomenona. This terminology seems to be gaining wider acceptance.

tion. The motion of the bands is easy to see because we see the bars as separate objects. We perceive these objects because of their local texture pattern, not because of any luminance variation. Computational theorists have not come to a consensus on how to represent objects and surfaces. Thus, the motion of these second-order stimuli cannot be easily explained by conventional theory. We might take the existence of these second-order stimuli, then, as a reminder that we need to extend current theory to incorporate a notion of perceived motions that includes concepts that connect local variations to broader ideas concerning surfaces and objects (Fleet and Langley, 1994; Hildreth et al., 1995).

Because we perceive the motion of borders, including borders defined by texture and depth, we must find ways to include neural signals that represent borders in the general theory of motion perception. Cavanagh and Mather (1989) suggest that we might reformulate the classification into first- and second-order processes as a different and broader question: Can motion perception be explained by a single basic motion-detection system that receives inputs from several types of visual subsystems, or are there multiple motion sensing systems, each with their own separate input? There is no current consensus on this point. Some second-order phenomena can be understood by simple amendments to current theory (Fleet and Langley, 1994), but phenomena involving transparency, depth, and occlusion may require significant additions to the theory (Hildreth et al., 1995). At present, then, I view the classification into first- and second-order motion systems as a reminder that many different signals lead to motion perception, and that at present our analyses have only explored a few types of these signals.

Stereo Depth

Wheatstone (1838) was the first to analyze thoroughly the implications of the simple but powerful fact that each eye sees the world from a slightly different position (p. 66):

> It will now be obvious why it is impossible for the artist to give a faithful representation of any near solid object, that is, to produce a painting which shall not be distinguished in the mind from the object itself. When the painting and the object are seen with both eyes, in the case of the painting two *similar* pictures are projected on the retinae, in the case of the solid object the two pictures are *dissimilar*; there is therefore an essential difference between the impressions on the organs of sensation in the two cases, and consequently between the perceptions formed in the mind; the painting therefore cannot be confounded with the solid object.

For near objects, the different perspective obtained by each eye provides us with an important cue to depth, namely, **retinal disparity** (see Chapter 6). The differences between a pair of stereo images and the differences seen when the observer moves have much in common. In the case of stereo depth we refer to the differences as retinal disparity, and in the case of motion sequence we refer to the differences as a motion flow field. In both cases the differences between the two images arise due to translation and rotation of the viewpoint associated with the different images.

Depth without Edges

Just as there has been some debate concerning the role of surfaces and edges in motion perception, so too there has been a debate on the role of these different levels of representation in perceiving depth. Until the mid-1960s, psychologists generally supposed that the visual pathways first formed an estimate of surface and edge properties within each monocular image. It was assumed that disparity and, ultimately, stereo depth were calculated from the positions of the edge and surface locations estimated in each of the monocular images (Ogle, 1964).

Julesz (1961, 1971) introduced a stimulus, the **random-dot stereogram**, that proves that an object can be seen in stereo depth even though the object's edges are invisible in the monocular images. The random-dot stereogram consists of a pair of related random dot patterns as shown in Figure 10.15. Each image seen separately appears to be a random collection of black and white dots. Yet, when the two images are presented separately to the two eyes, the relationship between the two collections of dots is detected by the visual pathways, and the observer can perceive the surface of the object in depth.

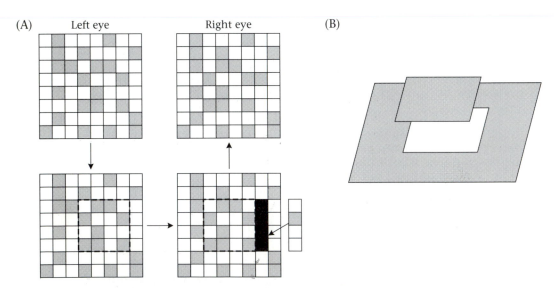

10.15 CONSTRUCTION OF A RANDOM-DOT STEREOGRAM. (A) First, a random dot pattern is created to present to, say, the left eye. The stimulus for the right eye is created by copying the first image, displacing a region horizontally, and then filling the gap with a random sample of dots. (B) When the right and left images are viewed simultaneously, the shifted region appears to be in a different depth plane from the other dots.

Figure 10.15 shows how to create the two images comprising a random-dot stereogram. First, create a sampling grid and randomly assign a black or white intensity to each position in the grid. This random image of black and white dots will be one image in the stereo pair. Next, select a region of the first image. Displace this region horizontally, overwriting the original dots. Displacing this region of dots leaves some unspecified positions; fill in these unspecified positions randomly with new black and white dots.

Random-dot stereograms provide a fascinating tool for vision science because the patterns we see in these stereo pairs are computed by signals that are carried separately by the two eyes. First, they demonstrate the simple but important point that, even though we cannot see any monocular edge or surface information of the object, we can still see the object based on the disparity cue. Second, they provide an interesting tool for anatomically localizing different types of perceptual computations. Recall that the earliest binocular cells are in the superficial layers of area V1 (Chapter 6). Hence, any part of the surface or edge computation that is performed in the monocular pathways prior to area V1 cannot play a role in the representation of edges and surfaces seen in random-dot stereograms.[9]

Depth with Edges

That observers perceive depth in random-dot stereograms does not imply that edge detection and surface interpretation play no role in depth perception. This is quite analogous to the experimental situation in motion perception. Observers perceive motion in random-dot kinematograms, but surfaces and edge representations appear to be an important part of how we perceive motion.

We can see the relationship between surface representations and depth by considering the role of surface **occlusion**. Occlusion is one of the most powerful monocular cues used to perceive depth, since when one object blocks the view of another, it is a sure sign of their depth relationship. Nakayama and Shimojo (1990) and He and Nakayama (1994a,b) have argued that occlusion relationships play an important role in judgments of binocular vision, too.

Their demonstrations of the role of occlusion in stereo depth are based on the simple physical observations shown in Figure 10.16A. Leonardo Da Vinci made use of this drawing in his *Trattato della Pittura* to describe the relationship between occlusion, half-occlusion, and transparency (quoted in Wheatstone, 1838):

> [I]f an object C be viewed by a single eye at A, all objects in the space behind it . . . are invisible to the eye at A; but when the other eye at B is opened, part of these objects become visible to it; those only being hid from both eyes that are included . . . in the double shadow CD

---

[9] Julesz (1971) calls the inference of anatomical localization from psychological study "psychoanatomy."

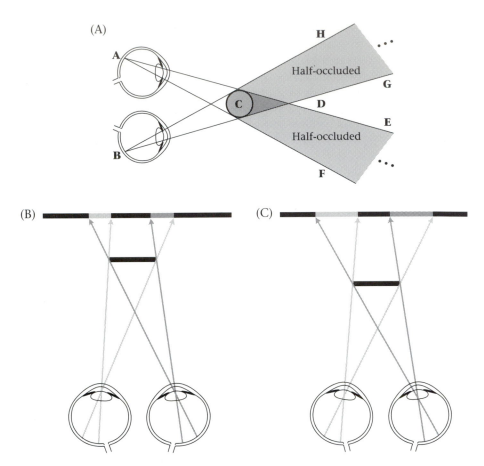

10.16 HALF-OCCLUDED REGIONS. In normal viewing, there will be regions of the image that are seen by both eyes, neither eye, or only one eye. (A) When viewing a small, nearby object, there is a fully occluded region just beyond the object (dark shading). There are two half-occluded regions (light gray shading). Well beyond the small object, both eyes see the image, so that the object is, effectively, transparent. The letters are from Da Vinci's description (see text). (B) The half-occluded regions seen by the right eye fall near the right edge of the near object, while the half-occluded regions seen by the left eye fall near the left edge of the near object. (C) The size of the half-occluded region depends on the distance between the observer, the near object, and the far object. After Da Vinci, reprinted in Wheatstone (1838).

cast by two lights at A and B . . . . [Because] the angular space EDG beyond D being always visible to both eyes . . . the object C seen with both eyes becomes, as it were, transparent, according to the usual definition of a transparent thing; namely, that which hides nothing beyond it.

Da Vinci points out that when an observer looks at an object, each eye encodes a portion of the scene that is not encoded by the other eye. These are called **half-occluded** regions of the image (Belhumeur and Mumford, 1992). When one looks beyond a small object, there is a small region that is fully occluded and another region that both eyes can see. When examining points in this farthest region, the small object is, effectively, transparent.

There are several simple rules that describe the location and properties of the half-occluded image regions. First, half-occluded regions seen by the left eye are always at the left edge of the near object, while half-occluded regions seen by the right eye are always at the right edge of the near object. The other two local possibilities (left eye sees an occlusion at the right edge, right eye sees an occluded region at the left edge) are physically impossible (Figure 10.16B).

Second, the relative size of the half-occluded regions varies systematically with the distances of the near and far objects. As the near object is placed closer to the observer, the half-occluded region becomes larger (Figure 10.16C). Hence, both the position and the size of half-occluded regions contain information that can be used to infer depth.[10]

Nakayama and Shimojo (1990) found that surface occlusion information influences observers' judgment of binocular depth. In their experiments, observers viewed a stereogram with physically unrealizable half-occlusions. They found that when the half-occlusion was, say, a pattern seen only by the right eye but near the left edge of a near object, the visibility of the pattern was suppressed. When they presented the same pattern at the right edge of the near object, where it could arise in natural viewing, the pattern was seen easily. Anderson and Nakayama (1994) summarize a number of related observations, and they conclude that occlusion configurations (i.e., a property of surfaces and objects) influence the earliest stages of stereo matching.

Perceived depth, like motion and color, is a visual inference. These results show that the visual inference of depth depends on a fundamental property of surfaces and objects, namely, that they can occlude one another.

Head and Eye Movements

Our eyes frequently move, smoothly tracking objects or jumping large distances as we shift our attention. To judge the motion of objects in the image, it is essential for the visual pathways to distinguish motion present in the image from motion due to eye movements.

Helmholtz (1865) distinguished two ways the visual system might incorporate information about eye position into judgments of motion (Figure 10.17). When we move our eyes, the motor system must generate a signal that is directed from the central nervous system to the

[10] Random-dot stereograms contain two half-occluded regions which are usually consistent with the image depth. When we displace the test region, we overwrite a portion of the original random dot image. The overwritten dots are half-occluded because they are only seen by the eye that views the first image. The dots that are added to complete the second image are half-occluded because they are only seen by the eye that views that second image.

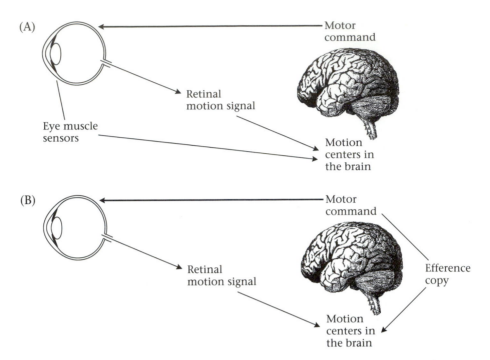

10.17 INFLOW AND OUTFLOW THEORIES FOR DISCOUNTING EYE MOVEMENT.
(A) According to inflow theory, signals from the retina and the muscles controlling eye
movement arrive at the motion centers in the brain. By comparing these two signals,
the motion centers discount eye movements and infer object motion. (B) According to
outflow theory, signals from the retina and an efference copy of the motor signal are
sent to motion centers in the brain. By comparing these two signals, the motion centers
discount eye movements and infer object motion.

eye muscles. This outgoing signal is one potential source of information
about eye movements. Helmholtz referred to this signal as denoting the
effort of will. He reasoned that a copy of this motor signal may be sent
to the brain centers responsible for motion perception, and that this
willful signal may be combined with retinal signals to estimate motion.
This hypothetical signal is called the *corollary discharge*. A second possible source of information involves nerve cells that are attached to the
muscles that control eye movements. Neural sensors may measure the
tension on the muscles, or the force exerted by the muscles, and the responses of these sensors may be sent to the brain centers responsible for
motion perception. These are incoming sources of information, so that
we can distinguish these two theories with the names **outflow theory**
and **inflow theory** (Gregory, 1990).

Helmholtz lists several simple experimental demonstrations in fa-
vor of outflow theory. First, when one rotates an eye by pushing on it
with a finger, the world appears to move. In this case, the retinal image moves, but there is no willful effort to rotate the eye. According to
outflow theory we should interpret the field as rotating, and it does.

Second, if one creates a stabilized retinal image, say, by creating an afterimage, rotating the eyeball does not make the afterimage appear to move. In this case there is no retinal image motion, and no willful effort to rotate the eye. Hence, no motion is expected according to outflow theory. Third, Helmholtz (1865) finds support for the outflow theory in the experience of patients whose eye muscles have been paralyzed. He writes (p. 245),

> . . . in those cases where certain muscles have suddenly been paralyzed, when the patient tries to turn his eye in a direction in which it's powerless to move any longer, apparent motions are seen, producing double images if the other eye happens to be open at the time.

There is good support, then, for the basic outflow theory. This raises a second interesting question concerning how the visual system infers the changing position of the eye. The nervous system has two types of information about eye position. One type of information is based on the retinal image and computed by the motion flow field. As discussed earlier in this chapter and in Appendix E, it is possible to estimate the observer's motion from the motion flow field. Now, we find that it is also possible to estimate the motion of the eye from an efferent signal from the motor pathways. Which does the visual system use?

The answer is very sensible. There are times when the information about eye position from the motor system is more reliable than information from the motion flow field. Conversely, sometimes motion flow information is more reliable. Experimental measurements suggest that under some conditions human observers use motion-flow information alone to estimate heading; under other conditions, extraretinal signals, presumably from the oculomotor pathways, are combined with motion-flow signals (Warren and Hannon, 1988; Royden et al., 1992).

Vision During Saccadic Eye Movements

There is an interesting and extreme case you can observe yourself in which the oculomotor system dominates retinal signals. First, find a small mirror and ask a friend to help you. Ask your friend to hold the mirror close to his or her eyes. Then, have your friend switch gaze between the left and right eye repeatedly. As your friend shifts gaze, you will see both eyes move. Then, change roles. While your friend watches you, shift your gaze in the mirror from eye to eye. Your friend will see your eyes shift, but you will not be able to see your own eyes move at all.

There have been several different measurements of sensitivity loss during rapid jumps of eye position, or **saccades**. To measure the loss of visual sensitivity, one needs to separate the visual effects from the simple effects having to do with the motion of the eye itself. The motion of the eye in, say, the horizontal direction changes the effective spatiotemporal signal in the direction of motion. By measuring sensitivity using horizontal contrast patterns, however, one can separate the effect of the eye movement on the signal from the suppression by the visual pathway. The suppressive effect caused by neural, rather than optical, factors is called **saccadic suppression**.

Sensitivity loss during saccades shows two main features that relate to the motion pathway. First, during saccades contrast sensitivity to low-frequency light–dark patterns is reduced strongly, while sensitivity to high-spatial-frequency patterns is not significantly changed (Volkman et al., 1978; Burr et al., 1994). Second, there is no sensitivity loss to colored edges during a saccade (Burr et al., 1994).

The curves in Figure 10.18 measure the probability of detecting a luminance grating as a function of the target contrast. The open circles show measurements made during steady fixation, and the filled circles show measurements made during a 6-degree saccade. To see the target during the saccade, subjects need to increase the target contrast. Plainly, the suppression is strongest for the low-spatial-frequency targets; also,

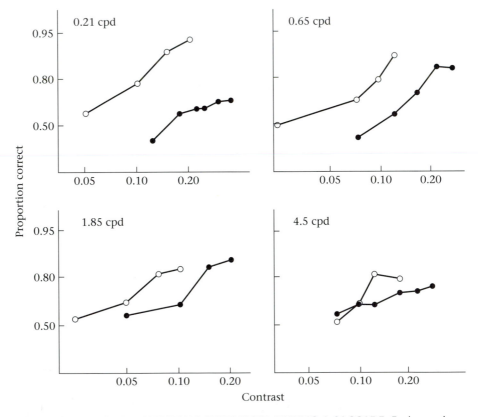

10.18 CONTRAST SENSITIVITY IS SUPPRESSED DURING A SACCADE. Each panel plots the probability of detection as a function of signal contrast while the observer is fixating (open circles) or executing a saccade (filled circles). The data are combined from three observers. The separate panels show measurements using patterns with different spatial frequencies. Source: Volkman et al., 1978.

there is little suppression of colored patterns. Lesion studies described in Chapter 5 suggested that these stimuli are detected mainly by signals on the magnocellular pathway. Based on the parallel loss of visual sensitivity from these lesions and during saccadic eye movements, Burr et al. (1994) suggested that saccadic suppression takes place within the magnocellular pathway.

The oculomotor and motion systems must work together to establish a visual frame of reference. Saccadic suppression illustrates that in some cases the visual system judges the retinal information to be unreliable and suppresses the retinal signal until a more stable estimate of the reference frame can be obtained. But the world remains visible when one's head turns, and observers can detect image displacements as small as 2–3%. Hence, although we suppress quite large displacements during saccades, we remain sensitive to displacements as we turn our heads or move about (Wallach, 1987).

The Cortical Basis of Motion Perception

More than any other visual sensation, motion seems to be associated with a discrete visual portion of the visual pathway. A visual stream that begins with the parasol cells in the retina and continues through cortical areas V1 and MT seems to have a special role in representing motion signals. This **motion pathway**[11] has been studied more extensively than any other portion of the visual pathways, and so most of this section of the chapter is devoted to a review of the responses of neurons in the visual stream from the parasol cells to area MT. Before turning to the physiological literature, however, I will describe an interesting clinical report of a patient who cannot see motion.

Acquired Motion Deficits

Zihl et al. (1983) described a patient (L.M.) who, following a stroke, had great difficulty in perceiving certain types of motion. There have been a few reports of individuals with a diminished ability to perceive motion as a consequence of stroke, and transient loss of motion perception can even be induced by magnetic stimulation of the brain (see also Vaina et al., 1990; Zeki, 1991; Beckers et al., 1992). But L.M. has been studied far more thoroughly than the others and so we will focus on her case.

L.M.'s color vision and acuity remain normal, and she has no difficulty in recognizing faces or objects. But she cannot see coffee flowing into a cup. Instead, the liquid appears frozen, like a glacier. Since she

---

[11] While I will call this visual pathway a "motion pathway," following common usage, the certainty implied by the phrase is premature. Other portions of the visual pathways may also be important for motion, and this pathway may have functions beyond motion perception.

cannot perceive the fluid rising, she spills while pouring. L.M. feels uncomfortable in a room with several moving people, or on a street, since she cannot track changes in positions: "People were suddenly here or there, but I have not seen them moving." She cannot cross the street for fear of being struck by a moving car: "When I'm looking at the car first, it seems far away. But then, when I want to cross the road, suddenly the car is very near" (Zihl et al., 1983).

There are very few patients with a specific motion loss, so few generalizations are possible.[12] Patient L.M. succeeds at certain motion tasks but fails at others. She has a difficult time segregating moving dots from stationary dots, or segregating moving dots from a background of randomly moving dots; but she has no difficulty with stereo (Zihl et al., 1983; Hess et al., 1989; Baker et al., 1991).

Patient L.M. has a lesion that extends over a substantial region of the visual cortex, so that this case does not localize sharply the regions of visual cortex that are relevant to her defects. However, it is quite surprising that the loss of motion perception can be dissociated from other visual abilities, such as color and pattern. This observation supports the general view that motion signals are represented on a special motion pathway. To consider the nature of the neural representation of motion further, we turn to experimental studies.

The Motion Pathway

The starting point for our current understanding of the motion pathway is Zeki's discovery that the preponderance of neurons in cortical area MT are direction-selective; they respond vigorously when an object or a field of random dots moves in one direction, and they are silent when the motion is in a different direction. These neurons are relatively unselective for other aspects of the visual stimulus, such as color or orientation (Dubner and Zeki, 1971; Zeki, 1974).

In visual areas prior to MT, direction-selective neurons represent only a fraction of the population. For example, about one-quarter of the neurons in area V1 are direction-selective, and these neurons fall within a subset of the cortical layers in V1 (Hawken et al., 1988). The proportion of direction-selective neurons appears to be even lower in area V2. Area MT appears to be the first area in which the vast majority of neurons, distributed throughout the anatomical area, are direction-selective.

The neurons in area MT are principally driven by signals originating in the magnocellular pathway (Figure 10.19). Recall from Chapters 5 and 6 that the magnocellular pathway terminates in layer 4Cα of the primary visual cortex. The output from 4Cα passes to layer 4B, and the output from 4B is communicated either directly to area MT, or first through regions within area V2 and then to area MT. The majority of

---

[12] Zeki (1991) calls the syndrome *akinetopsia*. His review makes clear that the evidence for the existence of this syndrome is much weaker than the evidence for dyschromatopsia.

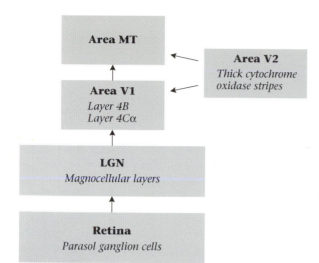

10.19 ANATOMY OF THE MOTION PATHWAY. The signal from parasol ganglion cells follows a discrete pathway into the brain. The signals can be traced through the parvocellular layers of the LGN and through area V1 to area MT. Neurons in area MT respond more strongly to signals from parasol ganglion cells than to signals from midget cells.

direction-selective neurons in area V1 fall within the same layers of V1 that communicate with area MT. Hence, the direction-selective neurons in area V1 appear to send their output mainly to area MT.[13]

There is one further piece of evidence concerning the significance of motion and area MT. The direction-selectivity of neurons within area MT is laid out in an organized fashion. Nearby neurons tend to be selective for motion in the same direction (Albright, 1984). This is analogous to the retinotopic organization evident in cortical areas V1 and V2 (see Chapter 6). Taken together, the evidence argues that area MT plays an important role in motion perception (Merigan and Maunsell, 1993).

As we measure from the periphery to visual cortex, we find that the receptive-field properties of the neurons within the motion pathway respond to increasingly sophisticated stimulus properties. The first major transformation is direction selectivity, which appears within neurons in layer 4B of area V1. Direction selectivity is a new feature of the receptive field, a feature which is not present in the earlier parts of the pathway.

Earlier in this chapter we saw that it is possible to estimate motion flow fields using neurons with receptive fields that are oriented in space–time (see Figure 10.7). DeAngelis et al. (1993a,b) measured the space–time receptive fields of neurons in cat visual cortex, and they found that some direction-selective neurons have linear space–time-oriented receptive fields (see also McLean et al., 1994). Some of their measurements are illustrated in Figure 10.20. The sequence of images in that figure shows the two-dimensional spatial receptive field of a neuron measured at different moments in time following the stimulus. Below the volume of measurements is the space–time receptive field for one-dimensional stimulation, shown in the (t, x) representation. This

---

[13] The parvocellular pathway does make some contribution to MT responses. This has been shown by blocking magnocellular-pathway responses and observing responses to signals in the parvocellular pathway. Nonetheless, by biological standards the separation is rather impressive (Maunsell et al., 1990).

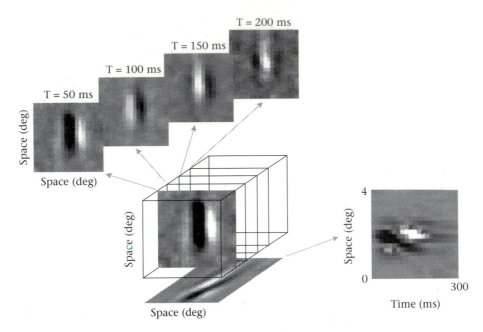

10.20   SPACE–TIME-ORIENTED RECEPTIVE FIELD IN CAT CORTEX. The images on the upper left show the spatial receptive field measured at different moments in time following stimulation. Taken together, these measurements form a space–time volume representation of the neural receptive field. The space–time receptive field for one-dimensional spatial stimulation is shown at the bottom of the volume and again on the right. In this (t, x) representation, the receptive field is oriented, implying that the neuron has a larger amplitude response to stimuli moving in some directions than others. After DeAngelis et al., 1993b.

receptive field is also shown at the right where it is easy to see that the receptive field is oriented in the space–time plot.

Movshon et al. (1985) discovered a novel feature of the receptive fields in some MT neurons that represents an additional property of motion analysis. They call the neurons that have this new receptive field property **pattern-selective** neurons, to distinguish them from simple direction-selective neurons, such as we find in area V1, which they call **component-selective**. They identified these two neuronal classes in area MT using a simple mixture experiment.

First they measured the direction-selective tuning curves of neurons in area MT using one-dimensional sinusoidal grating patterns. Figure 10.21 shows the tuning curves of two MT neurons. In these polar plots, the neuron's response to a stimulus is plotted in the same direction from the origin as the stimulus motion. A point's distance from the origin indicates the size of the neuron's response. The inner circle on the plot indicates the neuron's spontaneous firing rate. The direction-selective tuning curves of these neurons are similar to the tuning curves of neurons in area V1.

Having measured the tuning curve, Movshon and his colleagues asked the basic linear-systems question: can we use the tuning curve to

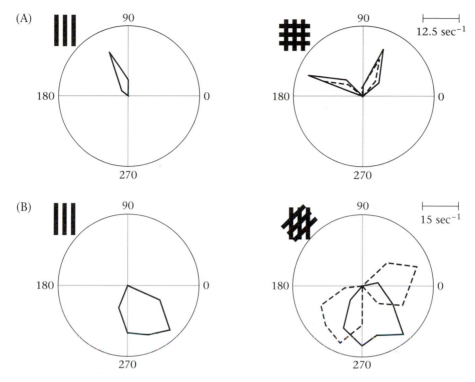

10.21 DIRECTION SELECTIVITY IN AREA MT. (A) The direction tuning of a component-selective neuron in area MT. (Left) The neuron responds to a grating moving up and to the left, but not to a plaid moving in the same direction (right). Instead, the neuron's responses to the plaid are predicted by its direction-selectivity to the components of the pattern. The predicted responses, based on the components, are shown as dashed lines. This response pattern is typical of direction-selective cells in area V1 and about half of the cells in area MT. (B) The direction tuning of a pattern-selective neuron in area MT (left). This neuron responded well to single gratings moving down and to the right. (Right) The cell also responded well to a plaid, whose components were separated by 135 degrees, moving down and to the right. Neither component of the plaid alone evokes a response from this neuron. Hence, this neuron responds to the direction of motion of the pattern, not to the direction of motion of the components. Source: Movshon et al., 1985.

predict the neuron's response to other patterns? To answer this question, they used new patterns formed by adding together individual grating patterns.

Consider the response of a component-selective MT neuron, such as that shown in Figure 10.21A. This type of neuron responds well only to a narrow range of directions of a sinusoidal pattern, upward and to the left. Movshon and his colleagues measured such a neuron's response to a plaid consisting of components separated in orientation by 90 degrees. This MT neuron responded well to the plaid stimulus whenever one of the plaid components moves upward and to the left. But the neuron did not respond well when the pattern as a whole was moving upward and to the left, since in that case neither of the plaid components is moving up and to the left.

Recall that when people view a moving plaid, it appears to move approximately in the direction predicted by the intersection of constraints (see Figure 10.11). The component-selective neuron's activity is not correlated with the perceived direction of motion. The component-selective neuron responds well only when the individual components appear to be moving upward and to the left. It does not respond well when the plaid as a whole appears to move in this direction.

The response of a pattern-selective neuron, as shown in Figure 10.21B, is correlated with the perceived direction of motion. In the study by Movshon et al., the pattern-selective neuron's response was large when a single sinusoidal grating moved down and to the right. The neuron also responded well to a 135-degree plaid pattern moving down and to the right. Remember, when the plaid is moving down and to the right, the plaid components are moving in directions that are outside of the response range of this neuron. If we isolate the components of the 135-degree plaid pattern moving down and to the right and present them to the neuron, neither will evoke a response. Yet, when we present them together they result in a powerful response from the neuron. The nonlinear neuron response correlates with the perceived direction of motion of the stimulus.

In their survey of area MT, Movshon and his colleagues found that approximately 25% of the neurons in area MT were pattern-selective, half the neurons were classified as component-selective, and the rest could not be classified. Having observed the signal transformation, we would like to understand the circuitry that implements the transformation.

Motion Perception and Brain Activity

LESION STUDIES. Lesion studies provide further evidence that area MT plays a role in motion perception. A lesion in area MT causes performance deficits in various motion tasks with no corresponding loss in visual acuity, color perception, or stereoscopic depth perception (Siegel and Anderson, 1986; Newsome and Paré, 1988; Schiller, 1993).

Newsome and Paré (1988) observed profound deficits when a monkey was forced to discriminate motion using the random-dot kinematogram shown in Figure 10.22. In this type of kinematogram, each dot is flashed briefly at random positions on the screen. The correlation of the dot positions from frame to frame is the independent variable. When the correlation is zero, a dot is equally likely to appear anywhere on the screen in the next frame. At this correlation level, there will be some local motion signals, by chance, but the average motion will be zero. The experimenter can introduce net motion in the stimulus by correlating some of the dot positions in adjacent frames. When the correlation is positive, some fraction of the dots, the correlated dots, reappear displaced by a fixed amount in one direction. Hence, the correlated dots introduce a net motion direction into the display.

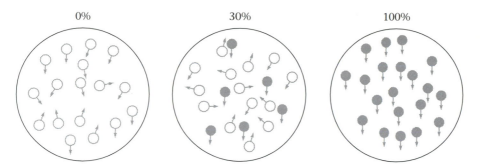

10.22 A RANDOM-DOT KINEMATOGRAM USED TO MEASURE MOTION SENSITIVITY. Each dot is flashed briefly at random positions on the screen. When the correlation is zero, a dot is equally likely to move in any direction in the next frame. The experimenter can introduce motion into the stimulus gradually by increasing the correlation between dots presented in successive frames. Because the correlated dots (shown as shaded circles) all move in the same direction, the fraction of correlated dots controls the net motion signal in the display. In the actual display, the correlated and uncorrelated dots in a frame appear the same; the filled and open dots are used in the figure only to explain the principle. Source: Newsome and Paré, 1988.

Ordinarily, the monkey is asked to discriminate whether the net direction of dot motions is in one of two directions. When few of the dot motions are correlated, performance is near chance (50% correct). When many of the dot motions are correlated, performance is nearly perfect (100% percent correct). The investigators measure threshold by varying the number of correlated dots required for the monkey to judge the correct direction of motion in 75% of the trials.

There are two MT areas, one on each side of the brain. Each area receives input from the opposite visual hemifield. After lesioning area MT on one side of the brain, Newsome and Paré found that threshold for detecting motion increased by a factor of roughly 4 for stimuli in the relevant hemifield. The threshold for stimuli in the other hemifield remained at preoperative performance levels, as does the animal's performance on nonmotion tasks, such as orientation discrimination (Newsome and Wurtz, 1988).

In Newsome and Paré's experiment, the motion deficit is transient; performance returns to preoperative levels within a week or two following the lesion. In other motion tasks, such as speed discrimination, the lesion-induced deficit can be permanent (Schiller, 1993). The transient loss of function in certain tasks affords the opportunity to study neural plasticity. Presumably, following removal of MT some of the functions of the lost area are taken over by existing areas. There is evidence of functional reorganization of many cortical functions. For example, Gilbert et al. (1992) have shown that after a retinal lesion that created a blind spot in the animal's visual field, the receptive fields of neurons within area V1 reorganize fairly quickly. Neurons whose receptive fields were driven by retinal signals originating in the lesioned area begin to respond to the signals from surrounding retinal areas. This plasticity seems to be a fundamental and special capability of the cortex, since this type of reorganization was not detected in the subcortical LGN. Probably, this ability to reorganize the visual pathways is a fundamental component of the visual system. We know, for example, that visual development depends upon receiving certain types of visual stimulation (e.g., Freeman et al., 1972; Stryker and Harris, 1986; Shatz, 1992). The recovery of the animals in the Newsome and Paré study and the rapid reorganization of receptive fields found by Gilbert et al. (1992) suggest that this reorganization may be a pervasive feature of visual systems in adult animals as well.

BEHAVIOR AND NEURAL ACTIVITY. The visual pathways constantly infer the properties of the objects we perceive. These algorithms are essential to vision, but mainly, they are hidden from our conscious awareness. We have spent most of this book trying to understand these algorithms, and how they are implemented in the visual pathway. There is a second important and intriguing question about the cortical representation of information: this is the question of our conscious experience. At some point, the visual inference is complete. Next, the motor pathways must act, and perhaps our conscious awareness must be informed about the visual inference. What is the nature of the representation that corresponds to the final visual inference? Which neural responses code this representation?

There is a growing collection of papers that probe the relationship between behavior and neural responses. An important part of the ability to perform such studies has been the development of techniques to measure the neural activity of alert, behaving monkeys. To obtain such measurements, the experimenter implants a small tube into the animal's skull. During experimental sessions the experimenter inserts a microelectrode through the tube to record neural activity. The electrode insertion is not painful, so there is no need to anesthetize the animal. In this way, the experimenter can measure neural activity while monkeys are engaged in performing simple perceptual tasks. These experiments provide an opportunity to compare behavior and neural activity within a single alert and behaving animal (Parker and Hawken, 1985; Britten et al., 1992).

The relationship between performance and neural activity has been studied for the detection of contrast patterns, orientation discrimination, and motion direction discrimination (e.g., Tolhurst, 1983; Parker and Hawken, 1985; Barlow et al., 1987; Hawken et al., 1990; Vogels, 1990; Britten et al., 1992). In the motion experiment reported by Britten et al. (1992), for example, the experimenters first isolated a neuron in area MT and determined the neuron's receptive field and best motion direction. The monkey was then shown a random-dot kinematogram moving in one of two directions within the receptive field of the neuron. The animal made a forced-choice decision concerning the perceived direction of motion, and at the same time the experimenters recorded the activity of the neuron. The response of individual neurons did not predict the animal's response on any single trial, but using a simple statistical model Britten et al. discovered that, on average, the response of a single MT neuron discriminated the motion direction as well as the animal could discriminate the motion direction.

Considerably more information is encoded by a single MT neuron about motion than is encoded by a single V1 neuron about pattern. For example, the sensitivity of individual V1 neurons to sinusoidal contrasting gratings is substantially lower than the animal's sensitivity. The similarity between behavioral and neural sensitivity on the motion task supports the view that area MT is specialized to represent motion perception. The finding also raises some interesting questions about how information is pooled within the nervous system to make behavioral decisions. In area MT alone there are many hundreds of neurons with equivalent sensitivity to this stimulus. If the responses of these neurons are largely independent, then pooling their outputs would improve performance substantially. Yet, the animal's performance is not much better than we would expect if the animal were simply using the output of a single neuron. Perhaps this is so because the neural responses are correlated (Zohary et al., 1994).

MICROSTIMULATION STUDIES. Generally, observations based on correlations are a weaker form of evidence than observations based on direct experimental manipulations. Newsome and his collaborators extended their analysis beyond correlation by manipulating the neural responses during behavioral trials (Salzman and Newsome, 1992).

As in the correlational experiments, the investigators first isolated a neuron in area MT. Within area MT, nearby neurons tend to have similar direction selectivity (Albright, 1984). The experimenters used a test stimulus whose direction corresponded to the best direction of the isolated neuron; the presumption is that this direction defines the best direction of the receptive field for most of the nearby neurons.

Again, the monkey made a forced-choice decision between kinematogram motion in the best direction of the neuron or in the opposite direction. In one half of the trials, randomly selected, the investigator injected a small amount of current into the brain, stimulating the neurons near the electrode. The microstimulation changed the monkey's performance, as if the current strengthened the motion signal in the direction of the local neurons' best direction sensitivity. The open and filled symbols in the Figure 10.23 show the monkey's performance on trials with and without the current injection, respectively. The monkey was more likely to behave as if the stimulus moved in the direction preferred by the neurons in the presence of microstimulation than in its absence. In this particular experimental condition, the microstimulation was equivalent to increasing the percentage of dots moving in the test direction by 10 percent.

There are two reasons why this experiment is very significant. First, the method involves a direct experimental manipulation of the animal's behavior, rather than an inference based on a correlation. The investi-

10.23 THE EFFECT OF ELECTRICAL STIMULATION IN AREA MT ON MOTION PERCEPTION. An alert behaving monkey judged the direction of motion of a random-dot kinematogram. Judgments made without electrical stimulation are shown by the filled circles; judgments made in the presence of small amounts of electrical stimulation within area MT are shown by the open triangles. In this experiment, the microstimulation had the same effect as increasing the fraction of correlated dots by 10 percent. Source: Salzman et al., 1992.

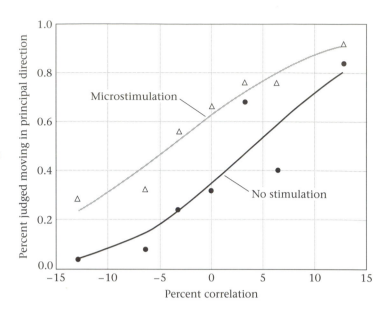

gator actively controls the state of the neurons and observes a change in the behavior. Second, the method reminds us of the hope of some-day designing visual prosthetic devices. By understanding the perceptual consequences of visual stimulation, we may be able to design visual prosthetic devices that generate predictable and controlled visual sensations.

Conclusion

Many important aspects of motion perception can be understood and predicted based on computations using only the local space–time variations of image intensities. Many of the computational elements of motion calculations, such as space–time-oriented linear filters and velocity-constraint lines, have a natural counterpart in the receptive fields of neurons within the motion pathway.

The results of many behavioral experiments suggest that the surface and object representations also provide a source of useful information for the computation of motion and depth. Observers see moving surfaces sliding transparently across one another; they see motions of texture elements defined by implicit edges; and they infer three-dimensional shapes and depth from the limited information in sets of random dots. It seems that we must understand how to incorporate surfaces in our computational theories, and we must understand how surfaces are represented in the neural pathways, to arrive at our next level of understanding of motion perception. The coupling of computational, behavioral, and neural measurements has served us well thus far, and I suspect that trying to incorporate surface representations using all of these methods will continue to be our best chance of understanding motion.

Taken together, it is evident that our inferences of motion and depth are not isolated visual computations, but rather are part of a web of visual judgments. We perceive motion in a way that depends on contrast, color, and other more abstract image features such as surface, edge, and transparency. Integrating this information requires some sophisticated neural processing, and we are just at the beginning of studying this process both behaviorally and neurophysiologically. In the next chapter, I will review some of the more interesting but complex aspects of how we integrate different types of visual cues in order to make sense of the retinal image.

Exercises

1. **(a)** Qualitatively, what will the response of a space–time-oriented linear filter be to a drifting sinusoidal pattern?

    (b) Suppose you know the response of a space–time-oriented linear filter to two stimuli. Will you be able to predict the filter's response to the superposition of the stimuli?

2. Different display technologies use different methods for temporal sampling of motion sequences. Several of these strategies are described in Footnote 1 in this chapter.

    (a) Represent the different sampling schemes used by television and by movies on a space–time diagram.

    (b) Represent these temporal sampling methods on a spatial-frequency versus temporal-frequency diagram, (f_t, f_x).

3. A square-wave grating consists of the weighted sum of a several sinusoidal components. It is possible to create an interesting motion illusion, called the *fluted square wave*, by sampling the motion of the square wave and removing the fundamental component (Adelson and Bergen, 1985; Georgeson and Harris, 1990).

    (a) Make an (f_t, f_x) drawing showing the locations of the Fourier components for a stationary square-wave grating. (See Chapter 7 if you do not know what the Fourier components of a square wave are.)

    (b) Make an (f_t, f_x) drawing showing the locations of the Fourier components for a square-wave grating drifting continuously to the right.

    (c) Make an (f_t, f_x) drawing showing the locations of the Fourier components of a *sampled* square-wave grating drifting to the right. Choose the temporal sampling interval so that the energy in the temporal replicas is aligned into a uniform grid.

    (d) Now, remove the components present in the original sinusoid from the drawing containing the sampled square wave. Examine the pattern of Fourier components that remain and predict the perceived motion of this pattern.

4. There is a classic visual illusion called the *Pulfrich effect* which illustrates the interconnection among motion, depth, and timing. Suppose you observe a pendulum that is swinging back and forth in a plane parallel to the front of your face. Now, cover one eye with with a dark filter, such as a half-log-unit neutral-density filter which you can purchase at a camera store. After a few moments, the pendulum will appear to be swinging outside of the plane, following an elliptical arc.

   (a) The Pulfrich effect is explained by assuming that (a) under normal viewing, temporal synchrony is used to identify corresponding signals from the two eyes, and (b) the signal from the eye whose light intensity is attenuated by the filter arrives later to the brain than the signal from the unattenuated eye. Make a diagram showing why this temporal lag can explain the perceived elliptical path of the swinging pendulum.

   (b) Read the articles by Thompson (1993) and Carney et al. (1989) for recent analyses of this phenomenon in terms of the visual pathways.

   (c) Read the article by Hofeldt and Hoefle (1993) for an application of the Pulfrich effect to predicting the performance of baseball players.

5. The following questions are meant to be thought-provoking, not to have simple answers. Write brief answers concerning how you might develop a research strategy to answer these questions.

   (a) Why should perceived velocity depend on the color or contrast of a moving stimulus? What implications does the existence of this relationship have for the way human motion detectors are organized? Is your hypothesis testable by experiment?

   (b) Very young infants cannot control their eye movements very well. What implication does this have for their ability to perceive motion? Answer using different assumptions concerning the quality of the efference copy signal and the retinal signals concerning motion flow fields.

   (c) Microstimulation experiments have been very useful in analyzing the relationship between area MT and motion perception. Design a microstimulation experiment to evaluate the relationship between a visual area and color perception.

11

Seeing

Seeing is a collection of inferences about the world. Motion, color, and depth are important individual judgments. To see, however, we must connect these inferences into a unified explanation of the image. Until we integrate the separate inferences of pattern, color, motion, and depth into a description of objects and surfaces, the world remains a disconcerting jumble of unconnected events.

It is easy to recognize the importance of integrating our visual inferences into a coherent view of the scene, but it is much harder to understand the process by which we perceive objects and surfaces. Because there is no current consensus on a theoretical approach to this topic, I have chosen to spend this chapter reviewing phenomena that I believe will be important in defining a computational theory of seeing.

In the first section, I will discuss clinical cases that illustrate the importance of being able to integrate information from different locations within an image and images acquired at different times. To those who are sighted from birth, the ability to integrate image information acquired from different viewpoints at different points in time is easy and automatic. As we walk about, we see single objects and not collections of independent images of the same objects. The computational complexity of the visual inference that integrates the different information is made quite plain, however, when we read about the difficulties of patients who were blind as infants but "cured" later in life. The tragic stories of these individuals, as they struggle to learn to see, provide us with some understanding of the complexity of object perception.

In the second section, I will review a set of visual illusions. Visual illusions help us understand how the visual pathways organize images into objects. I have selected a series of illusions that show how the visual system uses image information concerning occlusion, transparency, and boundaries to integrate judgments of brightness and shape. While I have mentioned the significance of many of these aspects of vision in earlier chapters, the illusions we will review here provide some clues about the rules for combining visual inferences into a complete description of the scene. And, there is a second reason for devoting this time to studying illusions: they are fun.

Miracle Cures

In 1963 Gregory and Wallace wrote a monograph describing a miracle cure. As an infant, the patient, S.B., had lost effective sight in both eyes from a corneal disease. At the age of 52, he received a corneal graft that restored his optics. After living most of his life without sight, S.B. looked upon his wife for the first time.

While the case of S.B. is one of the best studied, there have been a few similar cases described over the last few centuries. There is considerable uniformity (and some real surprises) concerning several aspects of these "miracle cures" (von Senden, 1960; Valvo, 1971; Sacks, 1991).

First, patients who have been blind most of their lives do not see well after their optics have been repaired. Even after months or years, they continue to struggle at tasks which those blessed with sight at birth find effortless. Some visual measures, such as acuity and color vision, can be within the normal range. But patients do not perceive depth, motion, or the relationship among features effortlessly. They have difficulty recognizing a face, or judging the movement of traffic. Their visual world is a jumble from which they can occasionally glean a useful pattern or bit of information. The descriptions of these cases suggest that many patients never acquire a good facility at grouping together features from different positions within the image, or features seen at different points in time from different perspectives. They have great difficulty integrating such information into a coherent description of the scene.

The difficulty in integrating information is not a small thing. The restoration of the elements of sight without this integrative ability is a disconcerting emotional experience. Most of the patients experience severe depression, and even those patients who overcome the depression wonder whether the returned sight was worth the effort. In summarizing the cases he studied, Valvo (1971, p. 4) wrote:

> The congenitally blind person especially, has to face the prospect of a difficult struggle before reaching a stage at which his vision permits him to understand the world around him. For a period of time varying with each patient, these people experience a confusing proliferation of perceptions, and they must learn to see as a child learns to walk. Moreover, personalities and character armors built up as a blind person have to be shed, and they often find it difficult to change their ways of liv-

ing. As one of our patients put it, "I had to die as a blind person to be reborn as a seeing person."

Gregory and Wallace heard about S.B.'s restoration of sight from a story in a London newspaper. They managed to get to the hospital after the first operation, in which the optics of one eye were repaired, but before the operation on the second eye.[1] They continued to visit with S.B. and examine his vision, when his health and mood permitted. Fairly quickly, S.B. managed to recognize various forms including uppercase letters and the face of a clock. His ability to recognize such patterns quickly was apparently due to his ability to transfer his understanding of these shapes based on touch into a corresponding visual sensation. This happened automatically and quickly, at a rate that astonished Gregory and Wallace. It suggested to them that he had a good facility for integrating information into objects and patterns when the information corresponded to his tactile experience.

Equally surprisingly, S.B. could recognize the shapes in the Ishihara color plates quite easily. He learned to identify color names, and in fact some colors were already known to him because, even though when blind he could not see pattern, he could detect the difference between light and dark. Also, the strong light used in opthalmological exams yields a red appearance that was probably familiar to him during his blindness.

Many of our most important perceptual abilities, however, were beyond S.B.'s reach. We take for granted our ability to judge the shape of objects as we change our viewpoint. As we walk around a house, or a tree, or a person, each image that we see is different. Yet, we integrate the information we acquire into a single unified description of an object or a person. But S.B. seemed to experience a different world as he moved around an object (Gregory, 1974, p. 111):

> Quite recently he had been struck by how objects changed their shape when he walked round them. He would look at a lamp post, walk round it, stand studying it from a different aspect, and wonder why it looked different and yet the same.

To see a moving object, we must also see the connection between the object at different moments in time. As the object moves, we often see it from different perspectives and we must be able to integrate the different retinal images of the object into a single coherent description. Patients with restored sight have a difficult time learning to perceive motion and depth. Sacks (1991) quotes from a patient with restored sight, Virgil, who wrote in his journal (May 10, 1993):

> During these first weeks [after surgery] I had no appreciation of depth or distance; street lights were luminous stains stuck to the window panes and corridors of the hospital were black holes. When I crossed the road the traffic terrified me, even when I was accompanied. I am

---

[1] The original monograph is difficult to obtain. But it is reprinted, along with additional material, in a collection of Gregory's writings entitled *Concepts and Mechanisms of Vision* (1974).

very insecure while walking; indeed I am more afraid now than before the operation.

Gregory's (1974) description of S.B. is striking in its similarity:

He [S.B.] found the traffic frightening, and would not attempt to cross even a comparatively small street by himself. This was in marked contrast to his former behaviour, as described to us by his wife, when he would cross any street in his own town by himself. In London, and later in his home town, he would show evident fear, even when led by a companion whom he trusted, and it was many months before he would venture alone. We heard that before the operation he would sometimes injure himself by walking briskly into a parked vehicle, or other unexpected obstruction, and he generally did not carry a white stick. As a blind man he was unusually active and aggressive. We began to see that this assurance had at least temporarily left him; he seemed to lack confidence and interest in his surroundings.

To perceive motion, the visual system must be able to integrate information over space and time. To perform this integration, one needs a means of short-term visual storage that can be used to represent recent information and visual inferences. If this visual storage fails, perhaps because it did not develop normally during early blindness, motion perception will be particularly vulnerable—more so, say, than color perception. One of Valvo's patients, H.S., described in his journal his difficulties with short-term visual memories as he learned to read (Valvo, 1971):

My first attempts at reading were painful. I could make out single letters, but it was impossible for me to make out whole words; I managed to do so only after weeks of exhausting attempts. In fact, it was impossible for me to remember all the letters together, after having read them one by one. Nor was it possible for me, during the first weeks to count my own five fingers: I had the feeling that they were all there, but . . . it was not possible for me to pass from one to the other while counting.

These clinical cases are important for the qualitative information they provide. We learn that patients can identify colors, or even individual letters. Yet, they have difficulty integrating their visual experiences into a single whole. As they walk around an object, it appears to be a series of different shapes, not a single unitary thing. Moving objects do not have any continuity of existence. Distance, which also requires a relative judgment, is impossible to judge accurately. The experiences of these patients show us how important the processes that integrate information over space and time are to seeing. To understand seeing, we must understand the processes that link our inferences of pattern, color, motion, and depth into a unified description of the world.

Illusions

For the vision scientist, illusions are fun. They draw people into our discipline, they inspire new algorithms, and they fill us with wonder. They are the children of our professional lives. And like children, illusions are a bit unruly. They do unpredictable things and defy a simple organization. You can try to insist that an illusion clean up its room, but a few minutes later you will discover another idea thrown haphazardly on the floor, or a theory turned upside down.

Of the many illusions known to vision scientists, only a few are suitable for the printed page. From those, I have selected mainly illusions that make some points about how we see objects.

Seeing the Three-Dimensional World

A central premise of object perception is that we see objects in a three-dimensional world. If there is an opportunity to interpret a drawing or an image as a three-dimensional object, we do. This principle is illustrated by the drawing created by Shepard (1990) shown in Figure 11.1. The two table tops have precisely the same two-dimensional shape on the page, except for a rigid rotation. Nobody believes this when first looking at the illusion. To convince yourself that the shapes of the table tops are are truly the same, trace one of them on an overhead transparency or tracing paper, and then rotate the tracing around. Or, make a cutout that covers one table top and then rotate it and place it on the other. The illusion shows that we do not see the two-dimensional shape drawn on the page, but instead we see the three-dimensional shape of

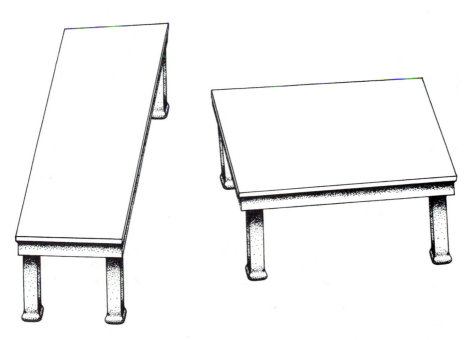

11.1 WE ASSUME THAT TWO-DIMENSIONAL SHAPES DESCRIBE THREE-DIMENSIONAL OBJECTS. Drawn on the two-dimensional page, the table tops are the same except for a rotation. Convince yourself that the shapes are the same on the page by making a cutout equal in size to one of the tabletops. Then, rotate the cutout and place it on the other tabletop. From Shepard, 1990.

the object in space. This experience, which is inescapable for us, appears to be unattainable for individuals like patient S.B., whose case was described in the previous section.

Boring (1964) illustrated the way we automatically interpret size and depth using an image like the one shown in Figure 11.2. When we copy the image of the distant figure and place it next to the closer figure, we are surprised to see the size of the distant figure on the page. Like Shepard's illusion, Boring's illusion shows that we interpret the size of the distant figure in terms of the three-dimensional cues in the image. It is hard for us to see the image on the page because, in most cases, we infer the size of things as if they were projections of three-dimensional objects.

Shadows and Edges

Not just size, but most visual inferences are based on the interpretation of image data as arising from objects in a three-dimensional world.

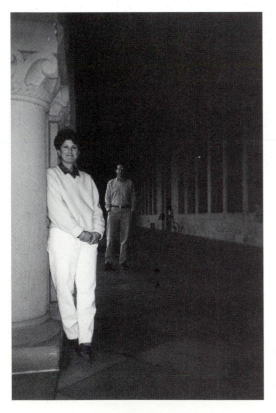 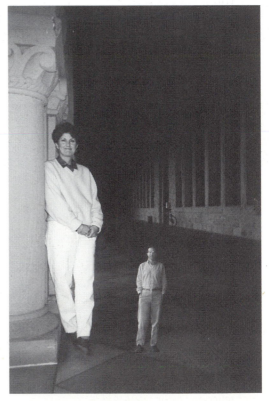

11.2 JUDGING SIZE. (Left) Seen in its proper context, the image can be used to infer the man's height accurately, and we are unaware of the size of the man's image on the page. We are made aware that the man's image is small when we translate the image to a new position with improper depth cues (right). After Boring, 1964.

Even judgments that seem simple, such as brightness, may depend on interpreting the scene as consisting of objects in a three-dimensional world.

Figure 11.3 is an example of a brightness judgment that depends on our interpretation of the objects in the image (Adelson, 1993). Consider the middle and right columns of diamond shapes in Figure 11.3A. The physical intensity of the light reflected from these two sets of diamonds is the same, but the diamonds in the middle column appear darker than the diamonds in the right column.

Adelson (1993) suggests that the brightness difference between the columns arises because of a transparency; that is, some columns appear to be seen through light and dark strips overlayed on the image. Another interpretation of the differences between the columns is that some of the columns are seen under a cast shadow (D. Marimont, personal communication). In either event, the brightness of the local regions appears to depend on the global interpretation of the image. This is shown by the images in panels B and C of Figure 11.3, which are variations of the image in panel A. The image in panel B has no shadow edge, while the image in panel C changes the image without destroying the perception of a shadow. The brightness difference is diminished when the shadow is destroyed, but the difference is maintained when the shadow is present.

As I described in Chapter 9, brightness and color appearance are better predicted by reflectance than by the light incident at the eye. If the visual system's objective is to associate brightness with reflectance, then the visual system should take transparency into account when judging an object's brightness. If the physical intensity of the light from a surface seen through the semitransparent object has the same intensity as light from a surface seen directly, then the surface behind the

(A)   (B)   (C)

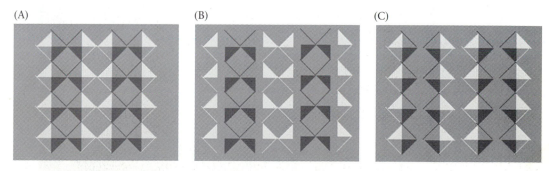

11.3 BRIGHTNESS AND SHADOWS. (A) Consider the bright column in the middle and the two flanking columns that appear to be in cast shadow. The intensity of the light reflected by the diamond-shaped regions in all three columns is the same, yet the diamonds in the bright middle column appear darker. (B) When we displace the columns and destroy the interpretation of the image as containing shadows, the brightness illusion is decreased greatly. (C) When we displace the columns but maintain the perceived shadows, the brightness illusion remains strong. After Adelson, 1993.

transparency (right columns 1 and 3 in Fig. 11.3A) must be more reflective and hence judged brighter. The example in Figure 11.3A shows that even image interpretations as complex as shadows or transparency can influence the brightness of a target.

The illusion in Figure 11.4 is named for three individuals who discovered it separately: the Craik-O'Brien-Cornsweet illusion. The illusion shows that surface boundaries influence brightness. The two areas on opposite sides of the border have the same physical intensity. Yet, the region on the right appears to be darker. The reason for this is that the intensity pattern at the border, shown at the bottom of the figure, suggests a spatial transition from a light to dark edge. This transition only occupies a small part of the image, and the intensity within the two regions away from the edge is the same. However, the visual system extends the inference from the boundary to a brightness judgment of the two large regions. It is quite surprising that the inference made using the boundary transition overrides the intensity levels within the individual regions. The inference from the boundary spreads across a large region and influences our perception of the entire object (O'Brien, 1958; Sherwood, 1966; Cornsweet, 1970; Burr, 1987).

Figures 11.3 and 11.4 show that judgments of transparency and boundaries can influence judgments of brightness. Figure 11.5 shows that brightness judgments can influence the perception of shape. Panel A shows an image containing a mound of dirt with a small dimple at the top. Panel B shows a second image containing a small crater with a mound at the bottom. The images in Figure 11.5 are the same except for being flipped (not rotated) up and down using a simple image-processing program.

11.4 EDGES CAN INFLUENCE THE BRIGHTNESS OF A LARGE REGION. The relative physical intensities of the images are shown by the trace. The intensities of the large regions are equal, but they are separated by an transient that defines an edge. Even though the intensities are equal, the region on the right appears to be darker. To confirm that the physical intensities of the areas are equal, cover the edge transient.

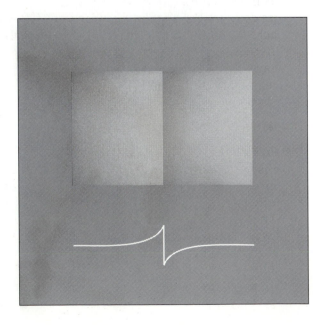

(A)

(B)

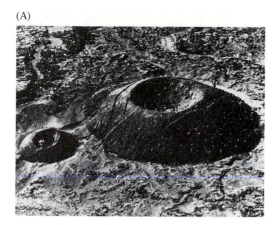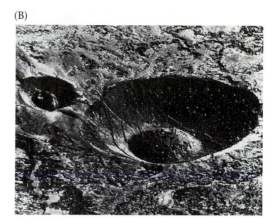

11.5 SHADING INFLUENCES SHAPE. The image in (A) is a photograph of two cinder cones in the K'au Desert lava fields of Hawaii. The image in (B) appears to contain craters with mounds in the center. Yet, the two images are the same except for an up-down flip. If you rotate the book 180 degrees, the image containing the mounds will now appear to contain craters, and conversely the image with craters will appear to contain mounds. The spatial relationship between the light and dark regions of the mound/crater is the main source of information defining it as convex or concave. Rotating the image rotates the shading cue and thus changes the shape we infer. After Rittenhouse, 1786.

If you rotate this book by 180 degrees, you will see that the mound in Figure 11.5A changes into a crater, and conversely the crater in Figure 11.5B changes into a mound. When we interpret these shapes, we assume that the illuminant is elevated. This assumption about the position of the illuminant guides our inference about the shape of objects in the image. The distinction between mound and crater in these images is mediated mainly by the shading differences. Hence, rotating the images changes the shading relationship, and we reinterpret the shape. Ramachandran (1988) has demonstrated this phenomenon in a number of different ways. He argues that the brain simplifies the interpretation of images by assuming that the illumination consists of a single light source (see also Knill and Kersten, 1991).

Shapes

The Fraser spiral is named after the *perceived* form in Figure 11.6. In fact, there is no spiral in the figure at all; the apparent spiral is really a set of concentric circles. (To persuade yourself of this, take your finger and carefully trace one of the patterns that you believe to be part of the spiral.) The light–dark structure of the patterns within each circle suggests an inward spiral, but this curvature is not present in the global shape. Visual inferencing mechanisms fail to notice that the local features do not join properly into a single global spiral. This image, like the many famous drawings by Escher (1967), show that the visual mechanisms for interpreting objects in images can yield globally inconsistent solutions.

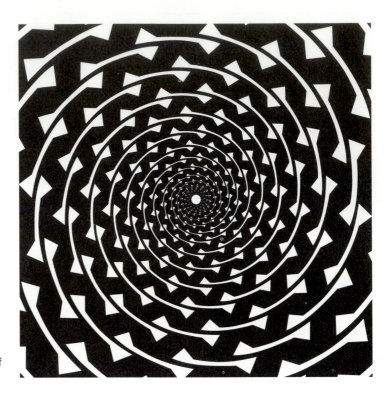

11.6 THE FRASER SPIRAL.
The figure consists of a set of concentric circles, not a spiral at all. Yet, because of the local pattern within the circles, we perceive the overall pattern as if it were a single spiral.

The objects you see in Figure 11.7 are visual inferences derived by integrating cues concerning occlusion and transparency. Figure 11.7A shows an image of a white triangle occluding three disks. We see the triangle even though no edges are present in the image to support the hypothesis that the triangle is present. Compare this figure with Figure 11.4. There, boundary information influenced the judgment of brightness. Here, occlusion information influences the judgment of a boundary and brightness. Figure 11.7A shows that the mechanisms for visual inferences accept the occlusion information as highly informative, even though there is missing edge and brightness information.

The transparency cues in Figure 11.7B are enough to infer the presence of a rectangle. Figure 11.7C shows that occlusion information can be used to infer rather complicated curved shapes, not just straight edges.

Figure 11.7D contains stereo pairs of the subjective contour in panel (A). When the depth cue is added, the subjective contour becomes somewhat more compelling (He and Nakayama, 1994b). Fusing a stereo pair takes some practice. Try placing a piece of paper perpendicular to the page and between the two images you wish to fuse. Put your noise against the edge of the paper so that each eye sees only one of the patterns. If you then relax, and look "through" the page, the two images will fuse into a single "depthful" image. If you see both dots on the two figures, you will know that you have merged the two images, not just

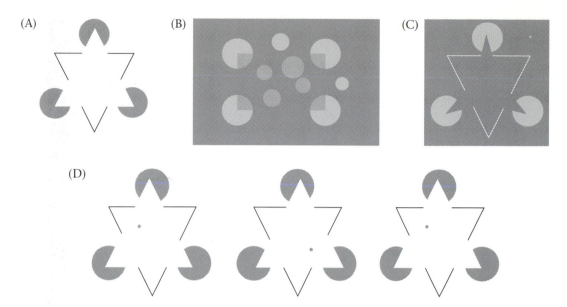

11.7 SUBJECTIVE CONTOURS. These subjective contours are inferred from occlusion and transparency cues in the images. (A) A triangle is suggested by occlusion, (B) a rectangle is suggested by transparency, and (C) a curved object is suggested by occlusion. (D) Stereo pairs of subjective contours. By diverging your eyes beyond the page, the image pair on the right (left) will fuse and you will see the subjective contours of a triangle in front (behind) of the circles. The subjective contour is somewhat more vivid when the depth cue is added. If you converge your eyes to fuse the images, the depth relationships will reverse. A–C after Kanizsa, 1976. D after He and Nakayama, 1994b.

suppressed one of them. If you fuse the pair on the right, the triangle will appear to be in a plane floating above the page. Fusing the pair on the left shows the subjective triangle behind the page.[2]

Normally, we think of occlusion as removing information, thereby making it harder to detect an object. However, the two examples in Figure 11.8 show that the presence of an occluding object can help us explain image information and see an object that might otherwise be difficult to discern. The pattern on the left of Figure 11.8A appears to be a set of two-dimensional drawings. When the gaps between the drawings are filled in by an occluding object, however, we can integrate the different drawings into a single three-dimensional shape of a cube. The only difference between the two drawings in panel A is that the white gaps separating the sections on the left have been filled in by the dark bars.

The patterns on the left of Figure 11.8B are drawn as if they were separate parts. Precisely the same patterns are present on the right, but this time they are separated by dark bars that suggest an occluding ob-

[2] If you fuse these stereo pairs by converging, rather than by diverging, your eyes, the depth relationships reverse.

(A)

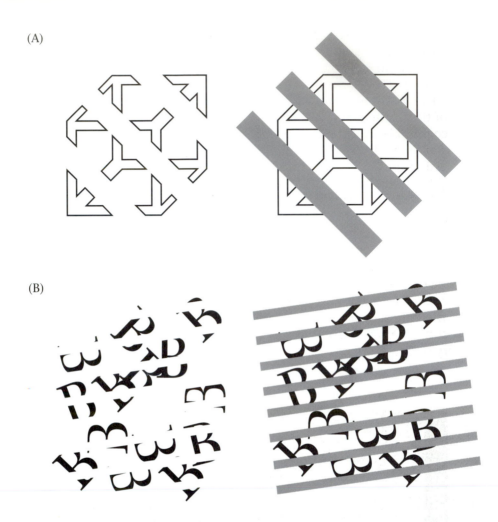

(B)

11.8 OCCLUSION AND OBJECT RECOGNITION. The presence of a clearly visible occluding surface helps us to integrate otherwise fragmentary image components. (A) When the line segments are seen without an occlusion cue, they appear as a set of uncorrelated two-dimensional patterns. By overlaying occluding boundaries, the pattern is seen as part of an object, namely, a three-dimensional cube. (B) When the pattern on the left is seen on its own, it appears as a jumble of unconnected curves and lines. By placing an occluding object over the white spaces, it is much easier to see that the occluded pattern is a collection of "B's." A after Kanizsa, 1979. B after Bregman, 1981.

ject. Again, it is much easier to recognize the pattern as a collection of letters when the occlusion is made visually explicit. Apparently, occlusion is a very important clue for visual inferences having to do with objects.

Integrating Cues

Much of object perception requires us to integrate image information for image features that are separated in space or in time. In some cases, when we integrate separate visual features into an object, we rely on certain implicit assumptions about the object. An interesting example that reveals our implicit assumptions can be revealed by the images in Figure 11.9. The image in panel A shows a face in its normal upright pose. The image in panel B shows the same face inverted and with several of the features, namely, the eyes and mouth, edited. In this form, it is recognizable as the same face, and it seems clear that there is something amiss with the individual features. But, we cannot infer what the expression on the face will be when the inverted face is rotated into the upright position (Thompson, 1980). You will be surprised at the appearance of the face in panel B when you rotate the book and see the face in its upright pose.

This may be an illusion that is specific to face perception. The clinical syndrome of prosopagnosia, the inability to recognize familiar faces, is further evidence that our brain has specialized circuitry for integrating the components of an image when we recognize and interpret faces. It seems more likely to me, however, that this illusion has to do with the integration of spatially segregated features. When we see a familiar object made up of many separate features in an unlikely orientation, it is very difficult to judge the object's structure (Kanizsa, 1979).

(A)

(B)

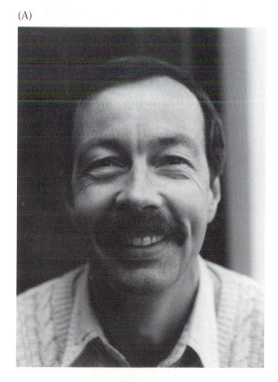
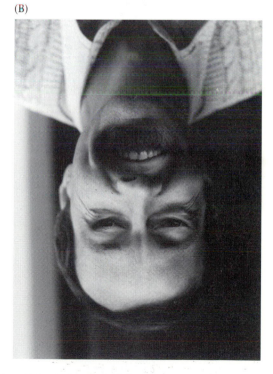

11.9 FACE RECOGNITION. (A) A face. (B) An edited and inverted version of the face. Can you integrate the features of the inverted face and predict the expression that will appear when you rotate the book? After Thompson, 1980.

Geometric Illusions

Gregory (1966) suggested that the simple and unassuming Müller–Lyer illusion, shown in Figure 11.10A, results from basic perceptual assumptions we make when we perceive depth. The two vertical lines shown in the illusion have the same length, but the line segment on the right

(A)

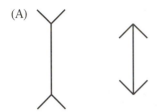

(B)

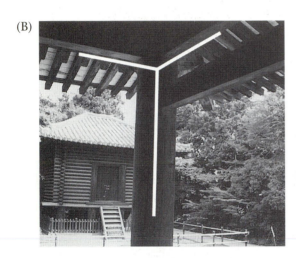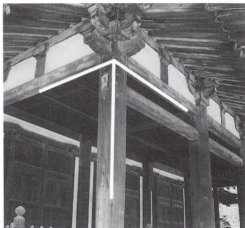

(C)

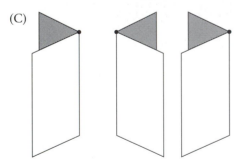

11.10 THE MÜLLER–LYER ILLUSION. (A) The classic Müller–Lyer illusion is shown. The line with the arrows pointed outward appears longer to most people, but the line lengths are the same. (B) The left and right parts of the image show two views of a corner of a building. From the inside, when the corner is relatively far from the viewer, the edges are oriented like open arrows. From the outside, when the corner is relatively close to the viewer, the edges between the corner and the ceiling are oriented like closed arrows. (C) A three-dimensional analogue of the Müller–Lyer illusion is shown. The separations between the middle dot and the dots on either side are the same. In this rendering of the illusion, the open and closed arrow shapes are not a cue for depth. Yet, the Müller–Lyer illusion is quite powerful. C after DeLucia and Hochberg, 1991.

appears to be longer. Gregory argues that the lines appear to be of different length because we cannot escape interpreting even such trivial images as three-dimensional objects. As the image in Figure 11.10B illustrates, in the natural environment the edges that define a near corner are similar to the lines on the left of Figure 11.10A. The edges that define a far corner are similar to the lines on the right. Gregory explains the illusion as a consequence of our relentless interpretation of images as arising from a three-dimensional world. Lines that sweep out equal retinal angle, but that are at different depths, must have different physical size. Gregory suggests that even the impoverished stimulus in the Müller–Lyer illusion invokes the visual system's inferences of objects and depth. The improper application of a good principle causes the equal line segments to appear different.

Gregory's hypothesis is important because it reminds us that the basic function of visual inferences is to see objects in three dimensions. The interpretation of visual illusions, however, is never straightforward. To test Gregory's suggestion, DeLucia and Hochberg (1991) created the version of the Müller–Lyer illusion shown in Figure 11.10C. The middle dot is equidistant from the right and left dots. Yet, just as in the Müller–Lyer illusion, the separation between the two dots attached by the closed arrow form appears smaller than the separation between the dots connected by the open arrow form. In this schematic three-dimensional image, there is little chance that the separations between the dots has to do with different depths. Gregory's hypothesis and this counterexample are a wonderful exchange that illustrates how qualitative hypotheses concerning the mechanisms of visual illusions can be tested and become part of the scientific study of vision.

Summary

Throughout this chapter, we have seen the importance of integrating separate visual inferences into a single explanation of the contents of a scene. Patients who cannot integrate visual information may identify color or a shape, but they feel that they cannot see because they cannot integrate the separate inferences into a sensible interpretation of the objects and surfaces in a scene. Many of the illusions we have reviewed show us that, to see as a whole, we must resolve conflicting information. We do not see a two-dimensional shape properly because we insist on interpreting the data as a three-dimensional shape. We do not see physical intensity properly because we insist on interpreting a shadow or an edge.

I have chosen the illusions here to emphasize several important principles that the visual system uses to combine different visual inferences. We integrate shape and depth cues by assuming that we are perceiving objects in a three-dimensional world; we use shadows, occlusions, and edges to interpret the properties of objects; we build up global interpretations from many local properties; yet, we also use familiar poses of objects and typical locations of illuminations to help us interpret ambiguous images.

The rules governing our sight reflect the physics of the world we see. These rules describe the interactions of objects at a physical scale within the domain of the psychologist and engineer—a human scale. This is not the physics of the subatomic or the physics of the galactic, but it is the physics of the world in which we live and interact. By studying the rules of this human-centered physics of perceived objects, we learn how we might see. By making neural and behavioral measurements of our brains and our perceptions, we learn how we do see.

Appendixes

A

Shift-Invariant Linear Systems

Many of the ideas in this book rely on properties of shift-invariant linear systems. In the text, I introduced these properties without any indication of how to prove that they are true. In this appendix, I will sketch proofs of several important properties of shift-invariant linear systems. Then I will describe convolution and the discrete Fourier series, two tools that help us take advantage of these properties.[1]

Shift-Invariant Linear Systems: Definitions

Shift-invariance is a system property that can be verified by experimental measurement. For example, in Chapter 2, I described how to check whether the optics of the eye are shift-invariant by the following measurements. Image a line through the optics onto the retina, and measure the linespread function. Then, shift the line to a new position, forming a new retinal image. Compare the new image with the original. If the images have the same shape, differing only by a shift in position, then the optics are shift-invariant over the measured range.

---

[1] The results in this appendix are expressed using real harmonic functions. This is in contrast to the common practice of using complex notation, specifically Euler's complex exponential, as a shorthand to represent sums of harmonic functions. The exposition using complex exponentials is brief and elegant, but I believe it obscures the connection with experimental measurements. For this reason, I have avoided the development based on complex notation.

We can express the empirical property of shift-invariance using the following mathematical notation. Choose a stimulus, p_i, and measure the system response, r_i. Now, shift the stimulus by an amount j and measure again. If the response is shifted by j as well, then the system may be shift-invariant. Try this experiment for many values of the shift parameter, j. If the experiment succeeds for all shifts, then the system is shift-invariant.

If you think about this definition as an experimentalist, you can see that there are some technical problems in making the measurements needed to verify shift-invariance. Suppose that the original stimulus and response are represented at N distinct points, $i = 1, \ldots, N$. If we shift the stimulus three locations so that now the fourth location contains the first entry, the fifth the second, and so forth, how do we fill in the first three locations in the new stimulus? And, what do we do with the last three values, $N - 2$, $N - 1$, N, which have nowhere to go?

Theorists avoid this problem by treating the real observations as if they are part of an infinite periodic set of observations. They assume that the stimuli and data are part of an infinite periodic series with a period of N, equal to the number of original observations. If the data are infinite, the first three entries of the shifted vector are the three values at locations -3, -2, and -1. If the data are periodic with period N, these three values are the same as the values at $N - 3$, $N - 2$, and $N - 1$.

The assumption that the measurements are part of an infinite and periodic sequence permits the theorist to avoid the experimentalist's practical problem. The assumption is also essential for obtaining several of the simple closed-form results concerning the properties of shift-invariant systems. The assumption is not consistent with real measurements, since real measurements cannot be made using infinite stimuli: there is always a beginning and an end to any real experiment. As an experimentalist you must always be aware that many theoretical calculations using shift-invariant methods are not valid near the boundaries of data sets, such as near the edge of an image.

Suppose we refer to the finite input as $\mathbf{r}$, and suppose that the measured output, $\mathbf{l}$, is finite. In the theoretical analysis we extend both of these functions to be infinite and periodic. We will use a hat symbol ($\hat{\ }$) to denote the extended functions,

$$\hat{l}_{i+N} = l_i \quad \text{and} \quad \hat{p}_{i+N} = p_i \tag{A.1}$$

The extended functions $\hat{\mathbf{l}}$ and $\hat{\mathbf{p}}$ agree with our measurements over the measurement range from 1 to N. By the periodicity assumption, the values outside of the measurement range are filled in by looking at the values within the measurement range. For example,

$$(\ldots, \hat{l}_{-1} = \hat{l}_{N-1}, \hat{l}_0 = \hat{l}_N, \hat{l}_1, \ldots, \hat{l}_N, \hat{l}_{N+1} = \hat{l}_1, \ldots)$$

Convolution

Next, I will derive some of the properties of linear shift-invariant systems. I begin by describing these properties in terms of the **system matrix** (see Chapter 2). Then I will show how the simple structure of the shift-invariant system matrix permits us to relate the input and output by a summation formula called **cyclic convolution**. The convolution formula is so important that shift-invariant systems are sometimes called **convolution systems**.[2]

In Chapter 2, I reviewed how to measure the system matrix of an optical system for one-dimensional input stimuli. We measure the image resulting from a single line at a series of uniformly spaced input locations. If the system is shift-invariant, then the columns of the system matrix are shifted copies of one another (except for edge artifacts). To create the system matrix, we extend the inputs and outputs to be periodic functions (Equation A.1). Then, we select a central block of size $N \times N$ to be the system matrix, and we use the corresponding entries of the extended stimulus. For example, if the input stimulus consists of six values, $\mathbf{p} = (0,0,0,1,0,0)$, and the response to this stimulus is the vector, $\mathbf{l} = (0.0, 0.3, 0.6, 0.2, 0.1, 0.0)$, then the 6×6 system matrix is

$$\hat{C} = \begin{pmatrix} 0.2 & 0.6 & 0.3 & 0.0 & 0.0 & 0.1 \\ 0.1 & 0.2 & 0.6 & 0.3 & 0.0 & 0.0 \\ 0.0 & 0.1 & 0.2 & 0.6 & 0.3 & 0.0 \\ 0.0 & 0.0 & 0.1 & 0.2 & 0.6 & 0.3 \\ 0.3 & 0.0 & 0.0 & 0.1 & 0.2 & 0.6 \\ 0.6 & 0.3 & 0.0 & 0.0 & 0.1 & 0.2 \end{pmatrix} \tag{A.2}$$

For a general linear system, we calculate the output using the summation formula for matrix multiplication in Equation 2.4,

$$\hat{r}_i = \sum_{j=1}^{N} \hat{C}_{ij} \hat{p}_j \tag{A.3}$$

When the linear system is shift-invariant, this summation formula simplifies for two reasons. First, because of the assumed periodicity, the summation is precisely the same when we sum over any N consecutive integers. It is useful to incorporate this generalization into the summation formula as

$$\hat{r}_i = \sum_{j=\langle N \rangle} \hat{C}_{ij} \hat{p}_j \tag{A.4}$$

---

[2] Since we use only cyclic convolution here, I will drop the word "cyclic" and refer to the formula simply as convolution. This is slightly abusive, but it conforms to common practice in many fields.

Appendix A

where the notation $j = \langle N \rangle$ means that summation can take place over any N consecutive integers. Second, notice that for whichever $N \times N$ block of values we choose, the typical entry of the system matrix will be

$$\hat{C}_{ij} = \hat{l}_{i-j} \qquad (A.5)$$

We can use this relationship to simplify the summation further:

$$\hat{r}_i = \sum_{j=\langle N \rangle} \hat{l}_{i-j} \hat{p}_j \qquad (A.6)$$

In this form, we see that the response depends only on the input and the linespread. The summation formula in Equation A.6 is called **cyclic convolution**. Hence, we have shown that, to compute the response of a shift-invariant linear system to any stimulus, we need measure only the linespread function.

Convolution and Harmonic Functions

Next, we study some of the properties of the convolution formula. Most important, we will see why harmonic functions have a special role in the analysis of convolution systems.

Beginning with our analysis of optics in Chapter 2, we have relied on the fact that the response of a shift-invariant system to a harmonic function at frequency f is also a harmonic function at f. In that chapter, the result was stated in two equivalent ways:

1. If the input is a harmonic at frequency f, the output is a shifted and scaled copy of the harmonic.

2. The response to a harmonic at frequency f will be the weighted sum of a sinusoid and cosinusoid at the same frequency (Equation 2.8).

We can derive this result from the convolution formula. Define a new variable, $k = i - j$, and substitute k into Equation A.6. Remember that the summation can take place over any adjacent N values. Hence, the substitution yields a modified convolution formula,

$$\hat{r}_i = \sum_{k=\langle N \rangle} \hat{l}_k \hat{p}_{i-k} \qquad (A.7)$$

Next, we use the convolution formula in Equation A.7 to compute the response to a sinusoidal input $\sin(2\pi f j / N)$. From trigonometry we have that

$$\sin\left(\tfrac{2\pi f(i+j)}{N}\right) = \sin\left(\tfrac{2\pi f i}{N}\right)\cos\left(\tfrac{2\pi f j}{N}\right) + \sin\left(\tfrac{2\pi f j}{N}\right)\cos\left(\tfrac{2\pi f i}{N}\right) \quad (A.8)$$

Substitute Equation A.8 into Equation A.7, remembering that $\sin(-k) = -\sin(k)$ and $\cos(-k) = \cos(k)$:

$$\hat{r}_i = \sum_{k=\langle N \rangle} \hat{l}_k \sin(\tfrac{2\pi f i}{N})\cos(\tfrac{2\pi f k}{N}) + \sum_{k=\langle N \rangle} \hat{l}_k \sin(-\tfrac{2\pi f k}{N})\cos(\tfrac{2\pi f i}{N})$$

$$= \sin(\tfrac{2\pi f i}{N}) \sum_{k=\langle N \rangle} \hat{l}_k \cos(\tfrac{2\pi f k}{N}) - \cos(\tfrac{2\pi f i}{N}) \sum_{k=\langle N \rangle} \hat{l}_k \sin(\tfrac{2\pi f k}{N}) \quad (A.9)$$

We can simplify this expression to the form

$$\hat{r}_i = a\,\sin(\tfrac{2\pi f i}{N}) - b\,\cos(\tfrac{2\pi f i}{N}) \quad (A.10)$$

where

$$a = \sum_{k=\langle N \rangle} \hat{l}_k \cos(\tfrac{2\pi f k}{N})$$

$$b = \sum_{k=\langle N \rangle} \hat{l}_k \sin(\tfrac{2\pi f k}{N})$$

We have shown that when the input to the system is a sinusoidal function at frequency f, the output of the system is the weighted sum of a sinusoid and a cosinusoid, both at frequency f. This is equivalent to showing that when the input is a sinusoid at frequency f, the output will be a scaled and shifted copy of the input, $s_f \sin(\tfrac{2\pi f i}{N} + \phi_f)$ (see Equation 2.8). As we shall see below, it is easy to generalize this result to all harmonic functions.

The Discrete Fourier Series: Definitions

In general, when we measure the response of a shift-invariant linear system we measure N output values. When the input is a sinusoid, or more generally a harmonic, we can specify the response using only the two numbers, a and b, in Equation A.10. We would like to take advantage of this special property of shift-invariant systems. To do so, we need a method of representing input stimuli as the weighted sum of harmonic functions.

The method used to transform a stimulus into the weighted sum of harmonic functions is called the **discrete Fourier transform (DFT)**. The representation of the stimulus as the weighted sum of harmonic functions is called the **discrete Fourier series (DFS)**. We use the DFS to represent an extended stimulus, $\hat{p}$:

$$\hat{p}_i = \sum_{f=0}^{N-1} a_f \cos(\tfrac{2\pi f i}{N}) + b_f \sin(\tfrac{2\pi f i}{N}) \quad (A.11)$$

We are interested in that part of the extended stimulus that coincides with our measurements. We can express the relationship between the harmonic functions and the original stimulus, **p**, using a matrix equation,

$$\mathbf{p} = \mathbf{Ca} + \mathbf{Sb} \tag{A.12}$$

which has the matrix tableau form

$$\left(\begin{array}{c} \mathbf{p} \end{array}\right) = \left(\begin{array}{c} \mathbf{C} \end{array}\right)\left(\begin{array}{c} \mathbf{a} \end{array}\right) + \left(\begin{array}{c} \mathbf{S} \end{array}\right)\left(\begin{array}{c} \mathbf{b} \end{array}\right)$$

The vectors **a** and **b** contain the coefficients a_f and b_f, respectively. The columns of the matrices **C** and **S** contain the relevant portions of the cosinusoidal and sinusoidal terms, $\cos(2\pi f i/N)$ and $\sin(2\pi f i/N)$, that are used in the DFS representation.

The DFS represents the original stimulus as the weighted sum of a set of harmonic functions (i.e., sampled sine and cosine functions). We call these sampled harmonic functions the **basis functions** of the DFS representation. The vectors **a** and **b** contain the basis functions' **weights** or **coefficients**, which specify how much of each basis function must be added in to recreate the original stimulus, **p**.

The Discrete Fourier Series: Properties

Figure A.1 shows the sampled sine and cosine functions for a period of $N = 8$. The functions are arrayed in a circle to show how they relate to one another. There are a total of 16 basis functions. But, as you can see from Figure A.1, they are redundant. The sampled cosinusoids in the

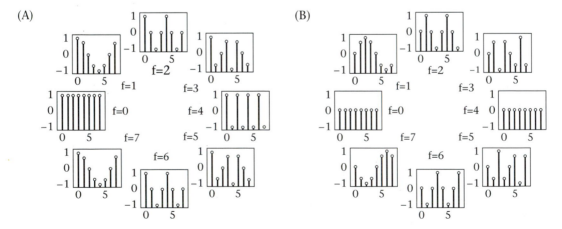

A.1 THE BASIS FUNCTIONS OF THE DISCRETE FOURIER SERIES. The cosinusoidal (A) and sinusoidal (B) basis functions of the DFS representation when $N = 8$ are shown. Notice the redundancy between the functions at symmetrically placed frequencies.

columns of **C** repeat themselves (in reverse order); for example, when $N = 8$ the cosinusoids for $f = 1, 2, 3$ are the same as the cosinusoids for $f = 7, 6, 5$. The sampled sinusoids in the columns of **S** also repeat themselves except for a sign reversal (multiplication by -1). There are only four independent sampled cosinusoids and four independent sampled sinusoids. As a result of this redundancy, neither the **S** nor the matrix **C** is invertible.

Nevertheless, the properties of these harmonic basis functions make it simple to calculate the vectors containing the weights of the harmonic functions from the original stimulus, **p**. To compute **a** and **b**, we multiply the input by the basis functions, as in

$$\mathbf{a} = \frac{1}{N}\mathbf{C}^T\mathbf{p} \quad \text{and} \quad \mathbf{b} = \frac{1}{N}\mathbf{S}^T\mathbf{p} \tag{A.13}$$

We can derive the relationship in Equation A.13 from two observations. First, the matrix sum, $\mathbf{H} = \mathbf{S} + \mathbf{C}$ has a simple inverse. The columns of **H** are orthogonal to one another, so that the inverse of **H** is simply:[3]

$$\mathbf{H}^{-1} = \frac{1}{N}\mathbf{H}^T = \frac{1}{N}(\mathbf{S} + \mathbf{C})^T$$

Second, the columns of the matrices **C** and **S** are perpendicular to one another: $\mathbf{0} = \mathbf{C}\mathbf{S}^T$. This observation should not be surprising, since continuous sinusoids and cosinusoids are also orthogonal to one another.

We can use these two observations to derive Equation A.13 as follows. Express the fact that **H** and $\frac{1}{N}\mathbf{H}^T$ are inverses as follows:

$$\mathbf{I}_{N\times N} = \mathbf{H}(\frac{1}{N}\mathbf{H}^T) \tag{A.14}$$

$$= \frac{1}{N}(\mathbf{C} + \mathbf{S})(\mathbf{C} + \mathbf{S})^T \tag{A.15}$$

$$= \frac{1}{N}(\mathbf{C}\mathbf{C}^T + \mathbf{S}\mathbf{S}^T) \tag{A.16}$$

where $\mathbf{I}_{N\times N}$ is the identity matrix. Then, multiply both sides of Equation A.14 by **p**:

$$\mathbf{p} = \frac{1}{N}(\mathbf{C}\mathbf{C}^T\mathbf{p} + \mathbf{S}\mathbf{S}^T\mathbf{p}) \tag{A.17}$$

Compare Equation A.17 and Equation A.12. Notice that the equations become identical if we make the assignments in Equation A.13. This completes the sketch of the proof.

---

[3] This observation is the basis of another useful linear transform method called the *Hartley transform* (Bracewell, 1986).

Measurements with Harmonic Functions

Finally, I will show how to predict the response of a shift-invariant linear system to any stimulus using only the responses to unit amplitude cosinusoidal inputs. This result is the logical basis for describing system performance from measurements of the response to harmonic functions. When the system is linear and shift-invariant, its responses to harmonic functions are a complete description of the system; but this is not true for arbitrary linear systems.

Because cosinusoids and sinusoids are shifted copies of one another, the response of a shift-invariant linear system to these functions is the same except for a shift. From a calculation like the one in Equation A.8, except using a cosinusoidal input, we can calculate the following result: if the response to a cosinusoid at f is the sum of a cosinusoid and sinusoid with weights (a_f, b_f), then the response to a sinusoid at frequency f will have weights $(b_f, -a_f)$. Hence, if we know the response to a cosinusoid at f, we also know the response to a sinusoid at f.

Next, we can use our knowledge of the response to sinusoids and cosinusoids at f to predict the response to any harmonic function at f. Suppose that the input is a harmonic function $a\cos(2\pi fi/N) + b\sin(2\pi fi/N)$, and the output is $a'\cos(2\pi fi/N) + b'\sin(2\pi fi/N)$. If the response to a unit amplitude cosinusoid is $u_f\cos(2\pi fi/N) + v_f\sin(2\pi fi/N)$, then the response to a unit amplitude sinusoid is $v_f\cos(2\pi fi/N) - u_f\sin(2\pi fi/N)$. Using these two facts and linearity, we calculate the coefficients of the response:

$$a' = au_f + bv_f$$

$$b' = av_f - bu_f \tag{A.18}$$

We have shown that if we measure the system response to unit amplitude cosinusoidal inputs, we can compute the system response to an arbitrary input stimulus as follows:

1. Compute the DFS coefficients of the input stimulus using Equation A.13.

2. Calculate the output DFS coefficients using Equation A.18.

3. Reconstruct the output using Equation A.11.

You will find this series of calculations used implicitly at several points in the text. For example, I followed this organization when I described measurements of the optical quality of the lens (Chapter 2) and when I described measurements of behavioral sensitivity to spatiotemporal patterns (Chapter 7).

B

Display Calibration

Visual displays based on a **cathode ray tube (CRT)** are used widely in business, education, and entertainment. The CRT reproduces color images using principles embodied in the color-matching experiment (Chapter 4).

The design of the color CRT is one of the most important applications of vision science; thus, it is worth understanding the design as an engineering achievement. Also, because the CRT is used widely in experimental vision science, understanding how to control the CRT display is an essential skill for all vision scientists. This appendix reviews several of the principles of monitor calibration.

An Overview of a CRT Display

Figure B.1A shows the main components of a color CRT display. The display contains a **cathode**, or **electron gun**, that provides a source of electrons. The electrons are focused into a beam whose direction is deflected back and forth in a raster pattern so that it scans the faceplate of the display.

Light is emitted by a process of absorption and emission that occurs at the faceplate of the display. The faceplate consists of a phosphor painted onto a glass substrate. The phosphor absorbs electrons from the scanning beam and emits light. A signal, generally controlled from a computer, modulates the intensity of the electron beam as it scans across the faceplate. The intensity of the light emitted by the phosphor

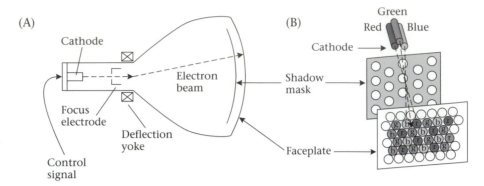

B.1   OVERVIEW OF A CRT DISPLAY. (A) A side view of the display showing the cathode, which is the source of electrons, and a method of focusing the electrons into a beam that is deflected in a raster pattern across the faceplate of the display. (B) The geometrical arrangement of the electron beams, shadow-mask, and phosphor allows each electron beam to stimulate only one of the three phosphors.

at each point on the faceplate depends on the intensity of the electron beam as it scans past that point.

Monochrome CRTs have a single electron beam and a single type of phosphor. In monochrome systems, the control signal only influences the intensity of the phosphor emissions. Color CRTs use three electron beams; each stimulates one of three phosphors. Each of the phosphors emits light of a different spectral power distribution. By separately controlling the emissions of the three types of phosphors, the user can vary the spectral composition of the emitted light. The light emitted from the CRT is always the mixture of three primary lights from the three phosphors, usually called the red, green, and blue phosphors.

In order that each electron beam stimulate emissions from only one of the three types of phosphors, a metal plate, called a **shadow-mask**, is interposed between the three electron guns and the faceplate. A conventional shadow-mask is a metal plate with a series of finely spaced holes. The relative positions of the holes and the electron guns are arranged, as shown in Figure B.1B, so that as the beam sweeps across the faceplate the electrons from a single gun that pass through a hole are absorbed by only one of the three types of phosphors; electrons from that gun that would have stimulated the other phosphors are absorbed or scattered by the shadow-mask.

The Frame-Buffer

In experiments, the control signal sent to the CRT display is usually created using computer software. There are two principal methods for creating these control signals. In one method, the user controls the three electron beam intensities by writing out the values of three matrices into three separate **video frame-buffers**. Each matrix specifies the control signal for one of the electron guns. Each matrix entry specifies the desired voltage level of the control signal at a single point on the faceplate. Usually, the intensity levels within each matrix are quantized to 8 bits, so this computer display architecture is called **24-bit color**, or **RGB color**.

In a second method, the user writes a single matrix into a single frame-buffer. The value at each location in this matrix is converted into three control signals sent to the display according to a code contained in in a **color look-up table**. This architecture is called **indexed color**. This method is cost-effective because it does away with two of the three frame-buffers. When using this method, the user can only select among 256 (8 bits) colors when displaying a single image.

The Display Intensity

Calibrating a visual display means measuring the relationship between the frame-buffer values and the light emitted by the display. In this section I will discuss the relationship between the frame-buffer values and the intensity of the emitted light. In the next section I will discuss the relationship between the frame-buffer values and the spectral composition of the emitted light.

We can measure the relationship between the value of a frame-buffer entry and the intensity of the light emitted from the display as follows. Set the frame-buffer entries controlling one of the three phosphor display intensities, say, within a rectangular region, to a single value. Measure the intensity of the light emitted from the displayed rectangle. Repeat this measurement at many different frame-buffer values for this phosphor, and then for the other two phosphors.

The dashed curve in Figure B.2 measures the ratio of the intensity at the highest frame-buffer level to the intensity at each of the other frame-buffer levels for the green phosphor. We can summarize the difference using this single ratio, the **relative intensity**, because over most of the range the spectral power distribution of the light emitted at one frame-buffer level is the same as the spectral power distribution of the light emitted from the monitor at maximum intensity, except for a scale factor. The insets in the graph show two examples of the spectral power distribution, measured when the frame-buffer was set to 255 and 190. These two curves have the same overall shape; they differ by a scale factor of one-half.

We can approximate the curve relating the relative intensity of the light emitted from this CRT display, I, and the frame-buffer value, v, by a function of the form

$$I = \alpha v^y + \beta$$

where α and β are two fitting parameters. For most CRTs, the exponent of the power function, y, has a value near 2.2 (see Brainard, 1989; Berns et al., 1993a, b).

(A)

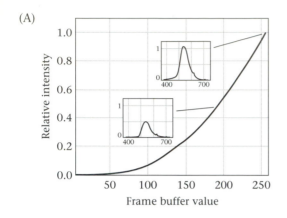

(B)

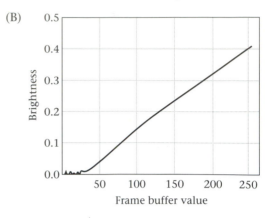

Frame buffer value

Frame buffer value

B.2 FRAME-BUFFER VALUE AND DISPLAY INTENSITY. (A) The dashed curve measures the intensity of the emitted light relative to the maximum intensity. The data shown are for the green phosphor. The insets in the graph show the complete spectral power distribution of the light at two different frame-buffer levels. (B) The dashed curve describing the relative intensities is replotted, using Stevens's power law, to show the linear relationship between the frame-buffer value and perceived brightness.

The nonlinear function relating the frame-buffer values and the relative intensity is due to the physics of the CRT display. While nonlinear functions are usually viewed with some dread, this particular nonlinear relationship is desirable because most users want the frame-buffer values to be linear with the brightness; they do not care how the frame-buffer values relate to intensity. As it turns out, perceived brightness, B, is related to intensity through a power-law relationship called **Stevens's power law** (Stevens, 1962; Sekuler and Blake, 1985; Goldstein, 1989), namely,

$$B = aI^{0.4}$$

where a is a fitting parameter. Somewhat fortuitously, the nonlinear relationship between frame-buffer values and intensity compensates for the nonlinear relationship between intensity and brightness. To show this, I have replotted Figure B.2A on a graph whose vertical scale is brightness, that is, relative intensity raised to the 0.4 power. Figure B.2B shows that the relationship between the frame-buffer value and brightness is nearly linear. This has the effect of equalizing the perceptual steps between different levels of the frame-buffer and simplifying certain aspects of controlling the appearance of the display.

The Display Spectral Power Distribution

The spectral power distribution of the light emitted in each small region of a CRT display is the mixture of the light emitted by the three phosphors. Since the mixture of lights obeys superposition, we can characterize the spectral power distributions emitted by a CRT using simple linear methods.

Suppose we measure the spectral power distribution of the red, green, and blue phosphors at their maximum intensity levels. We record these measurements in three column vectors, $\mathbf{m}_i$, $i = 1, 2, 3$.

By superposition, we know that light from the monitor screen is always the weighted sum of light from the three phosphors. For example, if all three of the phosphors are set to their maximum levels, the light emitted from the screen, call it $\mathbf{t}$, will have a spectral power distribution of

$$\mathbf{m}_1 + \mathbf{m}_2 + \mathbf{m}_3$$

More generally, if we set the phosphors to the three relative intensities $\mathbf{e} = (e_r, e_g, e_b)$, the light emitted by the CRT will be the weighted sum

$$\mathbf{t} = e_r\mathbf{m}_1 + e_g\mathbf{m}_2 + e_b\mathbf{m}_3$$

Figure B.3 is a matrix representation illustrating how to compute the spectral power distribution of light emitted from a CRT display. The vector $\mathbf{e}$ contains the relative intensity of each of the three phosphors. The three columns of a matrix, call it $\mathbf{M}$, contain the spectral power distributions of the light emitted by the red, green, and blue phosphors at maximum intensity. The spectral power distribution of light emitted from the monitor is the product $\mathbf{Me}$.

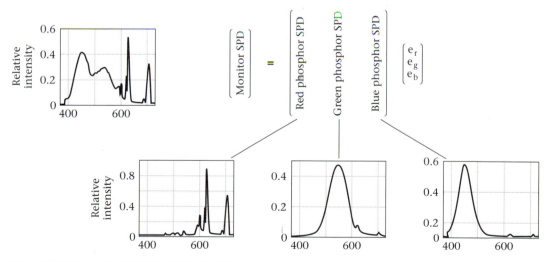

B.3 THE SPECTRAL POWER DISTRIBUTION OF LIGHT EMITTED FROM A CRT. The entries $\mathbf{e} = (e_r, e_g, e_b)$ are the relative intensity of the three phosphors. The columns of $\mathbf{M}$ contain the spectral power distributions (SPDs) at maximum intensity (graphs at bottom). The vector calculated by $\mathbf{Me}$ is the spectral power distribution of the light emitted by the CRT (graph at top left). The output shown in the figure was calculated for $\mathbf{e} = (0.5, 0.6, 0.7)^{\mathsf{T}}$.

The light emitted from a CRT is different from lights we encounter in natural scenes. For example, the spectral power distribution of the red phosphor, with its sharp and narrow peaks, is unlike the light we see in natural images. Nonetheless, we can adjust the three intensities of the three phosphors on a color CRT to match the appearance of most spectral power distributions, just as we can match appearance in the color-matching experiment by adjusting the intensity of three primary lights (see Chapter 4).

The Calibration Matrix

In many types of psychophysical experiments, we must be able to specify and control the relative absorption rates in the three types of cones. In this section, I show how to measure and control the relative cone absorptions when the phosphor spectral power distributions and the relative cone photopigment spectral sensitivities are known.

We use two basic matrices in these calculations. We have already created the matrix $\mathbf{M}$ whose three columns contain the spectral power distributions of the phosphors at maximum intensity. We also create a matrix, $\mathbf{B}$, whose three columns contain the cone absorption sensitivities (L, M, and S), measured through the cornea and lens (see Table 4.1). Given a set of relative intensities, $\mathbf{e}$, we calculate the relative cone photopigment absorption rates, $\mathbf{r}$, by the following matrix product:[1]

$$\mathbf{r} = \mathbf{B}^T\mathbf{M}\mathbf{e} = \mathbf{H}\mathbf{e} \qquad (B.1)$$

We call the matrix $\mathbf{H} = \mathbf{B}^T\mathbf{M}$, the monitor's **calibration matrix.** This matrix relates the linear phosphor intensities to the relative cone absorption rates.

As an example, I have calculated the calibration matrix for the monitor whose phosphor spectral power distributions are shown in Figure B.3, and for the cone absorption spectra listed in Table 4.1. The resulting calibration matrix is

$$\begin{pmatrix} 0.2732 & 0.9922 & 0.1466 \\ 0.1034 & 0.9971 & 0.2123 \\ 0.0117 & 0.1047 & 1.0000 \end{pmatrix}$$

Each column of the calibration matrix describes the relative cone absorptions caused by emissions from one of the phosphors: The absorptions from the red phosphor are in the first column, and absorptions due to the green and blue phosphors are in the second and third columns, respectively.

---

[1] This calculation applies to spatially uniform regions of a display, in which we can ignore the complications of chromatic aberration. Marimont and Wandell (1994) describe how to include the effects of chromatic aberration.

Suppose the red phosphor stimulated only the L-cones, the green the M-cones, and the blue the S-cones. In that case, the calibration matrix would be diagonal, and we could control the absorptions in a single cone class by adjusting only one of the phosphor emissions. In practice, the light from each of the CRT phosphors is absorbed in all three cone types, and the calibration matrix is never diagonal. As a result, to control the cone absorptions we must take into account the effect each phosphor has on each of the three cone types. This complexity is unavoidable because of the overlap of the cone absorption curves and the need to use phosphors with broadband emissions to create a bright display.

Example Calculations

Now, we consider two ways we might use the calibration matrix. First, we might wish to calculate the receptor absorptions to a particular light from the CRT. Second, we might wish to know how to adjust the relative intensities of the CRT in order to achieve a particular pattern of cone absorptions.

Using the methods described so far, you can calculate the relative cone absorption rates for any triplet of frame-buffer entries. Suppose the frame-buffer values are set to $(128, 128, 0)$. The pattern will look yellow, since only the red and green phosphors are excited. Assuming that the curves relating relative intensity to frame-buffer level are the same for all three phosphors (Fig. B.2), we find that the relative intensities will be $\mathbf{e} = (0.1524, 0.1524, 0.0)^T$. The product $\mathbf{Me}$ yields the relative cone absorption rates $\mathbf{r} = (0.1929, 0.1677, 0.0177)^T$. If we set the frame-buffer to $(128, 128, 128)$, which appears gray, the relative intensities are $(0.1524, 0.1524, 0.1524)$, and the relative cone absorption rates are $\mathbf{r} = (0.2152, 0.2001, 0.1702)^T$.

A second common type of calculation is used in behavioral experiments in which the experimenter wants to create a particular pattern of cone absorptions. To infer the relative display intensities necessary to achieve a desired effect on the cone absorptions, we must use the inverse of the calibration matrix, since

$$\mathbf{e} = \mathbf{H}^{-1}\mathbf{r} \tag{B.2}$$

To continue our example, the inverse of the calibration matrix is

$$\mathbf{H}^{-1} = \begin{pmatrix} 5.8677 & -5.8795 & 0.3876 \\ -0.6074 & 1.6344 & -0.2579 \\ -0.0049 & -0.1025 & 1.0225 \end{pmatrix}$$

Suppose we wish to display a pair of stimuli that differ only in their effects on the S-cones. Let us begin with a stimulus whose relative intensities are $\mathbf{e} = (0.5, 0.5, 0.5)^T$. Using the calibration matrix, we calculate that the relative cone absorption rates from this stimulus as $(0.706,$

0.656, 0.558). Now, let us create a second stimulus with a slightly higher rate of S-cone absorptions, say, $\mathbf{r} = (0.706, 0.656, 0.700)$. Using the inverse calibration matrix, we can calculate the relative display intensities needed to produce the second stimulus as (0.555, 0.4634, 0.645).

Notice that to create a stimulus difference seen only by the S-cones, we needed to adjust the intensities of all three phosphor emissions. This is because of the large overlap in wavelength sensitivity among the cone classes.

Color Calibration Tips

For most of us calibration is not, in itself, the point. Rather, we calibrate displays to describe and control experimental stimuli. If your experiments only involve a small number of stimuli, then it is best to calibrate those stimuli exhaustively. This strategy avoids making a lot of unnecessary assumptions, and your accuracy will be limited only by the quality of your calibration instrument.

In some experiments and most commercial applications, the number of stimuli is too large for exhaustive calibration. Brainard (1989) calculates that for the most extreme case, in which one has a 512×512 spatial array with RGB buffers at 8 bits of resolution there are $10^{1,893,917}$ different stimulus patterns. So many patterns, so little time.

Because of the large number of potential stimuli, we need to build a model of the relationship between the frame-buffer entries and the monitor output. The discussion of calibration in this appendix is based on an implicit model of the display. To perform a high-quality calibration, you should check some of the assumptions. What exactly are these implicit assumptions, and how close will they be to real performance?

Spatial Independence

First, we have assumed that the transfer function from the frame-buffer values to the monitor output is independent of the spatial pattern in the frame-buffer. Specifically, we have assumed that the light measurements we obtain from a region will be the same if the surrounding area is set to zero or set to any other intensity level.

In fact, the intensity in a region is not always independent of the spatial pattern in adjacent regions (see e.g., Lyons and Farrell, 1989; Naiman and Makous, 1992). It can be very difficult and impractical to calibrate this aspect of the display. As an experimenter, you should choose your calibration conditions to match the conditions of your experiment as closely as possible so that you do not need to model the variations with spatial pattern. For example, if your experiments will use rectangular patches on a gray background, then calibrate the display properties for rectangular patches on a gray background, not on a black or white background.

If you are interested in a harsh test to evaluate spatial independence of a display, try displaying a square pattern consisting of alternating pixels with frame-buffer entries set to 0 and 255. When you step away from the monitor, the pattern will blur; in principle, the brightness of this pattern should match the brightness of a uniform square of the same size all of whose values are set to the frame-buffer value whose relative intensity is 0.5. You can try the test using alternating horizontal lines, alternating vertical lines, or random dot arrays.

Phosphor Independence

As Brainard (1989) points out, the spatial-independence assumption reduces the number of measurements to approximately 1.6×10^7. This is still too many measurements to make; but at least we have reduced the problem so that there are fewer measurements than the number of atoms in the universe.

It is our second assumption, **phosphor independence**, that makes calibration practical. We have assumed that the signals emitted from three phosphors can be measured independently of one another. For example, we measured the relative intensities for the green phosphor and assumed that this curve is the same no matter what the state of the red and blue phosphor emissions. The phosphor-independence assumption implies that we need to make only 3×256 measurements, the relative intensities of each of the three phosphors, to calibrate the display (once the spectral power distributions of the phosphors are known; or equivalently, the entries of the calibration matrix).

Before performing your experiments, it is important to verify phosphor independence. Measure the intensity of the monitor output to a range of, say, red phosphor values when the green frame-buffer is set to zero. Then measure again when the green frame-buffer is set to its maximum value. The relative intensities of the red phosphor you measure should be the same after you correct for the additive constant from the green phosphor. In my experience, this property does fail on some CRT displays; when it fails your calibration measurements are in real trouble. I suspect that phosphor independence fails when the power supply of the monitor is inadequate to supply the needs of the three electron guns. Thus, when all three electron guns are being driven at high levels, the load on the power supply exceeds the compliance range and produces a dependence between the output levels of the different phosphors. This dependence violates the assumptions of our calibration procedure and makes calibration of such a monitor very unpleasant. Get a new monitor.

For further discussion of calibration, consult some papers in which authors have described their experience with specific display-calibration projects (e.g., Pekelsky et al., 1988; Brainard, 1989; Post and Calhoun, 1989; Berns et al., 1993a, b).

C

Classification

Many visual judgments are classifications: an edge is present, or not; a part is defective, or not; a tumor is present, or not. The threshold and discrimination performances reviewed in Chapter 7 are classifications as well: the subject saw it, or not; the stimulus was this one, or that. This appendix explains some of the basic concepts in classification theory and their application to understanding vision.

We will explore the issues in classification by analyzing some simple behavioral decisions, the kind that take place in many vision experiments. Suppose that, during an experimental trial, the observer must decide which of two visual stimuli, *A* or *B*, is present. Part of the observer's decision will be based on the pattern of cone absorptions during the experimental trial. We can list the cone absorptions in a vector, **d**, whose values represent the number of absorptions in each of the cones. Because there are statistical fluctuations in the light source, and variability in the image formation process, the pattern of cone absorptions created by the same stimulus varies from trial to trial. As a result, the pattern of cone absorptions from the two different stimuli may sometimes be the same, and perfect classification may be impossible.

What response strategy should a person use to respond correctly as often as possible? A good way to lead your life is this: *When you are uncertain and must decide, choose the more likely alternative.* We can translate this simple principle into a statistical procedure by the following set of calculations. Suppose that we know the probability of the signal being *A* when we observe **d**. This is called the **conditional probability**, $P(A \mid \mathbf{d})$, which is read as "the probability of *A* given **d**." Suppose we also know the conditional probability that the signal is B is $P(B \mid \mathbf{d})$. The observer should decide that the signal is the one that is more likely given the data, namely,

$$\text{if } P(A \mid \mathbf{d}) > P(B \mid \mathbf{d}) \text{ choose } A, \text{ else } B \tag{C.1}$$

We call the expression in Equation C.1 a **decision rule**. The decision rule in Equation C.1 is framed in terms of the likelihood of the stimulus (A or B) given the data ($\mathbf{d}$). This formulation of the probabilities runs counter to our normal learning experience. During training, we know that stimulus A has been presented, and we experience a collection of cone absorptions. Experience informs us about probability of the data given the stimulus, $P(\mathbf{d} \mid A)$, not the probability of the stimulus given the data, $P(A \mid \mathbf{d})$. Hence, we would like to reformulate Equation C.1 in terms of the way we acquire our experience.

Bayes's rule is a formula that converts probabilities derived from experience, $P(\mathbf{d} \mid A)$, into the form we need for the decision rule, $P(A \mid \mathbf{d})$. The expression for Bayes's rule is

$$P(A \mid \mathbf{d}) = P(\mathbf{d} \mid A)\frac{P(A)}{P(\mathbf{d})} \tag{C.2}$$

where $P(A)$ is the probability the experimenter presents signal A (in this case one-half) and $P(\mathbf{d})$ is the probability of observing $\mathbf{d}$ quanta. As we shall see, this second probability turns out to be irrelevant to our decision.

The probabilities on the right-hand side of Bayes's rule are either estimated from our experience, $P(\mathbf{d} \mid A)$, or they are a structural part of the experimental design $P(A)$. The probability that stimulus A or B is presented is called the **a priori probability**, or **base rate**. The probability $P(\mathbf{d} \mid A)$ is called the **likelihood** of the observation given the hypothesis. The probability $P(A \mid \mathbf{d})$ is called the **a posteriori probability**. Bayes's rule combines the base rate and the likelihood of the observation to form the a posteriori probability of the hypothesis.

We can use Bayes's rule to express the decision criterion in Equation C.1 in a more convenient form:

$$\text{if } P(\mathbf{d} \mid A)\frac{P(A)}{P(\mathbf{d})} > P(\mathbf{d} \mid B)\frac{P(B)}{P(\mathbf{d})} \text{ choose } A, \text{ else } B. \tag{C.3}$$

Since the probability of observing the data, $P(\mathbf{d})$, is in the denominator of both of sides of this inequality, this probability is irrelevant to the decision. Therefore, we can rewrite Equation C.3 as

$$\frac{P(\mathbf{d} \mid A)}{P(\mathbf{d} \mid B)} > \frac{P(B)}{P(A)} \tag{C.4}$$

The term on the left-hand side of the Equation C.4 is called the **likelihood ratio**. The quantity on the right is called the **odds ratio**. The formula tells us that we should select A when the likelihood ratio, which depends on the data, exceeds the odds ratio, which depends on the a priori knowledge. A system that uses this formula to classify the stimuli is called a **Bayes classifier**.

A decision-maker who follows the decision rule imposed by a Bayes classifier will make the smallest number of errors possible, given the uncertainty in the data. The reason is this: for each observation, **d**, the classification rule always selects the most likely response. This rule certainly minimizes the errors we make for that observation. The total number of errors equals the sum of the errors made across all possible observations, since the Bayes classifier minimizes the number of errors for all observations. For this reason, observers who use Bayes-classifier decision rules are called **ideal observers**.

A Bayes Classifier for an Intensity Discrimination Task

In this section we will devise a Bayes classifier for a simple experimental decision. Suppose that we ask an observer to decide whether we have presented one of two brief visual stimuli; the two stimuli are identical in all ways but their intensity. We suppose that the observer decides which stimulus was presented based on the total number of cone absorptions during the trial, $\sum_{i=1}^{N} d_i = d$, and without paying attention to the spatial distribution of the cone absorptions.

Across experimental trials, the number of absorptions from A will vary. There are two sources of this variability. One source of variability is in the stimulus itself. Photons emitted by a light source are the result of changes in the energy level of electrons within the source material. Each electron within the material has some probability of changing states and yielding some energy in the form of a photon. This change in excitation level is a purely statistical event and cannot be precisely controlled. The variability in the number of emitted photons, then, is inherent in the physics of light emission and cannot be eliminated.

A second source of variability is in the observer. On different experimental trials, the position of the eye, the accommodative state of the lens, and other optical factors will vary. As these image formation parameters vary, the chance that photons are absorbed within the photopigment will vary. These statistic fluctuations are unavoidable as well.

The physical variability is easy to model, while the biological variability is quite subtle. For this illustrative calculation, we will ignore the effects of biological variability and consider only the stimulus variability. In this case, the number of absorptions will follow the **Poisson distribution**. The formula for the Poisson probability distribution describes the probability of emitting d quanta given a mean level of μ,

$$P(d \mid \mu) = (\mu^d / d!)e^{-\mu} \tag{C.5}$$

The value μ is called the **rate-parameter** of the Poisson distribution. The variance of the Poisson distribution is also μ.

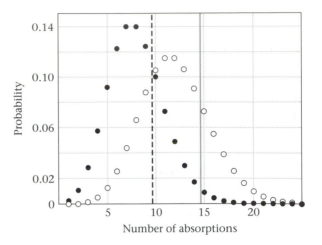

C.1   BAYES CLASSIFIER FOR INTENSITY DISCRIMINATION. The Poisson distributions of stimulus A with rate parameter $\mu_A = 8$ (filled circles) and and B with rate parameter $\mu_B = 12$ (open circles) are shown. When the a priori probabilities of seeing the stimuli are equal, the Bayes classifier selects B when the absorptions exceed the dashed line drawn through the graph. When the a priori probabilities are $P(A) = 0.75$ and $P(B) = 0.25$, the Bayes classifier selects B when the absorptions exceed the solid line drawn through the graph.

Figure C.1 shows the probability distributions of the number of cone absorptions from the two stimuli, A and B. For this illustration, I have assumed that the mean numbers of absorptions from the stimuli are $\mu_A = 8$ and $\mu_B = 12$. Since the a priori stimulus probabilities are equal, the observer will select stimulus A whenever $P(d \mid A)$ exceeds $P(d \mid B)$. For this pair of distributions, this occurs whenever the observation (number of cone absorptions) is less than 9.

Now, suppose that the experimenter presents A with probability 0.75 and B with probability 0.25. In this case, the subject can be right three-quarters of the time simply by always guessing A. Given the strong a priori odds for A, the Bayes classifier will only choose B if the likelihood exceeds 3 to 1. From the distributions in Figure C.1 we find that this occurs when there are at least 13 absorptions. The Bayes classifier uses the data and the a priori probabilities to make a decision.[1]

A Bayes Classifier for a Pattern-Discrimination Task

To discriminate between different spatial patterns, or stimuli located at different spatial positions, the observer must use the spatial pattern of cone absorptions. Consequently, pattern discrimination must depend

---

[1] In a classic paper, Hecht et al. (1942) measured the smallest number of quanta necessary for reliable detection of a signal. In the most sensitive region of the retina, under the optimized viewing conditions, they found that 100 quanta at the cornea, which corresponds to about 10 absorptions, are sufficient. The quanta are absorbed in an area covered by several hundred rods; hence, it is quite unlikely that two quanta will be absorbed by the same rod. They concluded, quite correctly, that a single photon of light can produce a measurable response in a single rod.

To find further support for their observation, Hecht et al. analyzed how the subject's responses varied across trials. They assumed that all of the observed variability was due to the stimulus and that none was due to the observer. Their account is repeated in a wonderful didactic style in Cornsweet (1970). I do not think this assumption is justified; a complete treatment of the data must take into account variability intrinsic to the human observer (e.g., Nachmias and Kocher, 1970).

on comparisons of a vector of measurements, **d**, not just a single value. In this section, we will develop a Bayes classifier that can be applied to a pattern-discrimination task.

Again, for illustrative purposes we assume that the variability is due entirely to the stimulus. Moreover, we will assume that the variability in light absorption at neighboring receptors is statistically independent. Independence means that the probability of d_i absorptions at the ith receptor and d_j at the jth is

$$P(d_i \, \& \, d_j \mid A) = P(d_i \mid A) \, P(d_j \mid A) \qquad \text{(C.6)}$$

We can extend this principle across all of the receptors to write the probability of observing **d** given signal A, namely,

$$L_A = \prod_{i=1}^{N} P(d_i \mid A) \qquad \text{(C.7)}$$

where L_A is the likelihood of observing **d** given the stimulus A.

Finally, we must specify the spatial pattern of two stimuli. The expected number of absorptions at the ith cone will depend on the spatial pattern of the stimulus. We will use $\mu_{A,i}$ and $\mu_{B,i}$ to refer to the mean intensities of the stimuli at location i.

We are ready to compute the proper Bayes classifier. The general form of the decision criterion is:

$$\text{if } \frac{P(\mathbf{d} \mid A)}{P(\mathbf{d} \mid B)} > \frac{P(B)}{P(A)} \quad \text{choose } A \text{, else } B \qquad \text{(C.8)}$$

If the two stimuli are presented in the experiment equally often, we can rewrite this equation as follows:

$$\text{if } P(\mathbf{d} \mid A) > P(\mathbf{d} \mid B) \quad \text{choose } A \text{, else } B \qquad \text{(C.9)}$$

Next, we can use independence to write:

$$\text{if } \prod_{i=1}^{N} P(d_i \mid A) > \prod_{i=1}^{N} P(d_i \mid B) \quad \text{choose } A \text{, else } B \qquad \text{(C.10)}$$

Now, we substitute the Poisson formula, take the logarithm of both sides, and regroup terms to obtain:

$$\text{if } \sum_{i=1}^{N} d_i \ln(\mu_{A,i}/\mu_{B,i}) > \sum_{i=1}^{N} \mu_{A,i} - \sum_{i=1}^{N} \mu_{B,i} \quad \text{choose } A \text{, else } B \qquad \text{(C.11)}$$

Equation C.11 can be interpreted as a very simple computational procedure. First, notice that the equation contains two terms. The first term is the weighted sum of the photopigment absorptions,

$$\sum_{i=1}^{N} d_i w_i \qquad\qquad (C.12)$$

where $w_i = \ln(\mu_{A,i}/\mu_{B,i})$. This is a very familiar computation; it is directly analogous to the calculation implemented by a linear neuron whose receptive-field sensitivity at position i is w_i (see Chapter 5).

The second term is the difference between the total number of photopigment absorptions expected from each stimulus:

$$\sum_{i=1}^{N} \mu_{A,i} - \sum_{i=1}^{N} \mu_{B,i}$$

This term acts as a normalizing criterion to correct for the overall response to the two stimuli. The decision rule in Equation C.11 compares a weighted sum of cone absorptions to the normalizing criterion: if the first term exceeds the second, then choose response A, else B.

We have learned that a Bayes classifier for pattern discrimination can be implemented using the results of simple linear calculations, like the calculations represented in the outputs of some peripheral neurons. In fact, making a decision like a Bayes classifier is equivalent to comparing the response of a linear neuron with a criterion value. If the response of the linear neuron with receptive field defined by w_i exceeds the criterion value, then choose stimulus A; otherwise choose B.

Figure C.2 shows an example of a Bayes classifier computed for a simple pattern-discrimination task. The two spatial patterns to be discriminated are shown in panels (A) and (B). The image in Figure C.2A is the retinal image of a line segment; Figure C.2B shows the retinal image of a pair of line segments, separated by 30 sec of arc. The grid marks on the image are spaced by 30 seconds of arc, essentially the same spacing as the cone inner segments. The curves below the images measure the intensity of the stimuli across a horizontal section.

Figure C.2C shows the weights of the Bayes classifier for discriminating the two images; the weights were computed using Equation C.12. In this image the gray level represents the value of the weight that should be applied to the individual cone absorptions: a medium gray intensity represents a zero weight, lighter values are positive weights, and darker values are negative weights. The spatial pattern of weights bears an obvious resemblance to the spatial patterns of receptive fields in the visual cortex.

The Bayes classifier specifies how to obtain the optimal discrimination performance when we know the signal and the noise. Apart from

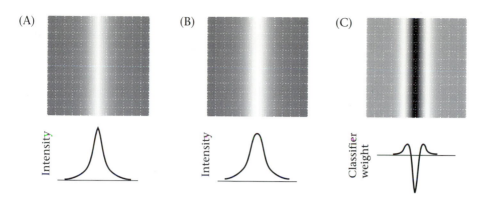

C.2 BAYES CLASSIFIER FOR A SPATIAL-DISCRIMINATION TASK. (A) The mean retinal image of a line. The grid lines are separated by 30 seconds of arc, approximately the spacing of the cone inner segments in the fovea. (B) The mean retinal image formed by a pair of lines separated by 30 seconds of arc. The intensity of each line is one-half the intensity of the line in panel A. (C) The weights for the Bayes classifier that should be used to discriminate the stimuli in (A) and (B), given the assumptions of independent Poisson noise. After Geisler, 1989.

the optimality of the Bayes classifier itself, observers in behavioral experiments can never know the true signal and noise perfectly. The performance of the Bayes classifier, therefore, must be equal or superior to human performance. In nearly all cases where a Bayes-classifier analysis has been carried out, the Bayes-classifier performance is vastly better than the performance of a human observer. Human observers usually fail to extract a great deal of information available in the stimulus. In general, then, the Bayes classifier does not model human performance (Banks et al., 1987).

Why, then, is the Bayes-classifier analysis important? The Bayes-classifier analysis defines what information is available to the observer. Defining the stimulus is an essential part of a good experimental design. The Bayes classifier defines what the observer can potentially do, and this serves as a good standard to use in evaluating performance. The Bayes classifier helps us to understand the task; only if we understand the task can we understand the observer's performance. As Geisler (1987, p. 30) notes:

> The real power of this approach is that the ideal discriminator [Bayes classifier] measures all the information available to the later stages of the visual system. I would like to suggest that measuring the information available in discrimination stimuli with a model of the sort I have described here should be done as routinely as measuring the luminances of the stimuli with a photometer. In other words, we should not only use a light meter but we should also use the appropriate information meter. It is simply a matter of following the first commandment of psychophysics: "know thy stimulus."

D

Signal Estimation: A Geometric View

This book is filled with calculations of the general form

$$\mathbf{a}^{\mathrm{T}}\mathbf{x} = \sum_{i=1}^{i=N} a_i x_i \qquad (D.1)$$

This formula is called the **dot product** of the vectors $\mathbf{a}$ and $\mathbf{x}$. It is so important that it is often given a special notation, such as $\mathbf{a} \cdot \mathbf{x}$. Every time we multiply a matrix by a vector, $\mathbf{A}\mathbf{x}$, we compute the dot product $\mathbf{x}$ with the rows of $\mathbf{A}$. In this section, I want to discuss some geometric intuitions connected with the dot-product operation.[1]

Although we used the dot-product calculation many times, I decided not to use dot-product notation in the main portion of the book because the notation treats the two vectors symmetrically; however, in most applications the vectors $\mathbf{a}$ and $\mathbf{x}$ had an asymmetrical role. The vector $\mathbf{x}$ was usually a stimulus, say, the wavelength composition of a light or a one-dimensional spatial pattern, and the vector $\mathbf{a}$ was part of the sensory apparatus, say, a photopigment wavelength sensitivity or a ganglion-cell receptive field. Because the physical entities we described were not symmetric, I felt that the asymmetric notation, $\mathbf{a}^{\mathrm{T}}\mathbf{x}$, was more appropriate.

---

[1] Physicists often refer to Equation D.1 as the scalar product because the result is a scalar; mathematicians often refer to the dot product as an inner product and write it using angle brackets: $\langle \mathbf{a}, \mathbf{x} \rangle$.

The scalar value of the dot product between two vectors is equal to

$$\mathbf{a} \cdot \mathbf{x} = \|\mathbf{a}\| \|\mathbf{x}\| \cos(\theta) \qquad (D.2)$$

where $\| \cdot \|$ is the vector length and θ is the angle between the vectors. To simplify the discussion in the remainder of this section, we will assume that the vector $\mathbf{a}$ has unit length.

Figure D.1A is a geometric representation of the dot-product operation. The unit vector $\mathbf{a}$ and the signal vector $\mathbf{x}$ are drawn as arrows extending from the origin. A dashed line is drawn from the tip of $\mathbf{x}$ (the signal) at right angles to the vector $\mathbf{a}$ (the sensor). The length of the vector from the origin to point of intersection between the perpendicular dashed line and $\mathbf{a}$ is called the **projection** of $\mathbf{x}$ onto $\mathbf{a}$. Because we have assumed that $\mathbf{a}$ has unit length, the length of the projection, $\|\mathbf{x}\| \cos(\theta)$, is equal to the dot product, $\mathbf{a} \cdot \mathbf{x} = \|\mathbf{a}\| \|\mathbf{x}\| \cos(\theta)$.

By inspecting Figure D.1B, you can see that there are many signal vectors, $\mathbf{x}$, that have the same dot product with $\mathbf{a}$. Specifically, all of the vectors whose endpoints fall along a line that is perpendicular to $\mathbf{a}$ have the same dot product with $\mathbf{a}$. Hence, any signal represented by a vector whose endpoint is on this line will cause the same response in the sensor represented by the vector $\mathbf{a}$.

The geometric intuition extends smoothly to vectors with more than two dimensions. Figure D.2A shows the dot product between a pair of three-dimensional vectors. In three dimensions, all of the vectors whose endpoints fall on a plane perpendicular to the unit-length vector $\mathbf{a}$ have the same dot product with that vector (Figure D.2B). In four or more dimensions the set of signals with a common dot-product value fall on a **hyperplane**.

Figures D.1B and D.2B illustrate the information that is preserved and that is lost in a dot-product calculation. When we measure the dot product of a pair of two-dimensional vectors, we learn that the signal must have fallen along a particular line; when we measure a three-dimensional dot-product, we learn that the signal must have fallen

D.1 A GEOMETRIC INTERPRETATION OF THE TWO-DIMENSIONAL DOT PRODUCT. (A) A geometrical view of the dot product of two vectors is shown. The dashed line is a perpendicular from the tip of vector **x** to the unit-length vector **a**. (B) Any vector whose endpoint falls along the dashed line yields the same scalar value when we compute the vector's dot product with **a**.

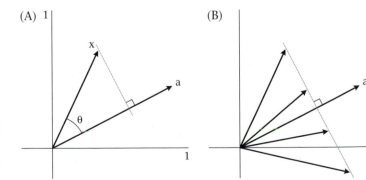

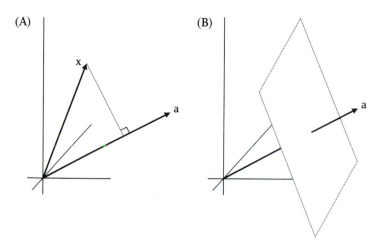

D.2 A GEOMETRIC REPRESENTATION OF THE THREE-DIMENSIONAL DOT PRODUCT. (A) The perpendicular from **x** to **a** is indicated by the dashed line. When **a** is a unit vector, the distance from the origin to the intersection of the dashed line with **a** is the scalar value of the dot product. (B) Any vector whose endpoint falls within the indicated plane yields the same scalar value when we compute the vector's dot with **a**.

within a certain plane. Hence, each dot product helps to define the set of possible input signals.

By combining the results from several dot products, we can estimate the input signal. We can use the geometric representation of the dot product in Figure D.1 to develop some intuitions about how to estimate the signal from a collection of sensor responses. This is a **signal-estimation** problem.

First, imagine that the response of each linear neuron is equal to the dot product of a vector describing the spatial contrast pattern of a stimulus with a vector describing the neuron's receptive field. Further, suppose that the input stimuli are drawn from a set of simple spatial patterns, namely, the weighted sums of two cosinusoidal gratings,

$$w_1 \cos(2\pi f_1 x) + w_2 \cos(2\pi f_2 x)$$

We can represent each of these spatial contrast patterns using a two-dimensional vector, $\mathbf{x} = (w_1, w_2)$, whose entries are the weights of the cosinusoids. We can represent the sensitivity of each linear neuron to these spatial patterns using a two-dimensional vector, $\mathbf{a}_i$, whose two entries define the neuron's sensitivity to each of the cosinusoidal terms. Because the neurons are linear, we can compute the ith neuron's response to any pattern in the set from the linear calculation in the dot product, namely, $\mathbf{a}_i^T \mathbf{x}$.

Figure D.3A shows geometrically how to use two responses to identify uniquely the two-dimensional input stimulus. Suppose that the response of the neuron with receptive field $\mathbf{a}_1$ is r_1. Then, we can infer that the stimulus must fall along a line perpendicular to the vector $\mathbf{a}_1$ and intersecting $\mathbf{a}_1$ at a distance $r_1 = \|\mathbf{x}\| \cos(\theta_i)$ from the origin.[2] If the response to the second neuron is r_2, we can draw a second line

[2] In general, we would place the perpendicular line at a distance of $\|\mathbf{x}\| \cos(\theta_i)/\|\mathbf{a}_i\|$, but we have assumed that $\mathbf{a}_i$ has unit length.

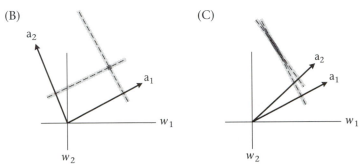

D.3 SIGNAL ESTIMATION FROM MULTIPLE LINEAR SENSORS. (A) We can infer the location of a two-dimensional signal vector from the responses of two linear sensors. (B) When the vectors representing the sensors are orthogonal, the estimation error is small. (C) When the vectors representing the sensors are nearly aligned, the estimation error tends to be quite large in the direction perpendicular to the sensor vectors.

that describes a second set of possible stimulus locations. The true stimulus must be on both lines, so it is located at the intersection of the two dashed lines.

When the sensor responses have some added noise, which is always the case in real measurements, some sensor combinations provide more precise estimates than others. Figure D.3B shows a pair of sensors whose vectors are nearly orthogonal to one another. Because of the sensor noise, the true identity of the signal is uncertain. The lightly shaded bands drawn around the perpendicular dashed lines show the effect of sensor noise on the estimated region from the individual measurements. The darkly shaded region is the intersection of the bands, showing the likely region containing the signal. For these orthogonal sensors, the dark band that is likely to contain the signal is fairly small.

Figure D.3C shows the same representation, but for a pair of sensors represented by nearly parallel vectors. Such sensors are said to be **correlated**. When the sensors are correlated in this way, the shaded region can be quite large in the direction perpendicular to the sensor vectors. In the presence of noise, correlated sensors provide a poor estimate of the signal.

Matrix Equations

Ordinarily, we use matrix multiplication to represent a collection of dot products. Many aspects of the signal-estimation problem can be expressed and solved using methods developed for matrix algebra.

To better appreciate the connection between matrix multiplication and the signal-estimation problem, consider the following example. Write the dot product of a two-dimensional signal and a sensor in the tableau format,

$$r_1 = (a_1 \quad a_2) \begin{pmatrix} x_1 \\ x_2 \end{pmatrix}$$

Now, suppose we have two sensors and two responses. Then, we can expand the tableau by adding more rows to represent the new measurements, as follows:

$$\begin{pmatrix} r_1 \\ r_2 \end{pmatrix} = \begin{pmatrix} a_{1,1} & a_{1,2} \\ a_{2,1} & a_{2,2} \end{pmatrix} \begin{pmatrix} x_1 \\ x_2 \end{pmatrix} \tag{D.3}$$

where $a_{i,\cdot}$ is a vector that represents the sensitivity of the ith sensor. In the usual signal-estimation problem, we know the properties of the sensors represented in the rows of the matrix, and we know the responses in $\mathbf{r}$. We wish to estimate the signal in $\mathbf{x}$. The pair of sensor vectors represented in the rows of the matrix, call it $\mathbf{A}$, are the counterpart of the vectors shown in Figure D.3A. Our ability to estimate the signal from the resposnes depends on the correlation between the rows of the matrix.

The matrix tableau in Equation D.3 shows a special case in which there are two sensors and two unknown values of the signal. In general, we might have more sensors or more unknowns in the signal. Having more sensors would force us to add more rows to the matrix; having more unknowns in the signal would force us to change the lengths of the sensor and signal vectors. Each of these changes might change the general shape of the matrix tableau. We can write the general case, without specifying the number of sensors or unknowns, using the following concise representation:

$$\mathbf{r} = \mathbf{Ax} \tag{D.4}$$

Again, in the (linear) signal-estimation problem we know the responses ($\mathbf{r}$) and the sensors in the rows of $\mathbf{A}$, and we wish to estimate the signal ($\mathbf{x}$).

Many topics we have reviewed in the text can be framed as linear estimation problems within the matrix in Equation D.4. For example, you might imagine that the rows of the matrix are retinal-ganglion receptive fields, the responses are neural firing rates, and the input is a spatial contrast pattern (Chapter 5). The brain may then need to estimate various properties of the contrast pattern from the neural firing patterns. Or, you might imagine that the rows of the matrix represent the spectral responsivities of the three cone types, the responses are the cone signals, and the signal is a spectral power distribution (Chapters 4 and 9). Or, you might imagine that the each row of the matrix represents the receptive field of a space–time-oriented neuron, the output is the neuron's response, and the signal comprises the two velocity components of the local motion flow field (Chapter 10).

There are many matrix-algebra tools that are useful for solving matrix equations like Equation D.4. To choose the proper tool for a problem, one must take into account a variety of specific properties of the measurement conditions. For example, in some cases there are more sensors than there are unknown entries in the vector **x**. We can represent this estimation problem using a matrix tableau as follows:

$$\begin{pmatrix} \\ \mathbf{r} \\ \\ \\ \end{pmatrix} = \begin{pmatrix} \\ \quad \mathbf{A} \quad \\ \\ \\ \end{pmatrix} \begin{pmatrix} \\ \mathbf{x} \\ \\ \end{pmatrix}$$

The shape of the tableau makes it plain that there are more responses in the vector **r** than there are unknowns in the vector **x**. This type of estimation problem is called **overconstrained**. When there is noise in the measurements, no exact solution to the overconstrained problem may exist; that is, there may be no vector **x** such that the equality shown in the tableau is perfectly satisfied. Instead, we must define an error criterion and try to find a "best" solution, that is, a solution that minimizes the error criterion.

In general, the best solution will depend on the noise properties and the error criterion. In some cases, say, when the noise is Gaussian and the error is the sum of the squared difference between the observed and predicted responses, there are good closed-form solutions to the linear estimation problem. That is, one can find an estimate of the signal by direct computation, without using any search algorithms. If one has other error criteria or noise, a search may be necessary.

A full discussion of the problems involved in signal estimation and matrix algebra would take us far beyond the scope of this book, but there are several excellent textbooks that explain these ideas (e.g., Lawson and Hanson, 1974; Vetterling et al., 1992; Strang, 1993). Also, the manuals for several computer packages, such as Matlab and Mathematica, contain useful information about using these methods and further references. To see how some of these tools have been applied to vision science, you might consult some of the following references: Wandell (1987); Nielsen and Wandell (1988); Tomasi and Kanade (1991); Heeger and Jepson (1992); Marimont and Wandell (1992); Brainard (1995); or Thomas et al. (1994).

E

Motion-Flow-Field Calculation

The motion flow field describes how an image point changes position from one moment in time to the next, say, as an observer changes viewpoint. I reviewed several properties of the motion flow field in Chapter 10, and I also reviewed how to use the information in a motion flow field to estimate scene properties, including observer motion and depth maps.

Here I describe how to compute a motion flow field. There are various reasons one might need to calculate a motion flow field. For example, motion flow fields are used as experiment stimuli to analyze human performance (e.g., Warren and Hannon, 1990; Royden et al., 1992). Also, algorithms designed to estimate depth maps from motion flow fields must be tested using artificial motion flow fields (e.g., Heeger and Jepson, 1992; Tomasi and Kanade, 1992).

To calculate the motion flow field, we will treat the eye as a pinhole camera, and we will define the position of the points in space relative to the pinhole. Based on this framework, we will derive two formulas. First, we will derive the **perspective-projection formula**. This formula describes how points in space project onto locations in the image plane of the pinhole camera. Second, we will derive how translating and rotating the position of the pinhole camera, i.e., the **viewpoint**, changes the point coordinates in space. Finally, we will combine these two formulas to predict how changing the viewpoint changes the point locations in the image plane, thus creating the motion flow field.

Imaging Geometry and Perspective Projection

We base our calculations on ray-tracing from points in the world onto an image plane in a pinhole camera (see Chapter 2). To simplify some of the graphics calculations, it is conventional to place the pinhole at the origin of the coordinate frame and the imaging plane in the positive quadrant of the coordinate frame. Figure E.1A shows the geometric relationship between a point in space, the pinhole, and the image plane.

The image plane is parallel to the x–y plane at a distance f along the z-axis. A ray from $\mathbf{p} = (p_1, p_2, p_3)$ passes toward the pinhole and intersects the image-plane location (u, v, f). Since the third coordinate, f, is the same for all points in the image plane, we can describe the image-plane location using only the first two coordinates, (u, v).

Parts A and B of Figure E.1 show the geometric relationship between a point in space and its location in the image plane from two different points of view: looking down the y-axis and x-axis, respectively. From both views, we can identify a pair of similar triangles that relate the po-

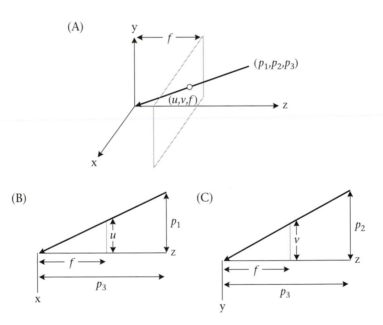

E.1 PERSPECTIVE CALCULATIONS FOR A PINHOLE CAMERA. The coordinate frame is centered at the pinhole, and the image plane is located at a distance f in front of the pinhole parallel to the x–y plane. (A) A ray from a point (p_1, p_2, p_3) that passes through the pinhole will intersect the image plane at location (u, v). (B) From a view along the y-axis we find a pair of similar triangles. These triangles define an equation that relates the image-plane coordinate, u, the point coordinates, and the distance from the pinhole to the image plane, f. (C) From a view along the x-axis, we find an analogous pair of similar triangles and an analogous equation for v.

sition of the point in three-dimensional space and the image point position. There are two equations that relate the point coordinates, $\mathbf{p} = (p_1, p_2, p_3)$, the distance from the pinhole to the image plane f, and the image-plane coordinates (u, v):

$$u = (p_1/p_3)f \quad \text{and} \quad v = (p_2/p_3)f \tag{E.1}$$

Imaging Geometry: Camera Translation and Rotation

The coordinate frame is centered at the pinhole. Hence, when the pinhole camera moves, each point in the world is assigned a new position vector. Here, we calculate the change in coordinates of the points for each motion of the pinhole optics. We will use the new coordinates to calculate the change in the point's image position, and then the motion-flow-field vectors.

At each moment in time we can describe the motion of the camera using two different terms. First, there is a translational component that describes the direction of the pinhole motion. Second, there is a rotational component that describes how the camera rotates around the pinhole. We use two vectors to represent the camera's velocity. The vector $\mathbf{t} = (t_1, t_2, t_3)^{\mathrm{T}}$ represents the translational velocity. Each term in this vector describes the velocity of the camera in one of the three spatial dimensions. The vector $\mathbf{r} = (r_x, r_y, r_z)^{\mathrm{T}}$ represents the angular velocity. Each term in this vector describes the rotation of the camera with respect to one of the three spatial dimensions. The six values in these vectors completely describe the rigid motion of the camera.

We can compute the coordinate change $\Delta\mathbf{p} = (\Delta p_1, \Delta p_2, \Delta p_3)^{\mathrm{T}}$, given the translation, rotation, and point coordinates as follows:

$$\Delta p_1 = r_x p_2 - r_y p_3 - t_1$$

$$\Delta p_2 = r_x p_3 - r_x p_1 - t_2$$

$$\Delta p_3 = r_y p_1 - r_x p_2 - t_3$$

These formulas apply when the rotation and translation are small quantities, measuring the instantaneous change in position.

Motion Flow

Finally, we compute motion flow by using Equation E.1 to specify how the change in position in space maps into a change in image position. The original point $\mathbf{p}$ mapped into an image position (u, v); after the observer moves, the new coordinate, $\mathbf{p} + \Delta\mathbf{p}$ maps into a new image position, (u', v'). The resulting motion flow is the difference in the two image positions, $\mathbf{m}(u, v) = (u - u', v - v')^{\mathrm{T}}$.

The following equation defines how the motion of the pinhole camera and the depth map combine to create the motion flow field (Heeger and Jepson, 1992):

$$\mathbf{m}(u,v) = \frac{1}{p_3(u,v)}\mathbf{A}(u,v)\mathbf{t} + \mathbf{B}(u,v)\mathbf{r} \qquad (\text{E.2})$$

The term $p_3(u,v)$ is the value of p_3 for the point in three-dimensional space with image position (u,v). The entries of the 2×3 matrices $\mathbf{A}(u,v)$ and $\mathbf{B}(u,v)$ depend only on known quantities, namely, the distance from the pinhole to the image plane and the image position, (u,v):

$$\mathbf{A}(u,v) \begin{pmatrix} -f & 0 & u \\ 0 & -f & v \end{pmatrix}$$

$$\mathbf{B}(u,v) = \begin{pmatrix} -(uv)/f & -(f+u^2/f) & v \\ (f+v^2/f) & -(uv)/f & -u \end{pmatrix}$$

Equation E.2 expresses a relationship we have seen already: the local motion flow field is the sum of two vectors (see Fig. 10.10). One vector describes a component of the motion flow field caused by viewpoint translation, $\mathbf{t}$. The second vector describes a component of the motion flow field caused by viewpoint rotation, $\mathbf{r}$. Only the first component, caused by translation, depends on the distance to the point, $p_3(u,v)$. The rotational component is the same for points at any distance from the viewpoint. Hence, all of the information concerning the depth map is contained in the motion-flow-field component that is caused by viewpoint translation.

F

A Sampling and Aliasing Demonstration

The following PostScript code was written by Arturo Puente, a former student of mine. Sending the code to a PostScript printer will produce square-wave patterns like those in Figure 3.12. If you print the patterns on transparent material, you can perform the demonstration described in the text.

```
%!PS-Adobe-1.0
% Description: Create bar patterns
% Parameters: Width of light and dark bars
%
/widthx1  10 def  % <- Value to change
/widthx2   2 def  % <- Value to change

/x1    90 def
/y1   180 def
/x2    { x1 widthx1 add } def
/y2   612 def
/numx     {432 widthx1 widthx2 add idiv} def

/form
{
 newpath
 x1 y1 moveto
 x1 y2 lineto
 x2 y2 lineto
 x2 y1 lineto
```

```
 closepath
 fill
/x1 x1 widthx1 widthx2 add add def
} def

numx {form} repeat

/Helvetica findfont 10 scalefont setfont
72 84 moveto
(Width solid lines =) show
widthx1 dup 3 string cvs show
72 72 moveto
(Width white lines =) show
widthx2 dup 3 string cvs show
showpage

%!PS-Adobe-1.0
% Description: Create sampling array
% Parameters: Sample spacing and separation width
%
/widthx    20 def  % <- Value to change
/widthy    10 def  % <- Value to change
/wall    1 def  % <- Value to change

/x1     90 def
/y1     180 def
/x2     { x1 widthx add } def
/y2     { y1 widthx add } def
/numx    {432 widthx idiv} def
/numy    {432 widthy idiv} def

/form {
 newpath
 x1 y1 moveto
 x2 y1 lineto
 x2 y2 lineto
 x1 y2 lineto
 x1 y1 lineto
 x1 wall add y1 wall add lineto
 x1 wall add y2 wall sub lineto
 x2 wall sub y2 wall sub lineto
 x2 wall sub y1 wall add lineto
 x1 wall add y1 wall add lineto
 closepath
 fill
/x1 x1 widthx add def
} def
```

```
/fileform
{
 numx {form} repeat
 /x1  90 def
 /y1 y1 widthy add def
} def

numy {fileform} repeat


%
%  Write out parameters
%
/Helvetica findfont 10 scalefont setfont
72 96 moveto
(Width of the rectangle in the x-axis = ) show
widthx dup 3 string cvs show
72 84 moveto
(Width of the rectangle in the y-axis = ) show
widthy dup 3 string cvs show
72 72 moveto
(Thickness of the wall = ) show
wall dup 3 string cvs show

showpage
%
```

Bibliography

Addams, R. 1834. An account of a peculiar optical phaenomenon seen after having looked at a moving body, etc. *Lond. and Edinburgh Phil. Mag. and J. Science,* 5:373–374.

Adelson, E. H. and Movshon, J. A. 1982. Phenomenal coherence of moving visual patterns. *Nature,* 300:523–525.

Adelson, E. H. 1993. Perceptual organization and the judgment of brightness. *Science,* 262:2042–2044.

Adelson, E. H. and Bergen, J. R. 1985. Spatiotemporal energy models for the perception of motion. *J. Opt. Soc. Am. (A),* 2:284–289.

Ahnelt, P., Keri, C., and Kolb, H. 1990. Identification of pedicles of putative blue-sensitive cones in the human retina. *J. Comp. Neurol.,* 293:39–53.

Ahnelt, P. K., Kolb, H., Pflug, R. 1987. Identification of a sub-type of cone photoreceptor, likely to be blue sensitive, in the human retina. *J. Comp. Neurol.,* 255:18–34.

Albers, J. 1975. *Interaction of Color.* Yale University Press, New Haven.

Albrecht, D. G. and Geisler, W. S. 1991. Motion sensitivity and the contrast-response function of simple cells in the visual cortex. *Visual Neurosci.,* 7:531–546.

Albrecht, D. G. and Hamilton, D. B. 1982. Striate cortex of monkey and cat: Contrast response function. *J. Neurophysiol.,* 48:217–237.

Albright, T. 1984. Direction and orientation selectivity of neurons in visual area MT of the macaque. *J. Neurophysiol.,* 52:1106–1130.

Alpern, M. 1974. What is it that confines in a world without color? *Inv. Opthalmol. Vis. Sci.,* 13:647–674.

Anderson, B. L. and Nakayama, K. 1994. Toward a general theory of stereopsis: Binocular matching, occluding contours, and fusion. *Psych. Review,* 101:414–445.

Anstis, S. M. 1980. The perception of apparent movement. *Proc. R. Soc. Lond. Ser. B,* 290:153–168.

Artal, P., Marcos, S., Navarro, R., and Williams, D. 1995. Odd aberrations and double-pass measurements of retinal image quality. *J. Opt. Soc. Am. (A),* 12:195–201.

Artal, P., Santamaria, J., and Bescos, J. 1989. Optical-digital procedure for the determination of white-light retinal images of a point test. *Opt. Eng.,* 28:687–690.

Ayama, M. and Ikeda, M. 1989. The dependence of chromatic valence functions on chromatic standards. *Vision Res.,* 29:1233–1244.

Azzopardi, P. and Cowey, A. 1993. Preferential representation of the fovea in the primary visual cortex. *Nature,* 361:719–721.

Baizer, J. S., Ungerleider, L. G., and Desimone, R. 1991. Organization of visual inputs to the inferior temporal and posterior parietal cortex in macaques. *J. Neurosci.,* 11:168–190.

Bak, M., Girvin, J. P., Hambrecht, F. T., Kufta, C. V., Loeb, G. E., and Schmidt, E. M.

1990. Visual sensations produced by intracortical microstimulation of the human occipital cortex. *Medical and Biological Engineering and Computing,* 28:257–259.

Baker, C. L., Jr., Hess, R. F., and Zihl, J. 1991. Residual motion perception in a "motion-blind" patient, assessed with limited-lifetime random dot stimuli. *J. Neurosci.,* 11:454–461.

Banks, M. S., Geisler, W. S., and Bennett, P. J. 1987. The physical limits of grating visibility. *Vision. Res.,* 27:1915–1924.

Barlow, H. B. 1972. Single units and sensation: A neuron doctrine for perceptual psychology? *Perception,* 1:371–394.

Barlow, H. B., Blakemore, C., and Pettigrew, J. D. 1967. The neural mechanism of binocular depth discrimination. *J. Physiol.,* 193:327–342.

Barlow, H. B., Fitzhugh, R., and Kuffler, S. W. 1957. Change of organization in the receptive fields of the cat's retina during dark adaptation. *J. Physiol.,* 137:338–345.

Barlow, H. B. and Foldiak, P. F. 1989. Adaptation and decorrelation in the cortex. In R. Durbin, C. Miall, and G. Mitchison, (eds.), *The Computing Neuron.* Addison-Wesley, MA.

Barlow, H. B., Kaushal, T. P., Hawken, M., and Parker, A. J. 1987. Human contrast discrimination and the threshold of cortical neurons. *J. Opt. Soc. Am. (A),* 4:2366–2371.

Baylor, D. A. 1987. Photoreceptor signals and vision. *Inv. Opthlamol. Vis. Sci.,* 28:34–49.

Baylor, D. A., Nunn, B. J. and Schnapf, J. L. 1987. Spectral sensitivity of cones of the monkey *Macaca Fascicularis. J. Physiol.,* 390:145–160.

Beckers, G., et al. 1992. Cerebral visual motion blindness: Transitory akinetopsia induced by transcranial magnetic stimulation of human area V5. *Proc. R. Soc. Lond. Ser. B,* 249:173–178.

Bedford, R. E. and Wyszecki, G. 1957. Axial chromatic aberration of the human eye. *J. Opt. Soc. Am.,* 47:564–565.

Belhumeur, P. N. and Mumford, D. 1992. A Bayesian treatment of stereo correspondence problem using half-occluded regions. In *Proc. Inst. Electrical Electronics Engrs. Conference on Computer Vision and Pattern Recognition,* pp. 506–512. Los Alamitos, CA.

Berlin, B. and Kay, P. 1969. *Basic Color Terms: Their Universality and Evolution.* Univ. of Calif. Press, Berkeley, CA.

Berns, R. S., Motta, R. J., and Gorzynski, M. E. 1993a. CRT colorimetry. Part I: Theory and practice. *Color Res. Appl.,* 18:299–314.

Berns, R. S., Gorzynski, M. E., and Motta, R. J. 1993b. CRT colorimetry. Part II: Metrology. *Color Res. Appl.,* 18:315–325.

Bishop, P. O. 1973. Neurophysiology of binocular single vision and stereopsis. In R. Jung (ed.), *Handbook of Sensory Physiology: Central Processing of Visual Information,* pp. 255–304. Springer-Verlag, Germany.

Bishop, P. O. 1979. Stereopsis and the random element in the organization of the striate cortex. *Proc. R. Soc. Lond. Ser. B,* 204:415–434.

Bishop, P. O. 1984. Processing of visual information within the retinostriate system. In I. Darien-Smith (ed.), *Handbook of Physiology: The Nervous System,* Vol. 3, pp. 257–316. Easton, NY.

Blakemore, C. and Campbell, F. W. 1969. On the existence of neurons in the human visual system selectively sensitive to the orientation and size of retinal images. *J. Physiol.,* 203:237–260.

Blakemore, C., Nachmias, J., and Sutton, P. 1970. The perceived spatial frequency shift: Evidence for frequency-selective neurons in the human brain. *J. Physiol.,* 210:727–750.

Blakemore, C. and Sutton, P. 1969. Size adaptation: A new aftereffect. *Science,* 166:245–247.

Blasdel, G. G. 1992. Differential imaging of ocular dominance and orientation selectivity in monkey striate cortex. *J. Neurosci.,* 12:3115–3138.

Boring, E. G. 1964. Size constancy in a picture. *Am. J. Psy.,* 77:494–498.

Born, R. T. and Tootell, R. B. H. 1992. Segregation of global and local motion processing in primate middle temporal visual area. *Nature,* 357:497–499.

Bowne, S. F. 1990. Contrast discrimination cannot explain spatial frequency, orientation or temporal frequency discrimination. *Vision Res.,* 30:449–461.

Boycott, B. B. and Dowling, J. 1969. Organization of the primate retina: Light microscopy. *Phil. Trans. R. Soc. B,* 255:109–184.

Boycott, B. B. and Wässle, H. 1974. The morphological types of ganglion cells of the domestic cat's retina. *J. Physiol.,* 240:397–419.

Boynton, R. M., Ikeda, M., and Stiles, W. S. 1964. Interactions among chromatic mechanisms as inferred from positive and negative increment thresholds. *Vision Res.,* 4:87–117.

Boynton, R. M. and Olson, C. X. 1987. Locating basic colors in the OSA space. *Col. Res. Appl.,* 12:94–105.

Bracewell, R. N. 1986a. *The Hartley Transform.* Oxford University Press, NY.

Bracewell, R. N. 1986b. *The Fourier Transform and Its Applications.* (2nd ed.) McGraw-Hill, NY.

Braddick, O. 1974. A short-range process in apparent motion. *Vision Res.*, 14:519–527.

Braddick, O. 1980. Low-level and high-level processes in apparent motion. *Phil. Trans. R. Soc. Lond. Series B*, 280:137–151.

Brainard, D. H. 1989. Calibration of a computer controlled color monitor. *Col. Res. Appl.*, 14:23–34.

Brainard, D. H. 1995. Colorimetry. In M. Bass (ed.), *Handbook of Optics. Vol. 1, Fundamentals, Techniques, and Design*, pp. 26.1–26.54. McGraw-Hill, Inc., NY.

Brainard, D. H. and Wandell, B. A. 1986. Analysis of the retinex theory of color vision. *J. Opt. Soc. Am.*, 3:1651–1661.

Brainard, D. H. and Wandell, B. A. 1990. Calibrated processing of image color. *Color Res. and Appl.*, 15:266–271.

Brainard, D. H. and Wandell, B. A. 1991a. A bilinear model of the illuminant's effect on color appearance. In J. A. Movshon and M. S. Landy (eds.), *Computational Models of Visual Processing*, pp. 171–187. MIT Press, Cambridge, MA.

Brainard, D. H. and Wandell, B. A. 1991b. The illuminant's effect on color appearance. In J. A. Movshon and M. S. Landy (eds.), *Cold Spring Harbor Symposium on Computational Models*, pp.169–186. The MIT Press, Cambridge, MA.

Brainard, D. H. and Wandell, B. A. 1992. Asymmetric color-matching: How color appearance depends on the illuminant. *J. Opt. Soc. Am.*, 9:1433–1448.

Bregman, A. S. 1981. Asking the "what for" question in auditory perception. In M. Kubovy and J. R. Pomerantz (eds.), *Perceptual Organization*, pp. 99–118. Lawrence Erlbaum Assoc., NJ.

Brewer, W. L. 1954. Fundamental response functions and binocular color matching. *J. Opt. Soc. Am.*, 44:207–212.

Brindley, G. S. 1970. *Physiology of the Retina and Visual Pathway*. Williams and Wilkins, Baltimore, MD.

Brindley, G. S. and Lewin, W. S. 1968. The sensations produced by electrical stimulation of the visual cortex. *J. Physiol.*, 196:479–493.

Britten, K. H., Shadlen, M. N., Newsome, W. T., and Movshon, J. A. 1992. The analysis of visual motion: A comparison of neuronal and psychophysical performance. *J. Neurosci.*, 12:4745–4765.

Bruner, J. S. and Potter, M. C. 1964. Interference in visual recognition. *Science*, 144:424–425.

Buchsbaum, G. 1980. A spatial processor model for object color perception. *J. Franklin Inst.*, 310:1–26.

Buchsbaum, G. and Gottschalk, A. 1984. Chromaticity coordinates of frequency-limited functions. *J. Opt. Soc. Am.*, 1:885–887.

Burkhalter, A. and Bernardo, K. L. 1989. Organization of corticocortical connections in human visual cortex. *Proc. Natl. Acad. Sci., U.S.A.*, 86:1071–1075.

Burkhalter, A., Bernardo, K. L., and Charles, V. 1993. Development of local circuits in human visual cortex. *J. Neurosci.*, 13:1916–1931.

Burnham, R. W., Evans, R. M., and Newhall, S. M. 1957. Prediction of color appearance with different adaptation illumination. *J. Opt. Soc. Am.*, 47:35–42.

Burns, S., Elsner, A. E., Pokorny, J., and Smith, V. C. 1984. The Abney effect: Chromaticity coordinates of unique and other constant hues. *Vision Res.*, 24:479–489.

Burr, D. C. 1987. Implications of the Craik-O'Brien illusion for brightness perception. *Vision Res.*, 27:1903–1913.

Burr, D. C., Morrone, M. C., and Ross, J. 1994. Selective suppression of the magnocellular visual pathway during saccadic eye movement. *Nature*, 371:511–513.

Burt, P. J. 1988. Smart sensing within a pyramid vision machine. *Proc. Inst. Electrical Electronics Engrs.*, 76:1006–1015.

Burt, P. J. and Adelson, E. J. 1983a. The Laplacian Pyramid as a compact image code. *Inst. Electrical Electronics Engrs. Trans. on Communications*, 31:532–540.

Burt, P. J. and Adelson, E. J. 1983b. A multiresolution spline with applications to image mosaics. *ACM Transactions on Graphics*, 2:217–236.

Byram, G. M. 1944. The physical and photochemical basis of resolving power. Part II. Visual acuity and the photochemistry of the retina. *J. Opt. Soc. Am.*, 34:718–738.

Campbell, F. W. and Green D. G. 1965. Optical and retinal factors affecting visual resolution. *J. Physiol.*, 181:576–593.

Campbell, F. W. and Gubisch, R. W. 1966. Optical quality of the human eye. *J. Physiol.*, 186:558–578.

Campbell, F. W. and Robson, J. G. 1968. Applications of Fourier analysis to the visibility of gratings. *J. Physiol.*, 197:551–566.

Carlbom, I., Terzopoulos, D., and Harris, K. M. 1994. Computer-assisted registration, segmentation, and 3D reconstruction from images of neuronal tissue sections. *Inst. Electrical Electronics Engrs. Transactions on Medical Imaging*, 13:351–362.

Carney, T., Paradiso, M. A., and Freeman, M. A. 1989. A physiological correlate of the Pulfrich effect in cortical neurons of the cat. *Vision Res.*, 29:155–165.

Cavanagh, P. and Anstis, S. 1991. The contribution of color to motion in normal and color-deficient observers. *Vision Res.*, 31:2109–2148.

Cavanagh, P., Boeglin, J., and Favrea, E. 1985. Perception of motion in equiluminous kinematograms. *Perception*, 14:151–162.

Cavanagh, P. and Mather, G. 1989. Motion: The long and short of it. *Spatial Vision*, 4:103–129.

Cavanagh, P., Tyler, C. W., and Favreau, O. E. 1984. Perceived velocity of moving chromatic patterns. *J. Opt. Soc. Am. (A)*, 1:893–899.

Chang, J. J. and Julesz, B. 1983. Displacement limits for spatial frequency filtered rand-dot cinematograms in apparent motion. *Vision Res.*, 23:1379–1385.

Chichilnisky, E. J. 1995. *Perceptual Measurements of Neural Computations in Color Appearance*. Ph.D. Dissertation, Stanford University, Stanford, CA.

Chichilnisky, E. J. and Wandell, B. A. 1995. Photoreceptor sensitivity changes explain color appearance shifts induced by large uniform backgrounds in dichoptic matching. *Vision Res.*, 35:239–254.

Chubb, C. and Sperling, G. 1988. Drift-balanced random stimuli: A general basis for studying non-Fourier motion perception. *J. Opt. Soc. Am. (A)*, 5:1986–2007.

Cicerone, C. M. and Nerger, J. L. 1989. The relative numbers of long-wavelength-sensitive to middle-wavelength-sensitive cones in the human fovea centralis. *Vision Res.*, 29:115–128.

CIE Proc. 1931, p.19, Cambridge University Press, Cambridge, 1932.

Cohen, J. 1964. Dependency of the spectral reflectance curves of the Munsell color chips. *Psychonomic Sci.*, 1:369–370.

Coletta, N. H and Williams, D. J. 1987. Psychophysical estimate of extrafoveal cone spacing. *J. Opt. Soc. Am.*, 4:1503–1513.

Cornsweet, T. N. 1970. *Visual Perception*. Academic Press, NY.

Crick, F. 1993. *The Astonishing Hypothesis: The Scientific Search for the Soul*. Scribner, NY.

Critchley, M. 1965. Acquired anomalies of colour perception of central origin. *Brain*, 88:711–724.

Curcio, C. A., Allen, K. A., Sloan, K. R., Lerea, C. L., Hurley, J. B., Klock, I. B., and Milam, A. H. 1991. Distribution and morphology of human cone photoreceptors stained with anti-blue opsin. *J. Comp. Neurol.*, 312:610–624.

Curcio, C. A. and Sloan, K. R. 1992. Packing geometry of human cone photoreceptors: Variation with eccentricity and evidence for local anisotropy. *Vis. Neurosci.*, 9:169–180.

Curcio, C. A., Sloan, K. R., Kalina, R. E., and Hendrickson, A. E. 1990. Human photoreceptor topography. *J. Comp. Neurol.*, 292:497–523.

Curcio, C. A., Sloan, K. R., and Meyers, D. 1989. Computer methods for sampling, reconstruction, display and analysis of retinal whole mounts. *Vision Res.*, 29:529–540.

Curcio, C. A., Sloan, K. R., Packer, O., Hendrickson, A. E., and Kalina, R. E. 1987. Distribution of cones in human and monkey retina: Individual variability and radial asymmetry. *Science*, 236:579–582.

da Vinci, Leonardo. 1906. A Treatise on Painting. (J. F. Rigaud, Trans.), G. Bell, London.

Dacey, D. M. 1993. Morphology of a small-field bistratified ganglion cell type in the macaque and human retina. *Visual Neurosci.*, 10:1081–1098.

Dacey, D. M. and Lee, B. B. 1994. The "blue-on" opponent pathway in primate retina originates from a distinct bistratified ganglion cell type. *Nature*, 367:731–735.

Dacey, D. M. and Petersen, M. R. 1992. Dendritic field size and morphology of midget and parasol ganglion cells of the human retina. *Proc. Natl. Acad. Sci., U.S.A.*, 89:9666–9670.

Damasio, A., Yamada, T., Damasio, H., Corbett, J., and McKee, J. 1980. Central achromatopsia: Behavioral, anatomic, and physiologic aspects. *Neurology*, 30:1064–1071.

Daubechies, I. 1990. The wavelet transform, time-frequency localization and signal analysis. *Inst. Electrical Electronics Engrs. Trans. Inf. Theory*, 36:961–1005.

de Lange, H. 1958. Research into the dynamic nature of the human fovea-cortex systems with intermittent and modulated light. II. Phase shift in brightness and delay in color perception. *J. Opt. Soc. Am.*, 48:784–789.

Dean, P. 1991. Visual cortex ablation and thresholds for successively presented stimuli in rhesus monkeys: II Hue. *Exp. Brain Res.*, 35:69–83.

DeAngelis, G. C., Ohzawa, I., and Freeman, R. D. 1991. Depth is encoded in the visual cortex by a specialized receptive field structure. *Nature*, 352:156–159.

DeAngelis, G. C., Ohzawa, I., and Freeman, R. D. 1993a. Spatiotemporal organization of simple-cell receptive fields in the cat's striate cortex. I: General characteristics and postnatal development. *J. Neurophysiol.*, 69:1091–1117.

DeAngelis, G. C., Ohzawa, I., and Freeman, R. D. 1993b. Spatiotemporal organization of simple-cell receptive fields in the cat's striate cortex. II: Linearity of temporal and spatial summation. *J. Neurophysiol.*, 69:1118–1135.

DeLucia, P. R. and Hochberg, J. 1991. Geometrical illusions in solid objects under ordinary viewing conditions. *Perception and Psychophysics,* 50:547–554.

DeMarco, P., et al. 1992. Full-spectrum cone sensitivity functions for X-chromosome-linked anomalous trichromats. *J. Opt. Soc. Am. (A),* 9:1465–1476.

DeMonasterio, F., McCrane, E. P., Newlander, J. K., and Schein, S. 1985. Density profile of blue-sensitive cones along the horizontal meridian of macaque retina. *Inv. Opthalmol. Vis. Sci.,* 26:289–302.

Derrico, J. B. and Buchsbaum, G. 1991. A computational model of spatiochromatic image coding in early vision. *J. Vis. Comm. and Image Repr.,* 2:31–38.

Derrington, A. M. and Henning, G. B. 1989. Some observations on the masking effects of two-dimensional stimuli. *Vision Res.,* 28:241–246.

Derrington, A. M., Krauskopf, J., and Lennie. P. 1984. Chromatic mechanisms in lateral geniculate nucleus of macaque. *J. Physiol.,* 357:241–265.

Derrington, A. M. and Lennie, P. 1984. Spatial and temporal contrast sensitivities of neurons in lateral geniculate nucleus of macaque. *J. Physiol.,* 357:219–240.

Desimone, R. and Schein, S. 1987. Visual properties of neurons in area V4 of the macaque: Sensitivity to stimulus form. *J. Neurophysiol.,* 57:835–868.

Desimone, R., Schein, S., Moran, J. and Ungerleider, L. 1985. Contour color and shape analysis beyond the striate cortex. *Vision Res.,* 25:441–452.

DeValois, K. K. 1977a. Spatial frequency adaptation can enhance contrast sensitivity. *Vision Res.,* 17:1057–1065.

DeValois, K. K. 1977b. Independence of black and white: Phase-specific adaptation. *Vision Res.,* 17:209–215.

DeValois, R. L. 1965a. Behavioral and electrophysiological studies of primate vision. In S. D. Neff (ed.), *Contributions to Sensory Perception,* pp. 137–177. Academic Press, NY.

DeValois, R. L. 1965b. Analysis and coding of color vision in the primate visual system. *Cold Spring Harb. Symp. Quant. Biol.,* 30:565–579.

DeValois, R. L., Abramov, I., and Jacobs, G. H. 1966. Analysis of response patterns of LGN cells, *J. Opt. Soc. Am.,* 56:966–977.

DeValois, R. L., Albrecht, D. G., and Thorell, L. G. 1982. Spatial frequency selectivity of cells in the macaque visual cortex. *J. Opt. Soc. Am.,* 67:779–784.

DeValois, R. L. and DeValois, K. K. 1988. *Spatial Vision,* Oxford, NY.

DeValois, R. L., Morgan, H. C., Polson, M. C., Mead, W. R., and Hull, E. M. 1974. Psychophysical studies of monkey vision: I. Macaque luminosity and color vision tests. *Vision Res.,* 14:53–67.

DeValois, R. L., Smith, C. J., Karoly, A. J., and Kitai, S. T. 1958a. Electrical responses of primate visual system. I. Different layers of macaque lateral geniculate nucleus. *J. Comp. Physio. Psych.,* 51:662–668.

DeValois, R. L., Smith, C. J., Kitai, S. T., and Karoly, A. J. 1958b. Responses of single cells in different layers of the primate lateral geniculate nucleus to monochromatic light. *Science,* 127:238–239.

Deyoe, E. A., Felleman, D. J., Van Essen, D. C., and McClendon, E. 1994. Multiple processing streams in occipitotemporal visual cortex. *Nature,* 371:151–154.

Deyoe, E. A. and Van Essen, D. C. 1988. Concurrent streams in monkey visual cortex. *Trends Neurosci.,* 11:219–226.

Dixon, R. E. 1978. Spectral distribution of Australian daylight. *J. Opt. Soc. Am.,* 68:437–450.

Dobelle, W. H., Turkel, J., Henderson, D. C., and Evans, J. R. 1979. Mapping the representation of the visual field by electrical stimulation of human cortex. *Am J. Opthalmol.,* 88:727–735.

Drew, M. S. and Funt, B. V. 1992. Natural metamers. *Computer Vision, Graphics, and Image Proc.,* 56:139–151.

Dubner, R. and Zeki, S. M. 1971. Response properties and receptive fields of cells in an anatomically defined region of the superior temporal sulcus in the monkey. *Brain Res.,* 35:528–532.

D'Zmura, M. and Iverson, G. 1993a. Color constancy. I. Basic theory of two-stage linear recovery of spectral descriptions for lights and surfaces. *J. Opt. Soc. Am. (A),* 10:2148–2165.

D'Zmura, M. and Iverson, G. 1993b. Color constancy. II. Results for two-stage linear recovery of spectral descriptions for lights and surfaces. *J. Opt. Soc. Am. (A),* 10:2166–2180.

D'Zmura, M. and Lennie, P. 1986. Mechanisms of color constancy. *J. Opt. Soc. Am. (A),* 3:1662–1672.

Emerson, R. C., Bergen, J. R., and Adelson, E. H. 1992. Directionally selective complex cells and the computation of motion energy in cat visual cortex. *Vision Res.,* 32:203–218.

Engel, S. A., Rumelhart, D. E., Wandell, B. A., Lee, A. T., Shadlen, M., and Glover, G. 1994. fMRI of human visual cortex. *Nature,* 369:525.

Enroth-Cugell, C., Hertz, G., and Lennie, P. 1977. Cone signals in the cat's retina. *J. Physiol.,* 269:273–296.

Enroth-Cugell, C. and Pinto, L. H. 1970. Algebraic summation of centre and surround inputs to retinal ganglion cells of the cat. *Nature,* 226:458–459.

Enroth-Cugell, C. and Robson, J. G. 1966. The contrast sensitivity of retinal ganglion cells of the cat. *J. Physiol.,* 187:517–522.

Enroth-Cugell, C. and Robson, J. G. 1984. Functional characteristics and diversity of cat retinal ganglion cells. *Inv. Opthalmol. Vis. Sci.,* 25:250–267.

Enroth-Cugell, C., Robson, J. G., Schweitzer-Tong, D. E., and Watson, A. B. 1983. Spatiotemporal interactions in cat retinal ganglion cells showing linear spatial summation. *J. Physiol.,* 341:279–301.

Escher, M. C. 1967. *The Graphic Work of M. C. Escher.* Oldbourne, London.

Esteban, D. and Galand, C. 1977. Applications of quadruture mirror filters to split band voice coding schemes. *Proc. ICASSP,* pp. 191–195.

Exner, S. 1888. Ueber optische Bewegungsempfindungen. *Biologischess Centralblatt,* 8:144–150.

Fahle, M. and Poggio, T. 1981. Visual hyperacuity: Spatiotemporal interpolation in human vision. *Proc. R. Soc. Lond. Ser. B,* 213:451–477.

Farrell, J. E. and Desmarais, M. 1990. Equating character-identification performance across the visual field. *J. Opt. Soc. Am. (A),* 7:152–159.

Farrell, J. E. and Wandell, B. A. 1993. Scanner linearity. *J. Elect. Imaging,* 2:225–230.

Felleman, D. J. and Van Essen, D. C. 1991. Distributed hierarchical processing in the primate cerebral cortex. *Cereb. Cortex,* 1:1–47.

Fennema, C. L. and Thompson, W. B. 1979. Velocity determination in scenes containing several moving objects. *Comp. Graphics and Image Proc.,* 9:301–315.

Ferster, D. 1981. A comparison of binocular depth mechanism in areas 17 and 18 of the cat visual cortex. *J. Physiol.,* 311:623–655.

Fitzpatrick, D., Itoh, K., and Diamond, I. T. 1983. The laminar organization of the lateral geniculate body and the striate cortex in the squirrel monkey. *J. Neurosci.,* 3:673–702.

Flamant, F. 1955. Etude de lar repartition de lumiere dans l'image retinienne d'une fente. *Rev. Opt.,* 34:433–459.

Fleet, D. J. and Langley, K. 1994. Computation analysis of non-Fourier motion. *Vision Res.,* 34:3057–3079.

Foley, J. M. and Legge, G. E. 1981. Contrast detection and near-threshold discrimination in human vision. *Vision Res.,* 21:1041–1053.

Foster, D. H. and Nascimento, S. M. C. 1994. Relational colour constancy from invariant cone-excitation ratios. *Proc. R. Soc. Lond. Ser. B,* 257:115–121.

Fox, P. T., Miezin, F., Allman, J., Van Essen, D. C., and Raichle, M. E. 1987. Retinotopic organization of human visual cortex mapped with positron emission tomography. *J. Neurosci.,* 3:913–922.

Fox, P. T., Mintun, M., Raichle, M. E., Meizin, F., Allman, J. M., and Van Essen, D. C. 1986. Mapping human visual cortex with positron emission tomography. *Nature,* 323:806–809.

Freeman, R. D., Mitchell, D. E., and Moolodot, M. 1972. A neural effect of partial visual deprivation in humans. *Science,* 175:1384–1386.

Freeman, R. D. and Ohzawa, I. 1990. On the neurophysiological organization of binocular vision. *Vision Res.,* 30:1661–1676.

Freeman, W. T. and Brainard, D. H. 1994. Bayesian decision theory, the maximum local mass estimate, and color constancy. *Mitsubishi Electric Research Laboratories,* Cambridge, MA.

Gallego, A. and Gouras, P. (eds.) 1985. *Neurocircuitry of the Retina: A Cajal Memorial.* International Congress of Eye Research, Elsevier, NY.

Geisler, W. S. 1987. Ideal-observer analysis of visual discrimination. In The Committee on Vision, NAS (ed.) *Frontiers of Visual Science,* pp. 17-31. National Academy Press, Washington, DC.

Geisler, W. S. 1989. Sequential ideal-observer analysis of visual discriminations. *Psy. Rev.,* 96:267–314.

Georgeson, M. A. and Harris, M. G. 1990. The temporal range of motion sensing and motion perception. *Vision Res.,* 30:615–620.

Gibson, I. M. 1962. Visual mechanisms in a cone-monochromat. *J. Physiol.,* 161:10P.

Gibson, J. J. 1950. *The Perception of the Visual World.* Houghton-Mifflin, Boston.

Gilbert, C. D. 1993. Circuitry, architecture, and functional dynamics of visual cortex. *Cerebral Cortex,* 3:373–386.

Gilbert, C. D. and Wiesel, T. M. 1992. Receptive field dynamics in adult primary visual cortex. *Nature,* 356:150–152.

Gilinsky, A. S. 1968. Orientation-specific effects of patterns of adapting light on visual acuity. *J. Opt. Soc. Am.,* 58:13–18.

Goldstein, B. E. 1989. *Sensation and Perception.* (3rd ed.) Wadsworth Publishing Co., Belmont, CA.

Goodman, J. W. 1968. *Introduction to Fourier Optics.* McGraw-Hill, San Francisco.

Gouras, P. 1968. Identification of cone mechanisms in monkey ganglion cells. *J. Physiol.,* 199:533–547.

Gouras, P. (ed.). 1991. *The Perception of Color.* CRC Press, Boca Raton, FL.

Graham, N. 1989. *Visual Pattern Analyzers.* Oxford University Press, Oxford.

Graham, N., Robson, J. G., and Nachmias, J. 1978. Grating summation in fovea and periphery. *Vision Res., 18*:815–825.

Graham, N. and Nachmias, J. 1971. Detection of grating patterns containing two spatial frequencies: A comparison of single-channel and multiple-channel models. *Vision Res., 11*:251–259.

Granger, E. M. and Heurtley, J. C. 1973. Visual chromatic modulation transfer function. *J. Opt. Soc. Am., 63*:73–74.

Green, G. J. and Lesell, S. 1977. Acquired cerebral dyschromatopsia. *Arch. Opthalmol., 95*:121–128.

Gregory, R. L. 1974. *Concepts and Mechanisms of Perception.* Duckworth, London.

Gregory, R. L. 1990. *Eye and Brain.* Princeton University Press, Princeton, NJ.

Gregory, R. L. and Wallace, J. 1963. Recovery from early blindness: A case study. *Expl. Psychol. Soc. Monograph, 2.*

Hartline, H. K. 1940. The receptive fields of optic nerve fibers. *Am. J. Physiol., 130*:690–699.

Hawken, M. J. and Parker, A. J. 1990. Detection and discrimination mechanisms in the striate cortex of the Old World monkey. In C. Blakemore (ed.), *Vision: Coding and Efficiency; Conference Cambridge, England,* pp.103–116.

Hawken, M. J., Parker, A. J., and Lund, J. S. 1988. Laminar organization and contrast sensitivity of direction-selective cells in the striate cortex of the Old World monkey. *J. Neurosci., 10*:3541–3548.

He, Z. H. and Nakayama, K. 1994a. Apparent motion determined by surface layout not by disparity or three-dimensional distance. *Nature, 367*:173–175.

He, Z. H. and Nakayama, K. 1994b. Perceived surface shape not features determines correspondence strength in apparent motion. *Vision Res., 34*:2125–2135.

Hecht, S., Schlaer, S., and Pirenne, M. H. 1942. Energy, quanta, and vision. *J. Gen. Physiol., 25*:819–840.

Heeger, D. J. 1992. Normalization of cell responses in cat striate cortex. *Visual Neurosci., 9*:181–197.

Heeger, D. J. and Jepson, A. D. 1992. Subspace methods for recovering rigid motion. I: Algorithm and implementations. *Int. J. Computer Vision, 7*:95–117.

Helmholtz, H. von. 1866/1911. *Treatise on Physiological Optics.* Translated from the 3rd German ed. 1909–1911. (J. P. Southall, Ed. and Trans.). Optical Society of America, Rochester, NY.

Helson, H. 1938. Fundamental problems in color vision. I. The principle governing changes in hue, saturation and lightness of non-selective samples in chromatic illumination. *J. Exp. Psych., 23*:439–476.

Hendrickson, A. E. 1985. Dots, stripes and columns in monkey visual cortex. *Trends Neurosci., 8*:406–410.

Hendrickson, A. and Yuodelis, C. 1984. The morphological development of the human fovea. *Opthalmol., 91*:603–612.

Hendry, S. H. C. and Yoshioka, T. 1994. A neurochemically distinct third channel in the macaque dorsal lateral geniculate nucleus. *Science, 264*:575–577.

Hering, E. 1905. Grundzuge der Lehre vom Lichtsinn. In *Handbuck der gesammter Augenheilkunde,* Vol. 3, Ch. 13. Berlin.

Hering, E. 1964. *Outlines of a Theory of the Light Sense.* L. M. Hurvich and D. Jameson, Trans. Harvard Univ. Press, Cambridge, MA.

Hess, R. F., Baker, C. L., Jr., and Zihl, J. 1989. The "motion-blind" patient: Low-level spatial and temporal filters. *J. Neurosci., 9*:1628–1640.

Heywood, C. A., Cowey, A., and Newcombe, F. 1991. Chromatic discrimination in a cortically color blind observer. *Eur. J. Neurosci., 3*:802–812.

Heywood, C. A., Gadotti, A., and Cowey, A. 1992. Cortical area V4 and its role in the perception of color. *J. Neurosci., 12*:4056–4065.

Heywood, C. A., Wilson, B., and Cowey, A. 1987. A case study of cortical colour "blindness" with relatively intact achromatic discrimination. *J. Neurol. Neurosurg. Psychiatry, 50*:22–29.

Hildreth, E. C., Ando, H., Anderson, R. A., and Treue, S. 1995. Recovering three-dimensional structure from motion with surface reconstruction. *Vision Res., 35*:117–138.

Hofeldt, A. J. and Hoefle, F. B. 1993. Stereophotometric testing for Pulfrich's phenomenon in professional baseball players. *Perceptual and Motor Skills, 77*:407–416.

Holmes, G. 1918. Disturbances of vision by cerebral lesions. *Bre. J. Opthal., 2*:353–384.

Holmes, G. 1945. The organization of the visual cortex in man. *Proc. R. Soc. Lond. Ser. B, 132*:348–361.

Horton, J. C. and Hoyt, W. F. 1991. The representation of the visual field in human striate cortex: A revision of the classic Holmes map. *Arch. Opthalmol., 109*:816–824.

Horton, J. C. and Hubel, D. H. 1981. A regular patchy distribution of cytochrome-oxidase staining in primary visual cortex of the macaque monkey. *Nature, 292*:762–764.

Horton, J. C. and Stryker, M. P. 1993.

Amblyopia induced by anisometropia without shrinkage of ocular dominance columns in human striate cortex. *Proc. Natl. Acad. Sci., U.S.A.,* 90:5494–5498.

Hubbard, R. and Wald, G. 1951. The mechanism of rhodopsin synthesis. *Proc. Natl. Acad. Sci., U.S.A.,* 37:69–79.

Hubel, D. H. 1982. Exploration of the primary visual cortex 1955–1978. (Nobel Lecture). *Nature,* 299:515–524.

Hubel, D. H. 1988. *Eye, Brain and Vision.* W. H.Freeman, NY.

Hubel, D. H. and Livingstone, M. S. 1987. Segregation of form, color, and stereopsis in primate area 18. *J. Neurosci.,* 7:3378–3415.

Hubel, D. H. and Wiesel, T. N. 1959. Receptive fields of single neurons in the cat's striate cortex. *J. Physiol.,* 148:574–591.

Hubel, D. H. and Wiesel, T. N. 1962. Receptive fields, binocular interaction and functional architecture in the cat's visual cortex. *J. Physiol.,* 160:106–154.

Hubel, D. H. and Wiesel, T. N. 1965. Binocular interaction in striate cortex of kittens reared with artificial squint. *J. Neurophysiol.,* 26:1041–1059.

Hubel, D. H. and Wiesel, T. N. 1968. Receptive fields and functional architecture of monkey striate cortex. *J. Physiol.,* 195:215–243.

Hubel, D. and Wiesel, T. 1972. Laminar and columnar distribution of geniculo-cortical fibers in the macaque monkey. *J. Comp. Neurol.,* 146:421–450.

Hubel, D. and Wiesel, T. 1977. Functional architecture of macaque visual cortex. *Proc. R. Soc. Lond. Ser. B,* (The Ferrier Lecture) 198:1–59.

Hubel, D. and Wiesel, T. 1990. Brain mechanisms of vision. In I. Rock (ed.), *The Perceptual World,* pp. 3–24. W. H. Freeman, NY.

Hubel, D. H., Wiesel, T. N., and LeVay, S. 1977a. Plasticity of ocular dominance columns in monkey striate cortex. *Phil. Trans. R. Soc. Lond. Series B,* 278:131–163.

Hubel, D. H., Wiesel, T. N., and Stryker, M. P. 1977b. Orientation columns in macaque monkey visual cortex demonstrated by the 2-deoxyglucose autoradiographic technique. *Nature,* 269:328–330.

Hubel, D. H., Wiesel, T. N., and Stryker, M. P. 1978. Anatomical demonstration of orientation columns in macaque monkey. *J. Comp. Neurol.,* 177:361–380.

Humphrey, A. and Hendrickson, A. 1980. Radial zones of high metabolic activity in squirrel monkey striate cortex. *Soc. Neurosci. Abstr.,* 6:315.

Humphrey, N. K. 1974. Vision in a monkey without striate cortex: A case study. *Perception,* 3:241–255.

Hurvich, L. and Jameson, D. 1957. An opponent-process theory of color vision. *Psych Rev.,* 64:384–404.

IJspeert, J. K., Van Den Berg, T., and Spekreijse, H. 1993. A mathematical description of the foveal visual point spread function with parameters for age, pupil size and pigmentation. *Vision Res.,* 33:15–20.

Inouye, T. 1909. *Die Sehstorungen bei Schussverietzungen derk kortikalen Sehsphare.* Leipzig, Germany.

Jameson, D. and Hurvich, L. M. 1955. Some quantitative aspects of an opponent-colors theory. I. Chromatic responses and spectral saturation. *J. Opt. Soc. Am.,* 45:546–552.

Jameson, D. and Hurvich, L. M. 1959. Perceived color and its dependence on focal surrounding, and preceding stimulus variables. *J. Opt. Soc. Am.,* 49:890–898.

Jameson, D and Hurvich, L. M. 1964. Theory of brightness and color contrast in human vision. *Vision Res.,* 4:135–154.

Jenkins, F. A. and White, H. 1976. *Fundamentals of Optics.* (4th ed.) McGraw-Hill, NY.

Jennings, J. A. M. and Charman, W. N. 1981. Off-axis image quality in the human eye. *Vision Res.,* 21:445–455.

Joshua, D. E. and Bishop, P. O. 1970. Binocular single vision and depth discrimination. Receptive field disparities for central and peripheral vision and binocular interaction on peripheral single units in cat striate cortex. *Exp. Brain Res.,* 10:389–416.

Judd, D. B. 1940. Hue saturation and lightness of surface colors with chromatic illumination. *J. Opt. Soc. Am.,* 30:2–32.

Judd, D. B. 1951a. Basic correlates of the visual stimulus. In S. S. Stevens (ed.), *Handbook of Exp. sychology,* pp. 811–867. J. Wiley, NY.

Judd, D. B. 1951b. Report of U. S. Secretariat Committee on Colorimetry and Artificial Daylight. *Proc. CIE I,* (Stockholm) 7:11.

Judd, D. B. 1960. Appraisal of Land's work on two-primary color projections. *J. Opt. Soc. Am.,* 50:254–268.

Judd, D. B., MacAdam, D. L., and Wyszecki, G. W. 1964. Spectral distribution of typical daylight as a function of correlated color temperature. *J. Opt. Soc. Am.,* 54:1031–1040.

Judd, D. and Wyszecki, G. 1975. *Color in Business, Science, and Industry.* Wiley, NY.

Julesz, B. 1961. Binocular depth perception of computer-generated patterns. *Bell Syst. Tech. J.,* 39:1125–1162.

Julesz, B. 1971. *Foundations of Cyclopean Perception.* University of Chicago Press, IL.

Kalmus, H. 1965. *Diagnosis and Genetics of Defective Color Vision*. Pergamon Press, NY.

Kanade, T., Peolman, C. J., and Morita, T. 1993. A factorization method for shape and motion recovery. *Trans. Inst. Electronics, Information and Communication Engrs.*, J76D-II:1497–1505.

Kanizsa, G. 1979. *Organization in Vision*. Praeger, NY.

Kaplan, E. and Shapley, R. M. 1982. X and Y cells in the lateral geniculate nucleus of macaque monkeys. *J. Physiol.*, 330:125–143.

Kaplan, E. and Shapley, R. M. 1986. The primate retina contains two types of ganglion cells, with high and low contrast sensitivity. *Proc. Natl. Acad. Sci., U.S.A.*, 83:2755–2757.

Kelly, D. H. 1961. Visual responses to time-dependent stimuli. I. Amplitude sensitivity measurements. *J. Opt. Soc. Am.*, 51:422–429.

Kelly D. H. 1966. Frequency doubling in visual responses. *J. Opt. Soc. Am.*, 56:1628–1633.

Kelly, D. H. 1971a. Theory of flicker and transient responses. I. Uniform fields. *J. Opt. Soc. Am.*, 61:537–546.

Kelly, D. H. 1971b. Theory of flicker and transient responses. II. Counterphase gratings. *J. Opt. Soc. Am.*, 61:632–640.

Kelly, D. H. 1979a. Motion and vision. I. Stabilized images of stationary gratings. *J. Opt. Soc. Am.*, 69:1266–1274.

Kelly, D. H. 1979b. Motion and vision. II. Stabilized spatio-temporal threshold surface. *J. Opt. Soc. Am.*, 69:1340–1349.

Kelly, D. H. and Burbeck. C. 1984. Critical problems in spatial vision. *CRC Crit. Rev. Biomed. Eng.*, 10:125–177.

Kersten, D. 1987. Predictability and redundancy of natural images. *J. Opt. Soc. Am. (A)*, 4:2395–2400.

Klinker, G. J., Shafer, S. A., and Kanade, T. 1988. The measurement of highlights in color images. *Intl. J. Computer Vision*, 2:7–32.

Knill, D. C. and Kersten, D. 1991. Apparent surface curvature affects lightness perception. *Nature*, 351:228–230.

Knoblauch, K. and McMahon, M. 1993. A test of Maxwell's and Cornsweet's conjecture on the dimension of color discrimination of binocular color mixtures in dichromacy. *Inv. Opthalmol. Vis. Sci.*, 34:233.

Koenderink, J. J. 1990. Some theoretical aspects of optic flow. In R. Warren and A. H. Wertheim (eds.), *Resources for Ecological Psychology: Perception and Control of Self-Motion*, pp.53–68. Lawrence Erlbaum Assoc., Inc., Hinsdale, NJ.

Koenderink, J. J. and Van Doorn, A. J. 1975. Invariant properties of the motion parallax field due to the movement of rigid bodies relative to an observer. *Optica Acta*, 22:773–791.

Kolb, H. 1994. The architecture of functional neural circuits in the vertebrate retina. *Inv. Opthalmol. Vis. Sci.*, 35:2385–2403.

Kolers, P. 1972. *Aspects of Motion Perception*. Pergamon Press, NY.

Komatsu, H. and Wurtz, R. H. 1989. Modulation of pursuit eye movements by stimulation of cortical areas MT and MST. *J. Neurophysiol.*, 62:31–47.

Korte, A. 1915. Kinematosskpische Untersuchungen. *Zeitschrift für Psychologie*, 72:193–206.

Kouyama, N. and Marschak, D. W. 1992. Bipolar cells specific for blue cones in the macaque retina. *J. Neurosci.*, 12:1233–1252.

Kouyama, N., et al. 1992. Bipolar cells specific for blue cones in the macaque retina. *J. Neurosci.*, 12:1233–1252.

Kuffler, S. W. 1953. Discharge patterns and functional organization of mammalian retina. *J. Neurophysiol.*, 16:37–68.

Kwong, K. K., Belliveau, J. W., Chesler, D. A., Goldberg, I. E., Weisskoff, R. M., Poncelet, B. P., Kennedy, D. N., and Hoppel, B. E. 1992. Dynamic magnetic resonance imaging of human brain activity during primary sensory stimulation. *Proc. Natl. Acad. Sci., U.S.A.*, 89:5675–5679.

Lachica, E. A., Beck, P. D., and Casagrande, V. A. 1992. Parallel pathways in macaque monkey striate cortex: Anatomically defined columns in layer III. *Proc. Natl. Acad. Sci., U.S.A.*, 89:3566–3570.

Land, E. H. 1959. Color vision and the natural image, Part I. *Proc. Nat. Acad. Sci., U.S.A.*, 45:116–129.

Land, E. H. 1986. Recent advances in retinex theory. *Vision Res.*, 26:7–22.

Larimer, J., Krantz, D. H., and Cicerone, C. M. 1975. Opponent-process additivity. II. Yellow/blue equilibria and nonlinear models. *Vision Res.*, 15:723–731.

Lawden, M. C. and Cleland, P. G. 1993. Achromatopsia in the aura of migraine. *J. Neurol. Neurosurg. Psychiatr.*, 56:708–709.

Lawson, C. L. and Hanson, R. J. 1974. *Solving Least Squares Problems*. Prentice-Hall, Englewood Cliffs, NJ.

Lee, H. 1986. Method for computing the scene-illuminant chromaticity from specular highlights. *J. Opt. Soc. Am. (A)*, 3:1662–1672.

Legge, G. E. and Foley, J. M. 1980. Contrast making in human vision. *J. Opt. Soc. Am.*, 70:1458–1471.

Legge, G. E., Kersten, D., and Burgess, A. E. 1987. Contrast discrimination in noise. *J. Opt. Soc. Am. (A)*, 4:391–404.

Legrand. Y. 1937. Recherches sur la diffusion

de la lumière dans l'oeil humain. *Rev. d' Opt.,* 16:201–241.

Lehrer, N. 1985. The challenge of the cathode-ray tube. In L. E. Tannas, Jr. (ed.), *Flat-panel displays and CRTs.* Van Nostran Reinhold Co., NY.

Lennie, P. 1980. Parallel visual pathways: A review. *Vision Res.,* 20:561–594.

Lennie, P., Krauskopf, J., and Sclar, G. 1990. Chromatic mechanisms in striate cortex of macaque. *J. Neurosci.,* 2:649–669.

Lettvin, J. Y., Maturan, H. R., McCulloch, W. S., and Pitt, W. H. 1959. What the frog's eye tells the frog's brain. *Proc. Institute of Radio Engineers,* 47:1940–1951.

Leventhal, A. G., Rodieck, R. W., and Dreher, B. 1981. Retinal ganglion cell classes in the Old World monkey: Morphology and central projections. *Science,* 213:1139–1142.

Leventhal, A. G., Thompson, K. G., Liu, D., Neuman, L. M., and Ault, S. J. 1993. Form and color are not segregated in monkey striate cortex. *Inv. Opthalmol. Vis. Sci.,* 34:4 (Abstract No. 233).

Levi, D. M., Klein, S. A., and Aitsebaomo, A. P. 1985. Vernier acuity, crowding and cortical magnification. *Vision Res.,* 25:963–977.

Livingstone, M. S. and Hubel, D. H. 1982. Thalamic inputs to cytochrome oxidase-rich regions in monkey visual cortex. *Proc. Natl. Acad. Sci., U.S.A.,* 79:6098–7101.

Livingstone, M. S. and Hubel, D. H. 1984a. Anatomy and physiology of a color system in the primate visual cortex. *J. Neurosci.,* 4:309–356.

Livingstone, M. S. and Hubel, D. H. 1984b. Specificity of intrinsic connections in primate primary visual cortex. *J. Neurosci.,* 4:2830–2835.

Livingstone, M. S. and Hubel, D. H. 1987a. Connections between layer 4B of area 17 and the thick cytochrome oxidase stripes of area 18 in the squirrel monkey. *J. Neurosci.,* 7:3371–3377.

Livingstone, M. S. and Hubel, D. H. 1987b. Psychophysical evidence for separate channels for the perception of form, color, movement, and depth. *J. Neurosci.,* 7:3416–3468.

Livingstone, M. S. and Hubel, D. H. 1988. Segregation of form, color, movement, and depth: Anatomy, physiology, and perception. *Science,* 240:740–749.

Livingstone, M. S., Rosen, G. D., Drislane, F. W., and Galaburda, A. M. 1991. Physiological and anatomical evidence for a magnocellular defect in developmental dyslexia. *Proc. Natl. Acad. Sci., U.S.A.,* 88:7943–7947.

Longuet-Higgins, H. C. and Prazdny, K. 1980. The interpretation of a moving retinal image. *Proc. R. Soc. Lond.,* 208:385–397.

Lund, J. S., Lund, R. D., Hendrickson, A. E., Bunt, A. H., and Fuchs, A. F. 1975. The origin of efferent pathways from primary visual cortex, area 17, of the macaque monkey as shown by retrograde transport of horseradish peroxidase. *J. Comp. Neurol.,* 164:287–304.

Lynch, J. J., Silveira, L. C. L., Perry, V. H., and Merigan, W. H. 1992. Visual effects of damage to P ganglion cells in macaques. *Vis. Neurosci.,* 8:575–583.

Lyons, N. P. and Farrell, J. E. 1989. Linear systems analysis of CRT displays. *Soc. Inf. Display '89 Digest,* 20:220–223.

MacLeod, D. I. A., Williams, D. R., and Makous, W. 1992. A visual nonlinearity fed by single cones. *Vision Res.,* 32:347–364.

Mallat, S. G. 1989. A theory for multiresolution signal decomposition: The wavelet representation. *Inst. Electrical Electronics Engrs. Trans. on Pattern Analysis and Machine Intelligence,* 11:674–693.

Maloney, L. T. 1986. Evaluation of linear models of surface spectral reflectance with small numbers of parameters. *J. Opt. Soc. Am. (A),* 3:1673–1683.

Maloney, L. T. and Wandell, B. 1986. Color constancy: A method for recovering surface spectral reflectance. *J. Opt. Soc. Am. (A),* 1:29–33.

Malpeli, J. G., Schiller, P. H., and Colby, C. L. 1981. Response properties of single cells in monkey striate cortex during reversible inactivation of individual lateral geniculate laminae. *J. Neurophysiol.,* 46:1102–1119.

Marc, R. E. and Sperling, H. G. 1977. Chromatic organization of primate cones. *Science,* 196:454–456.

Mariani, A. P. 1984. Bipolar cells in the monkey retina selective for the cones likely to be blue-sensitive. *Nature,* 308:184–186.

Marimont, D. H. and Wandell, B. A. 1992. Linear models of surface and illuminant spectra. *J. Opt. Soc. Am. (A),* 9:1905–1913.

Marimont, D. and Wandell, B. 1993. Matching color images: The effects of axial chromatic aberration. *J. Opt. Soc. Am. (A),* 12:3113-3122.

Marr, D. 1982. *Vision.* W. H. Freeman, San Francisco.

Martin, K. A. C. 1992. Visual cortex parallel pathways converge. *Curr. Biol.,* 2:555–557.

Mather, G. 1989. Early motion processes and the kinetic depth effect. *Quart. J. Exp. Psych.: Human Exp. Psych.,* 41:183–198.

Maunsell, J. H. R., Nealey, T. A., Depriest, D. D. 1990. Magnocellular and parvocellular contributions to responses in the middle temporal visual area (MT) of the macaque monkey. *J. Neurosci.,* 10:3323–3334.

Maunsell, J. H. R., Sclar, G., Nealey, T. A., and Depriest, D. D. 1991. Extraretinal representations in area V4 in the macaque monkey. *Visual Neurosci.*, 7:561–574.

Maxwell, J. C. 1855. Experiments on colour, as perceived by the eye, with remarks on colour-blindness. *Trans. Roy. Soc. Edin.*, 21:275–298.

McCamy, C. S., Marcus, H., and Davidson, J. G. 1976. A color-rendition chart. *J. Appl. Phot.*, 48:777–784.

McCann, J. J., Hall, J. A., and Land, E. H. 1977. Color mondrian experiments: The study of average spectral distributions. *J. Opt. Soc. Am. (A)*, 67:1380.

McLean, J. and Palmer, L. A. 1989. Contribution of linear spatiotemporal receptive field structure to velocity selectivity of simple cells in area 17 of cat. *Vision Res.*, 29:675–680.

McLean, J., Raab, S., and Palmer, L. A. 1994. Contribution of linear mechanisms to the specification of local motion by simple cells in areas 17 and 18 of the cat. *Visual Neurosci.*, 11:271–294.

Meadows, J. 1974a. Disturbed perception of colours associated with localized cerebral lesions. *Brain*, 97:615–632.

Meadows, J. C. 1975. The anatomical basis of prosopagnosia. *J. Neurol. Neurosurg. Psychiatr.*, 37:489–501.

Merbs, S. L. and Nathans, J. 1992. Absorption spectra of human cone pigments. *Nature*, 356:433–435.

Merigan, W. H., Bryne, C. E., and Maunsell, J. H. R. 1991a. Does primate motion perception depend on the magnocellular pathway? *J. Neurosci.*, 11:3422–3429.

Merigan, W. H., Katz, L. M., and Maunsell, J. H. R. 1991b. The effects of parvocellular lateral geniculate lesions on the acuity and contrast sensitivity of macaque monkeys. *J. Neurosci.*, 11:994–1001.

Merigan, W. H. and Maunsell, J. H. R. 1993. How parallel are the primate visual pathways? *Annu. Rev. Neurosci.*, 16:369–402.

Milgram, D. L. 1975. Computer methods for creating photomosaics. *Inst. Electrical Electronics Engrs. Trans. Comput.*, ?C-24:1113–1119.

Miller, W. H. and Bernard, G. 1983. Averaging over the fovea receptor aperture curtails aliasing. *Vision Res.*, 23:1365–1369.

Milner, A. D., et al., 1991. Perception and action in visual form agnosia. *Brain*, 114:405–428.

Mitchell, D. E. 1988. Animal models of human strabismic amblyopia: Some observations concerning the interpretation of the effects of surgically and optically induced strabismus in cats and monkeys. In P. G. Shinkman (ed.), *Advances in Neural and Behavioral Development*, Vol. 3, pp. 209–269. Ablex, Norwood, NJ.

Mollon, J. D. and Bowmaker, J. K. 1992. The spatial arrangement of cones in the primate fovea. *Nature*, 360:677–679.

Mollon, J. D., Newcombe, F., Polden, P. G., and Ratcliff, G. 1980. On the presence of three cone mechanisms in a case of total achromatopsia. In G. Verriest (ed.), *Color Vision Deficiencies, V.* pp. 130–135. The Hague, Netherlands.

Mollon, J. D. and Polden, P. G. 1977. An anomaly in the response of the eye to light of short wavelengths. *Philos. Trans. R. Soc. Lond. Ser. B*, 278:207–240.

Moreland, J. D. 1982. Spectral sensitivity measured by motion photometry. In J. G. Verriest (ed.), *Colour Deficiencies*, Vol. 6, pp. 61–66. The Hague, Netherlands.

Mountcastle, V. B. 1957. Modality and topographic properties of single neurons of cat's somatic sensory cortex. *J. Neurophysiol.*, 20:408–434.

Movshon, J. A., Adelson, E. H., Gizzi, M. S., and Newsome, W. T. 1985. The analysis of moving visual patterns. In C. Chagas, R. Gattass, and C. Gross (eds.), *Pattern Recognition Mechanisms, (Pontificiae Academiae Scientarum Scripta Varia, 45)*, pp. 117–151. Vatican Press, Rome.

Movshon, J. A., Lisberger, S. G., and Krauzlis, R. J. 1990. Visual cortical signals supporting smooth pursuit eye movements. In *Cold Spring Harb. Symp. Quant. Biol., Vol. 55. The Brain.* Cold Spring Harbor Laboratory Press, Cold Spring Harbor, NY.

Movshon, J. A., Thompson, I. D., and Tolhurst, D. J. 1978a. Spatial summation in the receptive fields of simple cells in the cat's striate cortex. *J. Physiol.*, 283:53–77.

Movshon, J. A., Thompson, I. D., and Tolhurst, D. J. 1978b. Receptive field organization of complex cells in the cat's striate cortex. *J. Physiol.*, 283:79–99.

Movshon, J. A. and Van Sluyters, R. 1981. Visual neural development. *Annu. Rev. Psych.*, 32:477–522.

Mullen, K. 1985. The contrast sensitivity of human colour vision to red–green and blue–yellow chromatic gratings. *J. Physiol.*, 359:381–400.

Nachmias, J. and Kocher, E. C. 1970. Visual detection and discrimination of luminance increments. *J. Opt. Soc. Am.*, 60:382–389.

Nachmias, J. and Rogowitz, B. E. 1983. Masking by spatially-modulated gratings. *Vision Res.*, 23:1621–1630.

Nachmias, J., Sansbury, R., Vassilev, A., and Weber, A. 1973. Adaptation to square-wave gratings: In search of the elusive third harmonic. *Vision Res.*, 13:1335–1342.

Naiman, A. C. and Makous, W. 1992. Spatial non-linearities of grayscale CRT pixels. *SPIE Proceedings: Human Vision, Visual Processing, and Digital Display III*, Vol. 1666.

Naka, K.-I. and Rushton, W. A. H. 1966. An attempt to analyse colour reception by electrophysiology. *J. Physiol.*, 185:587–599.

Nakayama, K. 1985. Biological image motion processing: A review. *Vision Res.*, 25:625–660.

Nakayama, K. and Shimojo, S. 1990. Da Vinci stereopsis: Depth and subjective occluding contours from unpaired image points. (Special Issue: Optics, physiology and vision.) *Vision Res.*, 30:1811–1825.

Nathans, J., Merbs, S. L., Sung, C.-H., Weitz, C. J., and Wang, Y. 1992. Molecular genetics of human visual pigments. In A. Campbell (ed.), *Annu. Review of Genetics*, Vol. 26, pp.403–424. Annual Reviews, Inc., Palo Alto, CA.

Nayar, S. K. and Bolle, R. M. 1993. Computing reflectance ratios from an image. *Pattern Recognition*, 26:1529–1542.

Nealey, T. A. and Maunsell, J. H. R. 1994. Magnocellular and parvocellular contributions to the responses of neurons in macaque striate cortex. *J. Neurosci.*, 14:2069–2079.

Neitz, M., Neitz, J., and Jacobs, G. H. 1991. Spectral tuning of pigments underlying red-green color vision. *Inv. Opthalmol. Vis. Sci.*, 32:1092.

Neitz, J., Neitz, M., and Jacobs, G. H. 1993. More than three different cone pigments among people with normal color vision. *Vision Res.*, 33:117–122.

Nerger, J. L. and Cicerone, C. M. 1992. The ratio of L cones to M cones in the human parafoveal retina. *Vision Res.*, 32:879–888.

Newhall, S. M., Nickerson, D., and Judd, D. B. 1943. Final report of the O.S.A. subcommittee on spacing of the Munsell colors. *J. Opt. Soc. Am.*, 33:385.

Newsome, W. T. and Paré, E. B. 1988. A selective impairment of motion perception following lesions of the middle temporal visual area (MT).*J. Neurosci.*, 8:2201–2211.

Newsome, W. T. and Wurtz, R. H. 1988. Probing visual cortical function with discrete chemical lesions. *Trends Neurosci.*, 11:394–400.

Newton, I. 1704. *Optiks*. Smith and Walford, London.

Nicholls, J. G., Martin, A. R., and Wallace, B. G. 1992. *From Neuron to Brain: A Cellular and Molecular Approach to the Function of the Nervous System*. (3rd ed.), Sinauer Associates, Sunderland, MA.

Nielsen, K. R. and Wandell, B. A. 1988.

Discrete analysis of spatial-sensitivity models. *J. Opt. Soc. Am. (A)*, 5:743–755.

Noorlander, C. and Koenderink, J. J. 1983. Spatial and temporal discrimination ellipsoids in color space. *J. Opt. Soc. Am.*, 73:1533–1543.

Obermayer, K. and Blasdel, G. G. 1993. Geometry of orientation and ocular dominance columns in monkey striate cortex. *J. Neurosci.*, 13:4114–4129.

O'Brien, V. 1958. Contour perception, illusion and reality. *J. Opt. Soc. Am.*, 48:112–119.

Ogawa, S., Tank, D. W., Menon, R., Ellerman, J. M., Kim, S.-G., Merkle, H., and Ugurbil, K. 1992. Intrinsic signal changes accompanying sensory stimulation: Functional brain mapping with magnetic resonance imaging. *Proc. Natl. Acad. Sci., U.S.A.*, 89:5951–5955.

Ogle, K. 1964. *Research in Binocular Vision*. Hafner, NY.

Ohzawa, I., DeAngelis, G. C., and Freeman, R. D. 1990. Stereoscopic depth discrimination in the visual cortex: Neurons ideally suited as disparity detectors. *Science*, 249:1037–1041.

O'Keefe, L. P., Levitt, J. B., Kiper, D. C., Shapley, R. M., and Movshon, J. A. 1993. Functional organization of owl monkey LGN and visual cortex. *Inv. Opthalmol. Vis. Sci.*, 34:4 (Abstract No.1021).

Ono, H. and Barbeito, R. 1985. Utrocular discrimination is not sufficient for utrocular identification. *Vision Res.*, 25:289–299.

Oppenheim, A. V., Willsky, A. S., and Young, I. T. 1983. *Signals and Systems*. Prentice-Hall, NJ.

Oren, M. and Nayar, S. K. 1994. Generalization of Lambert's reflectance model. *Computer Graphics Proc. Annual Conf. Series*, pp. 239–246.

Packer, O. and Williams, D. R. 1992. Blurring by fixational eye movements. *Vision Res.*, 32:1931–1939.

Palmer, L. A. and Davis, T. L. 1981. Receptive-field structure in cat striate cortex. *J. Neurophysiol.*, 46:260–276.

Pantle, A. and Sekuler, R. W. 1968. Size-detecting mechanisms in human vision. *Science*, 162:1146–1148.

Parker, A. and Hawken, M. 1985. Capabilities of monkey cortical cells in spatial resolution tasks. *J. Opt. Soc. Am. (A)*, 2:1101–1114.

Parkkinen, J. P. S., Hallikainen, J., and Jaaskelainen, T. 1989. Characteristic spectra of Munsell colors. *J. Opt. Soc. Am.*, 6:318–322.

Pasternak, T. and Merigan, W. H. 1981. The luminance dependence of spatial vision in the cat. *Vision Res.*, 21:1333–1340.

Pavlidis, T. and Tanimoto, S. L. 1975. A hierarchical data structure for picture processing. *Comp. Gr. Image Proc.*, 4:104–119.

Pearson, D. E. 1975. *Transmission and Display of Pictorial Information.* Wiley, NY.

Pekelsky, J. R., Cowan, W. B., and Rowell, N. L. 1988. Real-time measurement systems for colour CRT characterization (human perceptual response). *Proc. SPIE - The Intl. Soc. Opt. Eng.*, 901:223–228.

Perkins, M. E. and Landy, M. S. 1991. Nonadditivity of masking by narrow-band noises. *Vision Res.*, 31:1053–1066.

Perry, V. H. and Cowey, A. 1980. The projection of the fovea to the superior colliculus in rhesus monkeys. *Vision Res.*, 5:53–61.

Perry, V. H. and Cowey, A. 1981. The morphological correlates of X- and Y-like retinal ganglion cells in the retina of monkeys. *Exp. Brain Res.*, 43:226–228.

Perry, V. H., Oehler, R., and Cowey, A. 1984. Retinal ganglion cells that project to the dorsal lateral geniculate nucleus in the macaque monkey. *Neurosci.*, 12:1101–1123.

Phillips, G. C. and Wilson, H. R. 1984. Orientation bandwidths of spatial mechanisms measured by masking. *J. Opt. Soc. Am. (A)*, 1:226–232.

Poggio, G. F. and Fischer, B. 1977. Binocular interaction and depth sensitivity in striate and prestriate cortex of behaving rhesus monkey. *J. Neurophysiol.*, 40:1392–1405.

Poggio, G. F., Gonzalez, F., and Krause, F. 1988. Stereoscopic mechanisms in monkey visual cortex: Binocular correlation and disparity selectivity. *J. Neurosci.*, 8:4531–4550.

Poggio, G. F. and Talbot, W. H. 1981. Mechanisms of static and dynamic stereopsis in foveal cortex of the rhesus monkey. *J. Physiol.*, 315:469–492.

Poirson, A. B. and Wandell, B. A. 1993. The appearance of colored patterns: Pattern-color separability. *J. Opt. Soc. Am.*, 12:2458–2471.

Pokorny, J. Smith, V. Verriest, G., and Pinckers, A. 1979. *Congenital and Acquired Color Vision Defects.* Grune and Stratton, NY.

Polyak, S. L. 1941. *The Retina.* University of Chicago Press, Chicago.

Polyak, S. L. 1957. The vertebrate visual system. Heinrick Kluver (ed.). Univ. of Chicago Press., Chicago.

Posner, M. I. and Raichle, M. E. 1994. *Images of Mind.* Scientific American Library, NY.

Post, D. L. and Calhoun, C. S. 1989. An evaluation of methods for producing desired colors on CRT monitors. *Col. Res. Appl.*, 14:172–186.

Prazdny, K. 1983. On the information in optical flows. *Computer Vision, Graphics, and Image Proc.*, 22:239–259.

Press, W. H., et al. 1992. *Numerical Recipes in C: The Art of Scientific Computing.* (2nd ed.) Cambridge University Press, NY.

Pugh, E. N. 1976. The nature of the π_1 mechanism of W. S. Stiles. *J. Physiol.*, 257:713–747.

Pugh, E. N. and Mollon, J. D. 1979. A theory of the π_1 and π_2 colour mechanisms of Stiles. *Vision Res.*, 19:293–312.

Ramachandran, V. S. 1988. Perceiving shape from shading. *Sci. Amer.*, 259:58–65.

Ramachandran, V. S., Cobb, S. Rogers-Ramachandran, D. 1988. Perception of 3-D structure from motion: The role of velocity gradients and segmentation boundaries. *Perception and Psychophysics*, 44:390–393.

Ramón y Cajal, S. 1892. The retina of vertebrates. In D. Maguire and R. W. Rodieck, (trans.), *The Vertebrate Retina*, pp.775–904. W. H. Freeman, San Francisco.

Reid, R. C. and Shapley, R. M. 1992. Spatial structure of cone inputs to receptive fields in primate lateral geniculate nucleus. *Nature*, 356:716–718.

Richards, W. 1971. Anomolous stereoscopic depth perception. *J. Opt. Soc. Am.*, 61:410–414.

Rittenhouse, D. 1786. Explanation of an optical deception. *Trans. Am. Phil. Soc.*, 2:37–42.

Robson, J. G. 1966. Spatial and temporal contrast sensitivity functions of the visual system. *J. Opt. Soc. Am.*, 56:583–601.

Robson, J. G. 1980. Neural images: The physiological basis of spatial vision. In C. S. Harris (ed.), *Visual Coding and Adaptability*, pp. 177–214. Erlbaum.

Rockland, K. S. and Lund, J. S. 1983. Intrinsic laminar lattice connections in primate visual cortex. *J. Comp. Neurol.*, 216:303–318.

Rockland, K. S. and Pandya, D. N. 1979. Laminar origins and terminations of cortical connections of the occipital lobe in the rhesus monkey. *Brain Res.*, 179:3–20.

Rodieck, R. W. 1965. Quantitative analysis of cat retinal ganglion cell responses to visual stimuli. *Vision Res.*, 5:583–601.

Rodieck, R. W. 1973. *The Vertebrate Retina.* W. H. Freeman, San Francisco.

Rodieck, R., Binmoeller, K. F., and Dineen, J. D. 1985. Parasol and midget ganglion cells of the human retina. *J. Comp. Neurol.*, 233:115–132.

Rodieck, R. and Watanabe, M. 1993. Survey of the morphology of macaque retinal ganglion cells that project to the pretectum, superior colliculus, and parvicellular laminae of the lateral geniculate nucleus. *J. Comp. Neurol.,* 338:289–303.

Rovamo, J. and Virsu, V. 1979. An estimation an application of the human cortical magnification factor. *Expl. Brain Res.,* 37:495–510.

Rovamo, J., Virsu, V., and Nasaren, R. 1978. Cortical magnification factor predicts the photopic contrast sensitivity of peripheral vision. *Nature,* 271:54–56.

Royden, C. S., Banks, M. S., and Crowell, J. A. 1992. The perception of heading during eye movements. *Nature,* 360:583–585.

Ruechardt, E. 1958. Light: *Visible and Invisible.* University of Michigan Press, Ann Arbor, MI.

Rushton, W. A. H. 1962. Visual pigments in man.In R. Held and W. Richards (eds.), *Perception: Mechanisms and Models.* W. H. Freeman, NY.

Rushton, W. A. H. 1965. Visual adaptation: The Ferrier Lecture, 1962. *Proc. R. Soc. Lond. Ser. B,* 162:20–46.

Sacks, O. May 10, 1992. To see and not see. *The New Yorker,* pp.59–72.

Salzman, C. D., Murasugi, C. M., Britten, K. H., and Newsome, W. T. 1992. Microstimulation in visual area MT: Effects on direction discrimination performance. *J. Neurosci.,* 12:2331–2355.

Sastri, V. D. P. and Das, S. R. 1965b. Typical spectral distributions and color for tropical daylight. *J. Opt. Soc. Am.,* 58:391–398.

Schade, O. H. 1956. Optical and photoelectric analog of the eye. *J. Opt. Soc. Am.,* 46:721–739.

Schade, O. 1958. On the quality of color-television images and the perception of colour detail, *J. Soc. Mot. Pict. Telev. Eng.,* 67:801–819.

Schein, S. J. 1988. Anatomy of macaque fovea and spatial densities of neurons in foveal representation. *J. Comp. Neurol.,* 269:479–505.

Schiller, P. H. 1993. The effects of V4 and middle temporal (MT) area lesions on visual performance in the rhesus monkey. *Visual Neurosci.,* 10:717–746.

Schiller, P. H. and Lee, K. 1991. The role of the primate extrastriate area V4 in vision. *Science,* 251:1251–1253.

Schiller, P. H. and Lee, K. 1994. The effects of lateral geniculate nucleus, area V4, and middle temporal (MT) lesions on visually guided eye movements. *Visual Neurosci.,* 11:229–241.

Schiller, P. H. and Logothetis, N. K. 1990. The color-opponent and brad-based channels

of the primate visual system. *Trends Neurosci.,* 10:392–398.

Schiller, P. and Malpeli, J. 1978. Functional specificity of lateral geniculate nucleus laminae of the rhesus monkey. *J. Neurophysiol.,* 41:788–797.

Schnapf, J. L., Kraft, T. W., and Baylor, D. A. 1987. Spectral sensitivity of human cone photoreceptors. *Nature,* 325:439–441.

Schnapf, J. L., Kraft, T. W., Nunn, B. J., and Baylor, D. A. 1989. Transduction in primate cones. *Neurosci. Res.,* 10:9–14.

Schnapf, J. L., Nunn, B. J., Meister, M., and Baylor, D. A. 1990. Visual transduction in cones of the monkey *Macaca Fascicularis. J. Physiol.,* 427:681–713.

Schrodinger, E. 1970. Measurement for daylight vision. In D. L. MacAdam (ed.), *Sources of Color Science,* pp.134–182. MIT Press, Cambridge, MA.

Schwartz, E. A. 1977. Voltage noise observed in rods of the turtle retina. *J. Physiol.,* 272:217–246.

Sekiguchi, N., Williams, D. R., and Brainard, D. H. 1993a. Aberration-free measurements of the visibility of isoluminant gratings. *J. Opt. Soc. Am. (A),* 10:2105–2117.

Sekiguchi, N., Williams, D. R., and Brainard, D. H. 1993b. Efficiency in detection of isoluminant and isochromatic interference fringes. *J. Opt. Soc. Am. (A),* 10:2118–2133.

Sekuler, R. and Blake, R. 1985. *Perception.* Alfred A. Knopf, NY.

Shadlen, M and Carney, T. 1986. Mechanisms of human motion perception revealed by a new cyclopean illusion. *Science,* 232:95–97.

Shafer, S. A. 1985. Using color to separate reflection components. *Color Res. Appl.,* 10:210–218.

Shapley, R. 1990. Visual sensitivity and parallel retinocortical channels. *Annu. Rev. Psy.,* 41:635–658.

Shatz, C. J. 1992. The developing brain. *Sci. Amer.,* 267:60–67.

Shatz, C. J. and Stryker, M. P. 1978. Ocular dominance in Layer IV of the cat's visual cortex and the effects of monocular deprivation. *J. Physiol.,* 281:267–283.

Shepard, R. N. 1990. *Mind Sights.* W. H. Freeman and Co., NY.

Sherman, S. M. and Koch, C. 1990. Thalamus. In Gordon M. Shepherd (ed.), *The Synaptic Organization of the Brain.* (3rd ed.), Oxford University Press, NY.

Sherwood, S. L. (ed.) 1966. *The Nature of Psychology: A Selection of Papers, Essays and Other Writings by the Late K. J. W. Craik.* Cambridge University Press, Cambridge.

Shimojo, S., Silverman, G. H., and Nakayama, K. 1988. An occlusion-related mechanism of depth perception based on motion and interocular sequence. *Nature,* 333:265–268.

Siegel, R. M. and Andersen, R. A. 1986. Motion perceptual deficits following ibotenic acid lesions of the middle temporal area (MT) in the behaving rhesus monkey. *Soc. Neurosci. Abstr.,* 12:1183.

Simoncelli, E. P. 1988. *Orthogonal Sub-band Image Transforms.* Unpublished Masters Thesis, Elect. Eng. and Comp. Sci., Massachusetts Institute of Technology.

Simoncelli, E. P. 1993. *Distributed representation and analysis of visual motion.* Vision and Modeling Group Tech. Rep. No. 209, MIT Medial Laboratory, Cambridge, MA.

Simoncelli, E. P. and Adelson, E. H. 1990. Non-separable extensions of quadrature mirror filters to multiple dimensions. *Proc. Inst. Electrical Electronics Engrs.,* 78:652–664.

Skottun, B. C., De Valois, R. L., Grosof, D. H., Movshon, J. A., Albrecht, D. G., and Bonds, A. B. 1991. Classifying simple and complex cells on the basis of response modulation. *Vision Res.,* 31:1079–1086.

Smith, A. T. and Edgars, G. K. 1990. The influence of spatial frequency on perceived temporal frequency and perceived speed. *Vision Res.,* 30:1467–1474.

Smith, V. C. and Pokorny, J. 1972. Spectral sensitivity of color-blind observers and the cone photopigments. *Vision Res.,* 12:2059–2071.

Sperling, G. 1989. Three stages and two systems of visual processing. *Spatial Vision,* 4:183–207.

Spillman, L. and Werner, J. (eds.) 1990. *Visual Perception: The Neurophysiological Foundations.* Academic Press, San Diego.

Sprague, J. M., Levy, J., DiBerardino, A., and Berlucchi, G. 1977. Visual cortical areas mediating form discrimination in the cat. *J. Comp. Neurol.,* 172:441–488.

Sterling, P., Calkins, D. J., Klug, K. J., Schein, S. J., and Tsukamoto, Y. 1994. Parallel pathways from primate fovea. *Inv. Opthalmol. Vis. Sci.,* 35:2001.

Sternheim, C. E., Stromeyer, C. F. III, and Khoo, M. C. K. 1979. Visibility of chromatic flicker upon spectrally mixed adapting fields. *Vision Res.,* 19:175–183.

Stevens, J. K. and Gerstein, G. L. 1976. Spatiotemporal organization of cat lateral geniculate receptive fields. *J. Neurophysiol.,* 39:213–238.

Stevens, S. S. 1951. *Handbook of Experimental Psychology.* J. Wiley, NY.

Stevens, S. S. 1962. The surprising simplicity of sensory metrics. *Am. Psy.,* 17:29–39.

Stiles, W. S. 1939. The directional selectivity of the retina and the spectral sensitivities of the rods and cones. *Proc. R. Soc. Lond. Ser. B,* 127:64–105.

Stiles, W. S. 1959. Color vision: The approach through increment-threshold sensitivity. *Proc. Nat. Acad. Sci., U.S.A.,* 45:100–114.

Stiles, W. S. 1978. *Mechanisms of Colour Vision.* Academic Press, London.

Stiles, W. S. and Burch, J. M. 1959. N. P. L. colour-matching investigation: Final report (1958). *Optica Acta,* 6:1.

Stockman, S., MacLeod, D. I., and Johnson, N. E. 1993. Spectral sensitivities of the human cones. *J. Opt. Soc. Am. (A),* 10:2491–2521.

Stone, L. S. and Thompson, P. 1992. Human speed perception is contrast dependent. *Vision Res.,* 32:1535–1549.

Stoner, G. R., Albright, T. D., and Ramachandran, V. S. 1990. Transparency and coherence in human motion perception. *Nature,* 344:153–155.

Strang, G. 1993. *Introduction to Linear Algebra.* Wellesley-Cambridge Press, Wellesley, MA.

Stromeyer, C. III, Cole, G. R., and Kronauer, R. E. 1985. Second-site adaptation in the red–green chromatic pathways. *Vision Res.,* 25:219–237.

Stryker, M. 1994. Precise development from imprecise rules. *Science,* 263:1244–1245.

Stryker, M. and Harris, W. 1986. Binocular impulse blockade prevents the formation of ocular dominance columns in cat visual cortex. *J. Neurosci.,* 6:2117–2133.

Svaetichin, G. 1956. Spectral response curves from single cones. *Acta Physiologica Scandinavica,* 134:17–46.

Svaetichin, G. and MacNichol, E. F. 1958. Retinal mechanisms for chromatic and achromatic vision. *Ann. N. Y. Acad. Sci.,* 74:385–404.

Teller, D. 1990. The domain of visual science. In L. Spillman and J. Werner (eds.), *Visual Perception: The Neurophysiological Foundations,* pp. 11–19. Academic Press, NY.

Teuber, H. L., Battersby, W. S., and Bender, M. B. 1960. *Visual Field Defects after Penetrating Missile Wounds of the Brain.* Harvard University Press, Cambridge, MA.

Thibos, L. N., Ming, Y., Xiaoxiao, Z., and Bradley, A. 1992. The chromatic eye: A new reduced-eye model of ocular chromatic aberration in humans. *Appl. Optics,* 31:3594–3600.

Thomas, I., Simoncelli, E., and Bajcsy, R. 1994. Spherical retinal flow for a fixating observer. In *Proceedings of the Workshop on Visual Behaviors,* pp. 37–44. Inst. Electrical Electronics Engrs. Computer Society Press, Los Alamitos, CA.

Thompson, P. 1980. Margaret Thatcher: A new illusion. *Perception,* 9:483–484.

Thompson, P. and Wood, V. 1993. The Pulfrich pendulum phenomenon in stereoblind subjects. *Perception,* 22:7–14.

Tolhurst, D. J. and Dean, A. F. 1987. Spatial

summation by simple cells in the striate cortex of the cat. *Exp. Brain Res.,* 66:607–620.

Tolhurst, D. J., Movshon, J. A., and Dean, A. F. 1983. The statistical reliability of signals in single neurons in cat and monkey visual cortex. *Vision Res.,* 23:775–785.

Tomasi, C. and Kanade, T. 1992. Shape and motion from image streams under orthography: A factorization method. *Int. J. Computer Vision,* 9:137–154.

Tomasi, C., et al. 1992. Shape and motion from image streams under orthography: A factorization method. *Int. J. Computer Vision,* 9:137–154.

Tominaga, S. and Wandell, B. A. 1989. The standard surface reflectance model and illuminant estimation. *J. Opt. Soc. Am. (A),* 6:576–584.

Tominaga, S. and Wandell, B. 1990. Component estimation of surface spectral reflectance. *J. Opt. Soc. Am. (A),* 7:312–317.

Tran, A., Liu, K., Tzou, K., and Vogel, E. 1987. An efficient pyramid image coding system. *Proc. ICASSP,* 18.6.1–18.6.4.

Treue, S., Andersen, R. A., Ando, H., and Hildreth, E. C. 1995. Structure-from-motion: Perceptual evidence for surface interpolation. *Vision Res.,* 35:139–148.

Treue, S., Husain, M., and Andersen, R. A. 1991. Human perception of structure from motion. *Vision Res.,* 31:59–76.

Ungerleider, L. G. and Mishkin, M. 1982. Two cortical visual systems. In D. J. Ingle, R. J. W. Mansfield, and M. S. Goodale, (eds.), *The Analysis of Visual Behavior,* pp. 549–586. MIT Press, Cambridge, MA.

Vaina, L. M., et al. 1990. Intact "biological motion" and "structure from motion" perception in a patient with impaired motion mechanisms: A case study. *Visual Neurosci.,* 5:353–369.

Valvo, A. 1971. *Sight Restoration after Long-Term Blindness: The Problems and Behavior Patterns of Visual Rehabilitation.* Am. Foundation for the Blind, NY.

Van Essen, D. C., et al. 1992. Information processing in the primate visual system: An integrated systems perspective. *Science,* 255:419–423.

van Nes, F. L. and Bouman, M. A. 1967. Spatial modulation transfer in the human eye. *J. Opt. Soc. Am.* 57:401–406.

Van Santen, J. and Sperling, G. 1985. Elaborated Reichardt detectors. *J. Opt. Soc. Am. (A),* 2:300–321.

Verrey, L. 1888. Hemiachromatopsie droite absolue. *Arch. d'Opthalmologie, Paris,* 8:289–301.

Vetterli, M. 1986. Filter banks allowing perfect reconstruction. *Sig. Proc.,* 10:219–244.

Vetterli, M. and Metin, U. K. 1992. Multiresolution coding techniques for digital television: A review. *Multidimensional Systems and Signal Processing,* 3:161–187.

Victor, J. D., Maiese, K., Shapley, R., Sidtis, J., and Gazzaniga M. 1987. Acquired central dyschromatopsia with presentation of color discrimination. *Clin. Vis. Sci.,* 3:183–196.

Virsu, V. and Rovamo, J. 1979. Visual resolution, contrast sensitivity, and the cortical magnification factor. *Exp. Brain Res.,* 37:475–494.

Vogels, R. and Orban, G. A. 1990. How well do response changes of striate neurons signal differences in orientation: A study in the discriminating monkey. *J. Neurosci.,* 10:3543–3558.

Volkman, F. C., Riggs, L. A., White, K. D., and Moore, R. K. 1978. Contrast sensitivity during saccadic eye movements. *Vision Res.,* 18:1193–1200.

von der Heydt, R., Adorjani, C., Hanny, P., and Baumgartner, G. 1978. Disparity sensitivity and receptive field incongruity of units in the cat striate cortex. *Exp. Brain Res.,* 31:523–545.

von Baumgarten, R. and Jung, R. 1952. Microelectrode studies on the visual cortex. *Rev. Neurol.,* 87:151–155.

von Kries, J. 1970a. Influence of adaptation on the effects produced by luminous stimuli. In D. L. MacAdam, (ed.), *Sources of Color Science,* pp. 120–127. The MIT Press, Cambridge, MA.

von Kries, J. 1970b. Chromatic adaptation. In D. L. MacAdam, (ed.), *Sources of Color Science,* pp. 109–119. The MIT Press, Cambridge, MA.

von Senden, M. 1960. Space and sight: The perception of space and shape in the congenitally blind before and after operation. Peter Heath (trans.) Free Press, Glencoe, IL.

Vrhel, M. J. and Trussell, H. J. 1994. Filter considerations in color correction. *Inst. Electrical Electronics Engrs. Trans. Image Proc.,* 3:147–161.

Wald, G. 1968. The molecular basis of visual excitation. *Nature,* 219:800–807.

Wald, G. and Brown, P. K. 1956. Synthesis and bleaching of rhodopsin. *Nature,* 177:174–176.

Wald, G. and Griffin, D. R. 1947. The change in refractive power of the human eye in dim and bright light. *J. Opt. Soc. Am.,* 37:321–336.

Wallach, H. 1987. Perceiving a stable environment when one moves. *Annu. Rev. Psych.,* 38:1–27.

Walls, G. L. 1960. "Land! Land!" *Psy. Bull.,* 57:29–48.

Wandell, B. A. 1985. Color measurement and discrimination. *J. Opt. Soc. Am. (A)*, 2:62–71.

Wandell, B. A. 1987. The synthesis and analysis of color images. *Inst. Electrical Electronics Engrs. PAMI*, 9:2–13.

Wandell, B. 1993. Color appearance: The effects of illumination and spatial resolution. *Proc. Natl. Acad. Sci., U.S.A.*, 90:1494–1501.

Wandell, B. A. and Pugh, E. N. 1980a. A field-additive pathway detects brief-duration, long-wavelength incremental flashes. *Vision Res.*, 20:613–624.

Wandell, B. A. and Pugh, E. N. 1980b. Detection of long-duration, long-wavelength incremental flashes by a chromatically coded pathway. *Vision Res.*, 20:625–636.

Warren, W. H. and Hannon, D. J. 1988. Direction of self-motion is perceived from optical flow. *Nature*, 336:162–163.

Warren, W. H., Jr. and Hannon, D. J. 1990. Eye movements and optical flow. *J. Opt. Soc. Am. (A)*, 7:160–169.

Wassef, E. G. T. 1952. Application of the binocular matching method to the study of the subjective appearance of surface colours. *Optica Acta*, 2:144–150.

Wassef, E. G. T. 1958. Investigation into the theory of prediction of the appearance of colors and its bearing on the theory of color vision. *Optica Acta*, 5:101–108.

Wassef, E. G. T. 1959. Linearity of the relationship between the tristimulus values of corresponding colours seen under different conditions of chromatic adaptation. *Optica Acta*, 6:378–393.

Wässle, H. and Boycott, B. B. 1991. Functional architecture of the mammalian retina. *Physiol. Rev.*, 71:447–480.

Wässle, H., Gruenert, U., Roehrenbeck, J., and Boycott, B. B. 1990. Retinal ganglion cell density and cortical magnification factor in the primate. *Vision Res.*, 30:1897–1912.

Watanabe, M. and Rodieck, R. 1989. Parasol and midget ganglion cells of the primate retina. *J. Comp. Neurol.*, 289:434–454.

Watson, A. B. 1983. Detection and recognition of simple spatial forms. In A. C. Slade (ed.), *Physical and Biological Processing of Images*, pp. 100–114. Springer-Verlag, Germany.

Watson, A. B. 1990. Perceptual-components architecture for digital video. *J. Opt. Soc. Am. (A)*, 7:1943–1954.

Watson, A. B. and Ahumada, A. J., Jr. 1985. Model of human visual-motion sensing. *J. Opt. Soc. Am. (A)*, 2:322–342.

Watson, A. B. and Ahumada, A. J., Jr. 1989. A hexagonal orthogonal-oriented pyramid as a model of image representation in visual cortex. *Inst. Electrical Electronics Engrs. Trans. on Biomed. Eng.*, 36:97–106.

Watson, A. B., Ahumada, A., and Farrell, J. E. 1983. *The window of visibility: A psychophysical theory of fidelity in time-sampled visual motion displays.* NASA Technical Paper 2211.

Watt, R. and Morgan, M. 1985. A theory of the primitive spatial code in human vision. *Vision Res.*, 25:1661–1674.

Weale, R. A. 1953. Cone-monochromatism. *J. Physiol.*, 121:548–569.

Weale, R. A. 1959. Photosensitive reactions in fovea of normal and cone-monochromatic observers. *Optica Acta*, 6:158–174.

Wertheimer, M. 1912. Experimentelle Studien uber das Sehen von Bewegung. *Zeitschrift für Psychologie*, 72:193–206.

Westheimer, G. 1960. Modulation thresholds for sinusoidal light distribution on the retina. *J. Physiol.*, 152:67–74.

Westheimer, G. 1979. The spatial sense of the eye. *Inv. Opthalmol. Vis. Sci.*, 18:893–912.

Westheimer, G. 1986. The eye as an optical instrument. In J. Thomas, et al., (ed.), *Handbook of Perception*, pp.4.1–4.20. Wiley, NY.

Westheimer, G. 1990. Relating neural mechanisms to visual perception: Historical and philosophical considerations. In L. Spillman and J. Werner (eds.), *Visual Perception: The Neurophysiological Foundations*, pp. 5–10. Academic Press, NY.

Westheimer, G. and McKee, J. 1977. Spatial configurations for visual hyperacuity. *Vision Res.*, 17:941–947.

Wheatstone, C. 1838. Contributions to the physiology of vision. Part I: On some remarkable, and hitherto unobserved, phenomena of binocular vision. *Phil. Trans. R. Soc. Lond.*, 128:371–394.

Wiesel, T. N. and Hubel, D. H. 1966. Spatial and chromatic interactions in the lateral geniculate body of the rhesus monkey. *J. Neurophysiol.*, 29:1115–1156.

Wikler, K. C., Williams, R. W., and Rakic, P. 1990. Photoreceptor mosaic: Number and distribution of rods and cones in the rhesus monkey retina. *J. Comp. Neurol.*, 297:499–508.

Williams, D. R. 1985a. Visibility of interference fringes near the resolution limit. *J. Opt Soc. Am. (A)*, 2:1087–1093.

Williams, D. R. 1985b. Aliasing in human foveal vision. *Vision Res.*, 25:195–295.

Williams, D. R. 1986. Seeing through the photoreceptor mosaic. *Trends Neurosci.*, 9:193–197.

Williams, D. R. 1988. Topography of the foveal cone mosaic in the living human eye. *Vision Res.*, 28:433–454.

Williams, D. R., Brainard, D. H., McMahon, M. J., and Navarro, R. 1994. Double-pass and interferometric measures of the optical quality of the eye. *J. Opt. Soc. Am. (A),* 11:3123–3135.

Williams, D. R. and Collier, R. J. 1983. Consequences of spatial sampling by a human photoreceptor mosaic. *Science,* 221:385–387.

Williams, D., MacLeod, D. I. A., and Hayhoe, M. 1981. Punctate sensitivity of the blue sensitive mechanism. *Vision Res.,* 21:1357–1375.

Wilson, H. R. and Gelb, D. J. 1984. Modified line-element theory for spatial-frequency and width discrimination. *J. Opt. Soc. Am.,* 1:124–131.

Wilson, H. R., McFarlane, D. K., and Phillips, G. C. 1983. Spatial frequency tuning of orientation selective units estimated by oblique masking. *Vision Res.,* 23:873–882.

Wilson, H. R. and Regan, D. 1984. Spatial-frequency adaptation and grating discrimination: Predictions of a line-element model. *J. Opt. Soc. Am.,* 1:1091–1096.

Wolff, L. B. 1994. Relative brightness of specular and diffuse reflection. *Opt. Engr.,* 33:285–293.

Wong-Riley, M. 1979. Changes in the visual system of monocularly sutured or enucleated cats demonstrated with cytochrome oxidase histochemistry. *Brain Res.,* 171:11–28.

Wulfing, E. 1892. Uber den kleinsten Gesichtswinkel. *Z. Biol.,* 29:199–202.

Wyszecki, G. and Stiles, W. S. 1982. *Color Science.* (2nd ed.) John Wiley and Sons, NY.

Yamashita, M. and Wässle, H. 1991. Responses of rod bipolar cells isolated from the rat retina to the glutamate agonist 2-amino-4-phosphonobutyric acid (APB). *J. Neurosci.,* 11:2372–2382.

Yap, Y. L., Levi, D. M., and Klein, S. A. 1987. Peripheral hyperacuity:; Three-dot bisection scales to a single factor from 0 to 10 degrees. *J. Opt. Soc. Am.,* 4:1557–1561.

Yellott, J. I. 1982. Spectral analysis of spatial sampling by photoreceptors: Topological disorder prevents aliasing. *Vision Res.,* 22:1205–1210.

Yellott, J. I., Wandell, B. A., and Cornsweet, T. N. 1984. The beginnings of visual perception: The retinal image and its initial encoding. In I. Darien-Smith (ed.), *Handbook of Physiology: The Nervous System.* Vol 3. pp. 257–316. Easton, NY.

Young, T. 1802. On the theory of light and colors. *Phil. Trans. R. Soc. Lond.,* 92:12–48.

Zeki, S. M. 1973. Colour coding in rhesus monkey prestriate cortex. *Brain Res.,* 53:422–427.

Zeki, S. M. 1974. Functional organisation of a visual area in the posterior bank of the superior temporal sulcus of the rhesus monkey. *J. Physiol.,* 236:549–573.

Zeki, S. 1977. Colour coding in the superior temporal sulcus of rhesus monkey visual cortex. *Proc. R. Soc. Lond. Ser. B,* 195:517–523.

Zeki, S. 1978. Uniformity and diversity of structure and function in rhesus monkey prestriate visual cortex. *J. Physiol.,* 277:273–290.

Zeki, S. M. 1980. The representation of colours in the cerebral cortex of the monkey. *Nature,* 284:412–418.

Zeki, S. M. 1983. The distribution of wavelength and orientation selective cells in different areas of monkey visual cortex. *Proc. R. Soc. Lond. Ser. B,* 217:449–470.

Zeki, S. 1985. Color pathways and hierarchies in the cerebral cortex. In D. Ottoson and S. Zeki (eds.), *Central and Peripheral Mechanisms of Color Vision,* pp. 19–44. MacMillan, London.

Zeki, S. 1990a. Parallelism and functional specialization in human visual cortex. *Cold Spring Harb. Symp. Quant. Biol.,* 55:651–661.

Zeki, S. 1990b. A century of cerebral achromatopsia. *Brain,* 113:1721–1777.

Zeki, S. 1991. Cerebral akinetopsia (visual motion blindness). *Brain,* 114:811–824.

Zeki, S. 1993. *A Vision of the Brain.* Blackwell Scientific Publications, Cambridge, MA.

Zihl, J., von Cramon, D., and Mai, N. 1983. Selective disturbance of movement vision after bilateral brain damage. *Brain,* 106:313–340.

Zohary, E., Shadlen, M. N., and Newsome, W. T. 1994. Correlated neuronal discharge rate and its implications for psychophysical performance. *Nature,* 370:140–143.

Author Index

Subject Index

About the Book

Type: Text, Stone Serif; Display, Stone Sans; Math, Lucida Bright
Editor: Peter Farley
Project Editor: Kathaleen Emerson
Copy Editor: J. David Baldwin
Production Manager: Christopher Small
Art: Line art by Nancy Haver, graphic art by Precision Graphics
Book Design: Peter Irvine, Steeple Desktop Publishing
Cover Design: Christopher Small
Composition: Paul C. Anagnostopoulos, MaryEllen Nauman Oliver,
    Windfall Software, using ZzTeX
Cover Manufacturer: Henry N. Sawyer Company
Book Manufacturer: Courier Companies, Inc.